METHODS IN MOLECULAR BIOLOGY™

Series Editor
**John M. Walker
School of Life Sciences
University of Hertfordshire
Hatfield, Hertfordshire, AL10 9AB, UK**

For further volumes:
http://www.springer.com/series/7651

Recombinant and In Vitro RNA Synthesis

Methods and Protocols

Edited by

Graeme L. Conn

Department of Biochemistry, Emory University School of Medicine, Atlanta, GA, USA

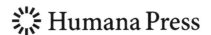

Editor
Graeme L. Conn
Department of Biochemistry
Emory University School of Medicine
Atlanta, GA, USA

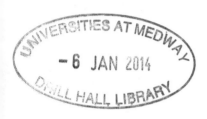

ISSN 1064-3745 ISSN 1940-6029 (electronic)
ISBN 978-1-62703-112-7 ISBN 978-1-62703-113-4 (eBook)
DOI 10.1007/978-1-62703-113-4
Springer New York Heidelberg Dordrecht London

Library of Congress Control Number: 2012947948

© Springer Science+Business Media, LLC 2012
This work is subject to copyright. All rights are reserved by the Publisher, whether the whole or part of the material is concerned, specifically the rights of translation, reprinting, reuse of illustrations, recitation, broadcasting, reproduction on microfilms or in any other physical way, and transmission or information storage and retrieval, electronic adaptation, computer software, or by similar or dissimilar methodology now known or hereafter developed. Exempted from this legal reservation are brief excerpts in connection with reviews or scholarly analysis or material supplied specifically for the purpose of being entered and executed on a computer system, for exclusive use by the purchaser of the work. Duplication of this publication or parts thereof is permitted only under the provisions of the Copyright Law of the Publisher's location, in its current version, and permission for use must always be obtained from Springer. Permissions for use may be obtained through RightsLink at the Copyright Clearance Center. Violations are liable to prosecution under the respective Copyright Law.
The use of general descriptive names, registered names, trademarks, service marks, etc. in this publication does not imply, even in the absence of a specific statement, that such names are exempt from the relevant protective laws and regulations and therefore free for general use.
While the advice and information in this book are believed to be true and accurate at the date of publication, neither the authors nor the editors nor the publisher can accept any legal responsibility for any errors or omissions that may be made. The publisher makes no warranty, express or implied, with respect to the material contained herein.

Printed on acid-free paper

Humana Press is a brand of Springer
Springer is part of Springer Science+Business Media (www.springer.com)

Preface

The discovery of catalytic RNAs in the mid-1980s marked the beginning of a new era in RNA biology and an ever-increasing appreciation of the diverse and critical roles played by this fascinating molecule. RNA structure—from primary sequence to complex tertiary folds with a rich landscape of posttranscriptional modifications—is intimately connected to its biological function. As a result, detailed molecular analyses of RNA molecules, their structures, modifications, conformational dynamics, stabilities, and interactions, are important challenges in the contemporary biological and biomedical sciences.

The essential foundation to such research is our ability to produce functional RNA molecules suitable for study in the laboratory. Many distinct approaches exist to overcome the various hurdles one might encounter, from initial construct design and synthesis through to the purification and other procedures that are critical to producing RNA samples that are chemically pure, conformationally homogeneous, and modified as required for the intended application. This book aims to provide a collection of approaches that guide the reader from the inception of a new RNA project to the final sample ready for analysis. These experimental protocols combine established work-horse approaches, developed over several decades in many labs around the world, with some of the latest innovative methods for RNA synthesis and purification.

Working with RNA presents significant challenges unique to this macromolecule; many of the necessary precautions and steps that should be taken when working with RNA are described in the individual chapters of this book. However, for the true RNA novice, the opening chapter of another recent volume of the MiMB series, "Working with RNA" (H. Neilson, in H. Neilsen Ed., *RNA*, Methods in Molecular Biology 703), is an excellent starting point.

Content and Organization of This Volume

The most common approaches to RNA synthesis for biochemical, biophysical, and structural studies are solid-phase automated chemical synthesis and enzymatic in vitro transcription. While each approach has its own set of capabilities, strengths, and limitations, today the former is largely the purview of commercial synthesis services and is therefore not a topic covered in depth in this book (though it is worth noting that many protocols, such as those for conjugation of fluorescent dyes to the RNA termini, are equally applicable, or could be readily adapted, for use with chemically synthesized RNA). Here, the focus will be largely on RNA in vitro transcription and the various ways this method can be adapted to produce highly purified, homogeneous, and, where required, specifically modified or functionalized RNAs for downstream experiments. We begin, however, with a new and quite different *recombinant* approach to RNA production in bacteria.

In the first two chapters, Ponchon and colleagues describe their recently developed "tRNA scaffold" approach for overexpression of defined RNA molecules in *Escherichia coli*. Target RNAs are embedded within a plasmid-encoded tRNA sequence so that they are expressed in a disguised form that the bacteria recognize and modify identically to endogenous tRNAs and do not target for degradation. This allows these engineered chimeric RNAs to accumulate in the cell, often in very large quantities. Chapter 1 introduces the tRNA scaffold system and describes protocols for pilot and large-scale RNA expression experiments and native purification of the chimeric RNAs by liquid chromatography. Next, Chapter 2 develops the approach through protocols that allow the target RNA to be accurately excised from its tRNA disguise using DNA oligonucleotides to direct RNase H cleavage of the chimeric RNA. Together these protocols provide a cost-effective means of producing large quantities of defined RNA sequences with the potential, for example, to directly incorporate isotopic labels simply by culturing the bacteria in medium containing appropriately labeled components.

In vitro transcription remains the predominant approach for RNA synthesis in the laboratory. All that is required is a DNA template encoding the RNA downstream of a suitable promoter sequence, the polymerase—typically T7 RNA polymerase (T7 RNAP)—and each ribonucleotide triphosphate (rNTP) building block. Polymerase and NTPs are both widely available from commercial sources and the enzyme can also be expressed and purified "in-house" (indeed, it is recommended that a T7 RNAP overexpression strain is obtained from one of the several sources cited in this book, particularly where large quantities of RNA are desired). This leaves only the template DNA to be obtained. For very short RNA fragments, chemically synthesized DNA oligonucleotides may be used directly for in vitro transcription. Alternatively, where a DNA template already exists, the promoter may be added via the primers in a polymerase chain reaction (PCR) and the product used directly for transcription or cloned into a suitable plasmid. The later approach has the advantage that new constructs can be sequence-verified, plasmid template can be simply and cheaply propagated in *E. coli* in large quantities, and additional sequences, such as ribozymes for transcript 3′-end processing, can be preloaded onto the plasmid to reduce the complexity of generating subsequent transcription constructs. But what if no template is available and the target is beyond the scope of a standard DNA oligonucleotide synthesis? While custom gene synthesis is an option, albeit an expensive one particularly if many variants of the sequence are needed, a versatile alternative is described in Chapter 3 by Bowman et al. that uses a "recursive PCR" protocol for long double-stranded DNA template synthesis. This ligation-free approach uses a series of tiled, partially complementary oligonucleotides of 50–70 nucleotides (nt) in length and can be simply adapted to produce sequence variants including mutations, insertions, or deletions, by substitution of just one oligonucleotide. The chapter covers all aspects of the approach: initial DNA design considerations including the approaches to create sequence variations, the recursive PCR reaction itself, product purification, and, finally, cloning into a destination vector for RNA in vitro transcription.

The next three chapters set out protocols for RNA in vitro transcription and established approaches to RNA purification by denaturing and native methods. These protocols should each serve as an excellent starting point for new RNA projects. While there is some overlap in the topics discussed in these three chapters, this serves to emphasize an important point: there is no single correct approach to follow—the best option for any given RNA may need to be teased from the details and additional suggestions provided in these chapters. Fortunately, the protocols described here should be readily adaptable to tackle any new RNA synthesis challenge.

Chapter 4 describes the in vitro transcription reaction in detail with basic protocols for plasmid template preparation, RNA synthesis, and denaturing purification. The chapter begins with a robust and scalable protocol for plasmid DNA purification, which removes the need for expensive commercial plasmid purification kits (which contain RNases!) or for CsCl gradients and their attendant large quantities of ethidium bromide. Next, a broadly applicable set of conditions for RNA in vitro transcription is described, followed by a protocol for RNA purification by denaturing polyacrylamide gel electrophoresis. In Chapter 5, Lu and Li continue this theme but with an emphasis on short RNA targets transcribed directly from chemically synthesized DNA oligonucleotides. This chapter also introduces native RNA purification by gel filtration chromatography and its application to studying RNA–protein interactions. Next, Chapter 6 by Booy et al. provides further exploration of the RNA in vitro transcription reaction coupled with detailed protocols for subsequent desalting/buffer exchange of synthesized RNA and its purification using Superdex 75 or 200 gel filtration chromatography columns on an FPLC system. This chapter closes with essential protocols and considerations for assessing RNA purity, concentration, and storage.

The next two chapters describe the use of ribozymes (RNA enzymes) to process RNA in vitro transcripts. Like other polymerases, T7 RNAP often adds additional nontemplated nucleotides to the 3′-end of its RNA transcripts and such heterogeneity can be a significant issue for some downstream applications. Heterogeneity can also occur at the 5′-end but, more commonly, issues here center on sequence limitations imposed by the promoter or difficulties encountered removing the 5′-end triphosphate for labeling or modification. Each of these problems can be circumvented using ribozymes to process the nascent transcript. First, in Chapter 7, Avis et al. describe the use of tandem 5′-hammerhead and 3′-hepatitis delta virus (HDV) *cis*-acting ribozymes. Detailed protocols guide the user from initial generation of new double ribozyme constructs—only the 3′-HDV can be preloaded on the plasmid—for their own target RNAs through to optimizing the balance between overall RNA yield and dual ribozyme cleavage efficiency. Chapter 8, by Szafraniec et al., describes the use of an antigenomic HDV ribozyme for *trans*-processing of target RNAs transcribed with a short (7 nt) sequence appended to their 3′-end. Subsequent precise cleavage of this tag by the *trans*-HDV ribozyme yields target RNAs with homogeneous 3′-ends. Unlike *cis*-acting ribozymes that are produced as a single transcript with the target RNA, here the ribozyme and target RNA are transcribed independently and the latter processed post-synthesis. This approach is therefore likely to be preferable where precious reagents are being used, such as selenium-derived (*see* Chapter 16) or isotopically labeled NTPs (*see* Chapters 17 and 18), since they are not incorporated into co-transcribed ribozyme sequences that are discarded.

In Chapter 9 Cheong et al. provide an alternative approach to transcript 3′-end processing using engineered DNAzymes (DNA enzymes). Protocols are provided detailing sequence specific DNA-affinity purification, transcript cleavage using the DNAzyme and removal of the cleaved tag and DNA to produce the final purified RNA. Affinity-based approaches for RNA purification are further developed in the next two chapters by DiTomasso et al. who describe a new system that exploits immobilization via an optimized λN-GST fusion bound to glutathione-sepharose. In Chapter 10, the expression and purification of the λN-GST fusion protein are described along with key quality control steps before use with RNA samples. Next, Chapter 11 outlines the synthesis of RNAs containing the "ARiBo" tag, comprising the activatable *glmS* ribozyme and λboxB RNA, at their 3′-end. The chapter covers all procedures from template preparation to small- and large-scale affinity purification and optimization of ribozyme cleavage. This scalable approach could potentially be adapted to be performed in a high-throughput manner, greatly simplifying the process of producing RNA construct libraries for biochemical/functional screening prior to more demanding structural or other biophysical experiments.

The remaining chapters deal with RNA modifications that facilitate specific downstream experiments including chemical or enzymatic probing of RNA structure and dynamics; analysis and quantification of RNA interactions; functional assays where specific modifications such as the 5′-cap, poly(A) tail or methylated nucleotides are critical; and, finally, for high-resolution structural studies by X-ray crystallography or NMR.

Chapter 12 describes a new plasmid system for synthesis of short RNAs within a "structure cassette" for enzymatic and chemical RNA structure probing experiments that use reverse transcription with a labeled DNA primer for readout. 5′- and 3′-flanking hairpin structures and an invariant 3′-end reverse transcription primer sequence are preloaded on the plasmid, thus simplifying the process of inserting new RNA-encoding sequences. Additional steps for analysis and quality control of RNAs transcribed within the structure cassette, which should be performed prior to probing experiments, are also described.

Co-transcriptional incorporation of modified nucleotides, at the RNA 5′-end and internally, are described by Moon and Wilusz in Chapter 13. A procedure is also detailed that allows the precise addition of a poly-A tail to transcribed RNAs. Collectively, these versatile protocols allow preparation of transcripts with a wide variety of modifications to facilitate downstream experiments that address diverse biological questions where such modifications play a critical role in the function or activity of the RNA. Many useful modifications can also be incorporated into the RNA post-synthesis. In Chapter 14, Zearfoss and Ryder describe their approaches for conjugating chemical tags to the 5′- and 3′-ends of RNA molecules (the approaches for 5′-end modification are also applicable to DNA oligonucleotides), including biotin and a wide variety of fluorescent dyes. In addition to detailed protocols for the labeling reactions, this chapter also provides a comprehensive survey of reagents available for RNA 5′- and 3′-end labeling, including the excitation and emission properties for each dye.

Chemical modifications of RNA, such as methylation of base or ribose, are common but their roles are often not well characterized. Essential to systematic and rigorous analyses of RNA modification functions are methods to purify modified RNAs away from unmodified transcripts. Chapter 15 describes a novel approach to isolate site-specifically modified RNAs using the N1-methyl-guanosine (m^1G) tRNA methylation as an example. Using selective DNA oligonucleotide hybridization, where the DNA binds only to unmodified RNA due to the disruption of normal base pairing by the base modification, unmodified transcripts are specifically targeted for degradation by RNase H. This novel approach should prove broadly applicable to other modifications and RNA types where suitably purified modification enzyme is available and Watson–Crick base pairing is disrupted in the modified RNA strand.

High-resolution structural studies of RNAs and RNA–protein complexes, by X-ray crystallography or NMR, are central to our understanding of RNA biology but remain a highly challenging undertaking. Many of the preceding chapters describe approaches that can produce RNA suitable for structural studies. However, for both X-ray crystallography and NMR specific hurdles exist in the process of structure determination that can be overcome through application of the approaches described in the next three chapters.

After obtaining suitably diffracting crystals, the major hurdle remaining in X-ray crystallographic structure determination is likely to be the "Phase Problem." This relates to the fact that in an X-ray diffraction experiment only the intensities of the diffracted X-rays are measured whereas the phase information is lost. Where a similar structure already exists, this information can be "recovered" by a process known as molecular replacement; otherwise, initial estimates must be experimentally obtained through some form of specific incorporation of electron-rich (or "heavy") atoms into the sample. For proteins, for example, structurally or functionally obligatory ions (e.g., Zn^{2+}) or those incorporated via trial-and-error soaking experiments (e.g., Hg^{2+}) can be used; most commonly today, however, direct protein derivatization is accomplished through selenomethionine addition to the medium for expression in an auxotrophic bacterial strain. Although some parallel approaches exist for nucleic acids, such as incorporation of halogen (bromide or iodide) derivatives of the nucleoside bases during solid-phase chemical synthesis, the options available for RNA are generally more limited. In Chapter 16, Lin and Huang address this deficiency with a description of the synthesis, purification, and use of selenium-derived rNTPs (Se-NTPs). These novel reagents allow the production, via in vitro transcription, of RNA molecules with selenium specifically incorporated into the RNA backbone that can be used for phasing of RNA or RNA–protein complex crystal structures using well-established single- or multiple-wavelength anomalous diffraction experiments.

NMR spectroscopy is a powerful approach for studying the dynamics, interactions, and structures of macromolecules, including RNA. However, multidimensional experiments using isotopically labeled samples are a prerequisite for NMR studies of all but the simplest of systems. Approaches for synthesis of isotopically labeled RNA samples are therefore essential and selective labeling of positions on the ribose or base moieties can greatly simplify NMR spectra and their analysis. Chemical synthesis has the advantage of allowing label incorporation at any desired nucleotide positions within an RNA chain but in vitro transcription provides a significantly more economical route to labeled RNA samples. In Chapter 17, Martino and Conte provide a detailed description of current approaches for producing isotopically labeled rNTPs for this purpose. As described in this chapter, through careful combination of the labeled medium component, the type of expression medium and the bacterial strain, a wide variety of uniform and different selective labeling regimes can be achieved. The protocols of this chapter carefully guide the user through the critical steps of RNA extraction and digestion, purification of 5′-ribonucleoside monophosphates (rNMPs) and their enzymatic phosphorylation to rNTPs for use in in vitro transcription reactions. The approaches described by Martino and Conte provide the user with a mixture of labeled rNTPs but NMR experiments may be further refined if the individual RNA building blocks can be isolated such that labels are incorporated only for selected nucleotides. A new method for preparative isolation of individual labeled rNMPs by ion-pair reversed-phase high performance liquid chromatography (HPLC) is provided by Dagenais and Legault in Chapter 18.

Finally, an approach known as RNA "splint ligation" is described by Kershaw and O'Keefe in Chapter 19. Here, T4 DNA ligase is used to efficiently join two RNA molecules using a DNA oligonucleotide bridge as a guide. Splint ligation can be used to incorporate a short isotopically labeled segment into a larger RNA for structural studies, or to produce RNAs with internal labels or cross-linking groups for analyses of RNA–RNA or RNA–protein interactions. The method thus adds a new dimension of versatility to many of the labeling and modification strategies described in the preceding chapters, as well as a cost-effective means to incorporate specific modifications, available only via chemical synthesis of a short RNA fragment, into RNA molecules of greater size, complexity, and functional utility.

In closing, I would like to express my sincere gratitude to all the authors who have contributed to this book for their outstanding efforts and patience throughout the long process of its preparation. Each deserves great credit for their willingness to invest the time to share these protocols and, in keeping with the tradition of the *MiMB* series, the detailed "tips and tricks" that can be crucial for their successful implementation in the laboratory. I hope that this new volume will live up to this tradition and, in doing so, help bring new investigators with fresh ideas to the fascinating world of RNA.

Atlanta, GA, USA *Graeme L. Conn*

Contents

Preface..		*v*
Contributors..		*xiii*

1	Purification of RNA Expressed In Vivo Inserted in a tRNA Scaffold........	1
	Luc Ponchon and Frédéric Dardel	
2	Selective RNase H Cleavage of Target RNAs from a tRNA Scaffold.........	9
	Luc Ponchon, Geneviève Beauvais, Sylvie Nonin-Lecomte,	
	and Frédéric Dardel	
3	Preparation of Long Templates for RNA In Vitro Transcription	
	by Recursive PCR..	19
	Jessica C. Bowman, Bahareh Azizi, Timothy K. Lenz, Poorna Roy,	
	and Loren Dean Williams	
4	General Protocols for Preparation of Plasmid DNA Template,	
	RNA In Vitro Transcription, and RNA Purification by Denaturing PAGE....	43
	Jo L. Linpinsel and Graeme L. Conn	
5	Preparation of Short RNA by In Vitro Transcription.............................	59
	Cheng Lu and Pingwei Li	
6	Native RNA Purification by Gel Filtration Chromatography..............	69
	Evan P. Booy, Hui Meng, and Sean A. McKenna	
7	*Cis*-Acting Ribozymes for the Production of RNA In Vitro	
	Transcripts with Defined 5′ and 3′ Ends...	83
	Johanna M. Avis, Graeme L. Conn, and Scott C. Walker	
8	*Trans*-Acting Antigenomic HDV Ribozyme for Production	
	of In Vitro Transcripts with Homogenous 3′ Ends....................................	99
	Milena Szafraniec, Leszek Blaszczyk, Jan Wrzesinski,	
	and Jerzy Ciesiolka	
9	Rapid Preparation of RNA Samples Using DNA-Affinity Chromatography	
	and DNAzyme Methods..	113
	Hae-Kap Cheong, Eunha Hwang, and Chaejoon Cheong	
10	Preparation of λN-GST Fusion Protein for Affinity Immobilization of RNA..	123
	Geneviève Di Tomasso, Philipe Lampron, James G. Omichinski,	
	and Pascale Legault	
11	Affinity Purification of RNA Using an ARiBo Tag.................................	137
	Geneviève Di Tomasso, Pierre Dagenais, Alexandre Desjardins,	
	Alexis Rompré-Brodeur, Vanessa Delfosse, and Pascale Legault	
12	Plasmid Template Design and In Vitro Transcription of Short RNAs	
	Within a "Structure Cassette" for Structure Probing Experiments..........	157
	Virginia K. Vachon and Graeme L. Conn	

13	In Vitro Transcription of Modified RNAs	171
	Stephanie L. Moon and Jeffrey Wilusz	
14	End-Labeling Oligonucleotides with Chemical Tags After Synthesis	181
	N. Ruth Zearfoss and Sean P. Ryder	
15	High-Purity Enzymatic Synthesis of Site-Specifically Modified tRNA	195
	Ya-Ming Hou	
16	Se-Derivatized RNAs for X-ray Crystallography	213
	Lina Lin and Zhen Huang	
17	Biosynthetic Preparation of $^{13}C/^{15}N$-Labeled rNTPs for High-Resolution NMR Studies of RNAs	227
	Luigi Martino and Maria R. Conte	
18	Preparative Separation of Ribonucleoside Monophosphates by Ion-Pair Reverse-Phase HPLC	247
	Pierre Dagenais and Pascale Legault	
19	Splint Ligation of RNA with T4 DNA Ligase	257
	Christopher J. Kershaw and Raymond T. O'Keefe	
Index		*271*

Contributors

JOHANNA M. AVIS • *Manchester Interdisciplinary Biocentre, Manchester, UK*
BAHAREH AZIZI • *School of Chemistry and Biochemistry, Georgia Institute of Technology, Atlanta, GA, USA*
GENEVIÈVE BEAUVAIS • *Laboratoire de Cristallographie et RMN biologiques, Université Paris Descartes CNRS, Paris, France*
LESZEK BLASZCZYK • *Institute of Bioorganic Chemistry, Polish Academy of Sciences, Poznan, Poland*
EVAN P. BOOY • *Department of Chemistry, University of Manitoba, Winnipeg, MB, Canada*
JESSICA C. BOWMAN • *School of Chemistry and Biochemistry, Georgia Institute of Technology, Atlanta, GA, USA*
CHAEJOON CHEONG • *Division of Magnetic Resonance Research, Korea Basic Science Institute, Ochang, Cheongwon, South Korea*
HAE-KAP CHEONG • *Division of Magnetic Resonance Research, Korea Basic Science Institute, Ochang, Cheongwon, South Korea*
JERZY CIESIOLKA • *Institute of Bioorganic Chemistry, Polish Academy of Sciences, Poznan, Poland*
GRAEME L. CONN • *Department of Biochemistry, Emory University School of Medicine, Atlanta, GA, USA*
MARIA R. CONTE • *Randall Division of Cell and Molecular Biophysics, King's College London, London, UK*
PIERRE DAGENAIS • *Département de Biochimie, Université de Montréal, Montreal, QC, Canada*
FRÉDÉRIC DARDEL • *Laboratoire de Cristallographie et RMN biologiques, Université Paris Descartes CNRS, Paris, France*
VANESSA DELFOSSE • *Département de Biochimie, Université de Montréal, Montreal, QC, Canada*
ALEXANDRE DESJARDINS • *Département de Biochimie, Université de Montréal, Montreal, QC, Canada*
GENEVIÈVE DI TOMASSO • *Département de Biochimie, Université de Montréal, Montreal, QC, Canada*
YA-MING HOU • *Department of Biochemistry and Molecular Biology, Thomas Jefferson University, BLSB, Philadelphia, PA, USA*
ZHEN HUANG • *Department of Chemistry, Georgia State University, Atlanta, GA, USA*
EUNHA HWANG • *Division of Magnetic Resonance Research, Korea Basic Science Institute, Ochang, Cheongwon, South Korea*
CHRISTOPHER J. KERSHAW • *The University of Manchester, Manchester, UK*
PHILIPE LAMPRON • *Département de Biochimie, Université de Montréal, Montreal, QC, Canada*

PASCALE LEGAULT • *Département de Biochimie, Université de Montréal, Montreal, QC, Canada*
TIMOTHY K. LENZ • *School of Chemistry and Biochemistry, Georgia Institute of Technology, Atlanta, GA, USA*
PINGWEI LI • *Department of Biochemistry and Biophysics, Texas A&M University, College Station, TX, USA*
LINA LIN • *Department of Chemistry, Georgia State University, Atlanta, GA, USA*
JO L. LINPINSEL • *Department of Biochemistry, Emory University School of Medicine, Atlanta, GA, USA*
CHENG LU • *Department of Biochemistry and Biophysics, Texas A&M University, College Station, TX, USA*
LUIGI MARTINO • *Randall Division of Cell and Molecular Biophysics, King's College London, London, UK*
SEAN A. MCKENNA • *Department of Chemistry, University of Manitoba, Winnipeg, MB, Canada*
HUI MENG • *Department of Chemistry, University of Manitoba, Winnipeg, MB, Canada*
STEPHANIE L. MOON • *Department of Microbiology, Immunology and Pathology, Colorado State University, Fort Collins, CO, USA*
SYLVIE NONIN-LECOMTE • *Laboratoire de Cristallographie et RMN biologiques, Université Paris Descartes, CNRS, Paris, France*
RAYMOND T. O'KEEFE • *The University of Manchester, Manchester, UK*
JAMES G. OMICHINSKI • *Département de Biochimie, Université de Montréal, Montreal, QC, Canada*
LUC PONCHON • *Laboratoire de Cristallographie et RMN biologiques, Université Paris Descartes, CNRS, Paris, France*
ALEXIS ROMPRÉ-BRODEUR • *Département de Biochimie, Université de Montréal, Montreal, QC, Canada*
POORNA ROY • *School of Chemistry and Biochemistry, Georgia Institute of Technology, Atlanta, GA, USA*
SEAN P. RYDER • *Department of Biochemistry and Molecular Pharmacology, University of Massachusetts Medical School, Worcester, MA, USA*
MILENA SZAFRANIEC • *Institute of Bioorganic Chemistry, Polish Academy of Sciences, Poznan, Poland*
VIRGINIA K. VACHON • *Department of Biochemistry, Emory University School of Medicine, Atlanta, GA, USA*
SCOTT C. WALKER • *Department of Biological Chemistry, University of Michigan, Ann Arbor, MI, USA*
LOREN DEAN WILLIAMS • *School of Chemistry and Biochemistry, Georgia Institute of Technology, Atlanta, GA, USA*
JEFFREY WILUSZ • *Department of Microbiology, Immunology and Pathology, Colorado State University, Fort Collins, CO, USA*
JAN WRZESINSKI • *Institute of Bioorganic Chemistry, Polish Academy of Sciences, Poznan, Poland*
N. RUTH ZEARFOSS • *Department of Biochemistry and Molecular Pharmacology, University of Massachusetts Medical School, Worcester, MA, USA*

Chapter 1

Purification of RNA Expressed In Vivo Inserted in a tRNA Scaffold

Luc Ponchon and Frédéric Dardel

Abstract

For structural, biochemical, or pharmacological studies, it is required to have pure RNA in large quantities. In vitro transcription or chemical synthesis are the principal methods to produce RNA. Here, we describe an alternative method allowing RNA production in bacteria and its purification by liquid chromatography. In a few days, between 10 and 100 mg of pure RNA are obtained with this technique.

Key words: Expression plasmid, Recombinant RNA, RNA expression, tRNA scaffold, Liquid purification

1. Introduction

The method of in vitro transcription has made a tremendous impact on the study of RNA. It is the most commonly used method; it allows pure RNA to be obtained quickly and does not require sophisticated equipment. Nevertheless, this method is a several-hour experiment during which RNAs can hydrolyze into cleaved products. Moreover, the T7 RNA polymerase used for in vitro transcription often adds additional, nontemplated nucleotide(s) at the 3′-terminus of the transcribed RNA (1). The RNAs are then traditionally purified by preparative electrophoresis followed by gel extraction. Although this approach can resolve RNA molecules up to 100 nucleotides in length, it is time-consuming and leads to acrylamide-associated impurities within the RNA (2–4). Here, we describe a novel alternative method based on a recombinant system.

Recombinant transfer RNA (tRNA) has been successfully expressed in vivo in *Escherichia coli* (5–8). This is possible because tRNAs are recognized and processed by a number of cellular enzymes. Furthermore, as a consequence of their three-dimensional structure, tRNAs are extremely stable to both heat-unfolding and nucleases (9). This allows them to escape degradation and accumulate in *E. coli* when overexpressed from a recombinant plasmid.

We took advantage of these specific features to express recombinant RNA as chimeras, by inserting them into the protective scaffold of a tRNA (10). Owing to their size, tRNA chimeras can easily be separated from bacterial tRNAs by chromatographic purification, which can be adapted to the large-scale purification of RNA (11). RNA yields depend on the nature of the transcript being produced. Expected yields are in the range of 10–100 mg of chimeric RNA per liter of culture but typically, longer RNAs are produced in lower amounts. We have now successfully applied this expression strategy to over 25 different RNAs. As an example of the approach, we describe here the production and the purification of the tRNA-HBV chimera corresponding to the epsilon domain of the hepatitis virus merged with human tRNALys (12).

2. Materials

Prepare all solutions using ultrapure water (prepared by purifying deionized water to attain a sensitivity of 15 MΩ cm at 25°C) and analytical grade reagents. Prepare and store all reagents at room temperature (unless indicated otherwise).

2.1. Pilot Expression Experiment

1. Chimeric RNA expression vector derived from the pBSTNAV plasmid (see Note 1).
2. Electroporator and electroporation cuvettes.
3. Electrocompetent JM101Tr *E. coli* cells (see Note 2).
4. 2× TY medium: Add 16 g tryptone, 10 g yeast extract, and 5 g sodium chloride to 1 L H_2O and sterilize by autoclaving.
5. 100 mg/mL Ampicillin. Filter-sterilize and store at 4°C.
6. Temperature-controlled shaking incubator.
7. Polypropylene conical tubes, 50 mL.
8. Lysis Buffer: 10 mM magnesium acetate and 10 mM Tris–HCl, pH 7.4.
9. Water-saturated phenol.
10. 5 M NaCl.
11. Ethanol.
12. 5× TBE: 54 g Tris base, 275 g boric acid, and 4.7 g EDTA per liter of water. TBE buffer is typically stored indefinitely at room temperature.
13. 40% Acrylamide/bis-acrylamide (19:1) solution.

14. 5× Loading Buffer: 50% (v/v) glycerol, 0.2% (w/v) xylene cyanol, and 1× TBE.
15. 10% Ammonium persulfate.
16. N,N,N,N'-tetramethyl-ethylenediamine (TEMED).
17. Urea–acrylamide gel running buffer: Mix 100 mL of 5×TBE and 900 mL of water.
18. Handheld UV lamp.
19. Kit for plasmid DNA Minipreps.

2.2. Large-Scale Cell Growth and RNA Purification

1. All components listed above for the pilot experiment (Subheading 2.1, items 1–19).
2. 1-L Culture flasks.
3. ÄKTA FPLC chromatography system (or equivalent).
4. Source 15Q column: Pack 50 mL of Source 15Q chromatographic medium in an XK26/40 column following the supplier's instructions (GE Healthcare).
5. Mono-Q HR 10/10 (GE Healthcare).
6. Apparatus for gel electrophoresis of RNA and protein.
7. 1 M Potassium phosphate, pH 7.0: Weigh out 107.12 g of K_2HPO_4 and 52.39 g of KH_2PO_4, transfer to a 1-L graduated cylinder, and add water to just under a volume of 1 L. Mix to dissolve completely and then adjust to a final volume of 1 L with additional water.
8. Buffer A: Transfer 40 mL of 1 M potassium phosphate, pH 7 to a 1-L graduated cylinder. Add water to a volume of 1 L. Mix.
9. Buffer B: Weigh out 58.44 g of NaCl and transfer to 1-L graduated cylinder. Add 40 mL of 1 M potassium phosphate, pH 7.0. Add water to a volume of 1 L and mix to dissolve.

3. Methods

Carry out all procedures at room temperature unless otherwise specified. We recommend two steps: a pilot expression experiment followed by a large-scale cell growth and RNA purification.

3.1. Pilot Expression Experiment

1. Transform 50 µl of electrocompetent JM101Tr with 10–100 ng chimeric RNA expression vector and inoculate 10 mL of 2×TY medium containing 100 µg/mL ampicillin in a culture flask. Shake overnight (16–18 h) at 220 rpm and 37°C.
2. Pellet 5 mL of saturated overnight culture by centrifugation for 10 min at $4,000 \times g$ and 4°C. Preserve 5 mL at 4°C for later plasmid DNA extraction.

3. Resuspend the cell pellet in 180 µL of Lysis Buffer. Add 200 µL of water-saturated phenol (see Note 3). Agitate gently for 20 min at room temperature in a polypropylene conical tube. Centrifuge for 10 min at $10,000 \times g$ and collect the 150 µL of aqueous phase.

4. Add 0.1 volume of 5 M NaCl and 2 volumes of ethanol. Centrifuge for 10 min at $10,000 \times g$ at 4°C in a polypropylene conical tube. Dissolve the pellet in 100 µL of water.

5. Prepare samples for 8% urea–acrylamide gel by mixing 40 µL of dissolved pellet with 10 µL of 5× Loading Buffer.

6. Mix 2 mL of 5×TBE, 2 mL of acrylamide mixture, and 5 g of urea, and add water to a volume of 10 mL in a 50 mL conical flask. Mix to dissolve the urea. Add 100 µL of ammonium persulfate, and 10 µL of TEMED, and cast gel within a 7.25×10 cm $\times 1$ mm gel cassette. Insert a ten-well gel comb immediately without introducing air bubbles.

7. Assemble the urea–acrylamide gel in the electrophoresis apparatus, fill with 0.5×TBE running buffer, and load the samples (20 µL each). Electrophorese at 80 V until the samples have entered the gel and then continue running at 200 V.

8. Following electrophoresis, pry the gel plates open with the use of a spatula. The gel will remain on one of the glass plates. Gently lift the gel from the glass plate and place it on shrink wrap (see Note 4) and place on a white paper. Reveal the RNA by UV shadowing with the handheld UV lamp placed above the gel (Fig. 1).

9. Purify the plasmid DNA from the reserved 5 mL of saturated overnight culture using a kit for plasmid DNA Miniprep, according to the manufacturer's instructions. Perform sequence analysis to confirm that the nucleotide sequence of the putative clone is correct. Plasmid DNA can be stored at −20°C for several months.

3.2. Large-Scale Cell Growth and RNA Purification

1. Transform 50 µL of electrocompetent JM101Tr (see Note 5) with 10–100 ng chimeric RNA expression vector and inoculate 1 L of 2×TY medium containing 100 µg/mL ampicillin in a culture flask. Shake overnight (16–18 h) at 220 rpm and 37°C.

2. Centrifuge the saturated 1 L culture for 30 min at $6,000 \times g$ and 4°C.

3. Dissolve the pellet in 8.6 mL of Lysis Buffer. Add 10 mL of water-saturated phenol (see Note 3). Agitate gently for 1 h at room temperature in a polypropylene conical tube.

4. Centrifuge for 30 min at $10,000 \times g$ and 4°C. Collect the aqueous phase and add 0.1 volume of 5 M NaCl and 2 volumes of ethanol to precipitate the RNA. Centrifuge for 30 min at

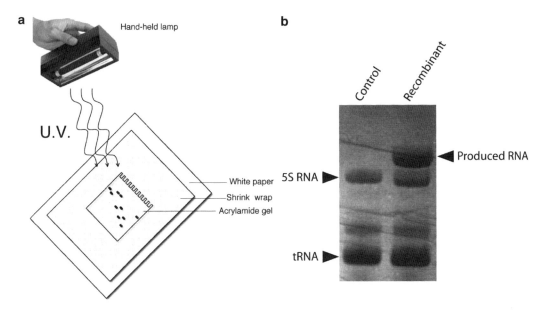

Fig. 1. The UV shadowing technique for visualizing nucleic acids separated on polyacrylamide gels. (**a**) Nucleic acid bands are visualized by shining a handheld shortwave UV light source (254 nm) on the surface of the gel. Nucleic acids will appear as *black bands* while the *white paper* will reflect the light through the shrink wrap. The detection limit of UV shadowing is approximately 0.3 μg of nucleic acid. (**b**) Crude RNA extracts from recombinant bacteria visualized by UV shadowing.

10,000 ×*g* and 4°C in a polypropylene conical tube. Dissolve the pellet in 40 mM potassium phosphate, pH 7.0 (Buffer A).

5. Equilibrate the anion exchange with Buffer A (see Note 6). Load the RNA extract onto the ion-exchange column. Wash the column with 70% buffer A:30% buffer B until a stable baseline is reached. Elute RNA with a 30–70% gradient of Buffer B over ten column volumes with a flow rate of 1 mL/min. Collect the eluant in fractions of 5 mL volume.

6. Analyze the fractions by electrophoresis on 8% urea–acrylamide gels and pool those containing the chimeric RNA. Recover the desired RNA by ethanol precipitation as described in step 4 (Fig. 2).

4. Notes

1. tRNA scaffold vectors derived from pBSTNAV can be obtained from the Laboratory of Biological Crystallography and NMR. To produce the tRNA chimeras in vivo, various options are available for the choice of the starting vector. The vectors we describe were derived from pBSTNAV. Six such vectors were constructed, based on either the human tRNALys3 (pBSK vectors) or on the *E. coli* initiator tRNAMet (pBSM vectors) (see ref. 12).

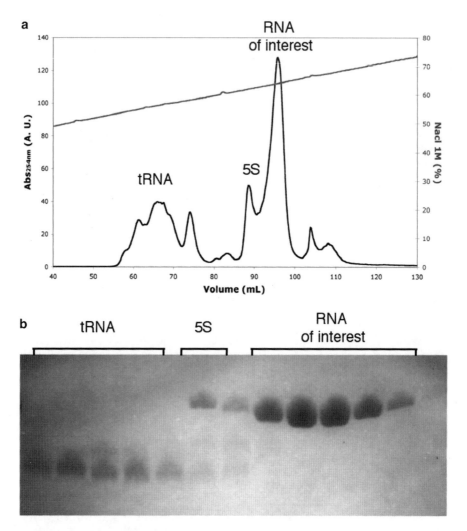

Fig. 2. Purification profile of the tRNA-HBV epsilon chimera by ion-exchange chromatography (Source 15Q column). (a) Source 15Q profile of the *Escherichia coli* RNA extraction purification. Eluent was 40 mM phosphate buffer (pH 7) with a salt gradient from 0.45 to 0.75 M NaCl. The major peak corresponds to the expressed RNA and the others to *E. coli* tRNAs and 5S ribosomal RNA (as labeled). (b) The fractions were analyzed by urea-PAGE, and RNA bands were visualized by UV shadowing. Successive fractions are shown from *left to right*. The various *E. coli* tRNA eluted first, followed by small amounts of 5S ribosomal RNA, whereas the tRNA-HBV chimera eluted last, at a sodium chloride concentration of about 600 mM.

2. As the lpp promoter on the expression vector is constitutive, there is no need for induction. RNA accumulates throughout the culture growth, up to the early stationary phase. Growing cells in rich medium is very important, as the expression of most tRNA-processing enzymes is growth rate dependent and thus tRNA chimera processing is also growth rate dependent (see ref. 13). For the same reason, it is important to use an "efficient" host strain, i.e., not carrying mutations affecting growth rate. Most standard laboratory *E. coli* strains used for protein expression were found to be efficient in this respect, e.g., BL21(DE3), DH5α, JM101, and other derivatives.

3. Phenol must be manipulated with caution. Phenol is toxic and corrosive; you should wear gloves and handle under a fume hood. Put Parafilm around each tube containing phenol, in particular for a centrifugation step.

4. You can use transparent film for wrapping food or any UV transparent support that prevents the adsorption of the wet gel on the white paper.

5. Always start with freshly transformed *E. coli* cells. As production of the RNA is strong and constitutive, mutations with lower expression yield tend to be selected over time, because strong overexpression slows growth. It is thus necessary to freshly transform with the plasmid every time to avoid this pitfall. A high transformation yield is desirable, as it minimizes the number of generations between transformation and saturation of the culture, and hence the risk of mutations.

6. We recommend using an anion exchange column. The anion exchange resin will bind RNA phosphate groups and allows separation of the larger chimeric RNA from most of the smaller host tRNA molecules. Elution is carried out with a salt gradient under native conditions. If a high purity is required, this purification step can be followed by a gel filtration step on a suitable chromatographic medium; typically, Superdex 75 can be used for small constructs (70–150 nt) and Superdex 200 for larger constructs (120–400 nt). In the rare cases where the size of the RNA of interest overlaps with an endogenous *E. coli* RNA (e.g., 5S rRNA), we found that this can usually be resolved by additional chromatographic steps, such as ion-exchange separation at two different pHs or by hydrophobic interaction chromatography (see ref. 14).

References

1. Schenborn ET, Mierendorf RC Jr (1985) A novel transcription property of SP6 and T7 RNA polymerases: dependence on template structure. Nucleic Acids Res 16:6223–6236
2. Lukavsky PJ, Puglisi JD (2004) Large-scale preparation and purification of polyacrylamide-free RNA oligonucleotides. RNA 10:889–893
3. Cheong HK, Hwang E, Lee C, Choi BS, Cheong C (2004) Rapid preparation of RNA samples for NMR spectroscopy and X-ray crystallography. Nucleic Acids Res 32:e84
4. Kieft JS, Batey RT (2004) A general method for rapid and nondenaturing purification of RNAs. RNA 10:988–995
5. Masson J-M, Miller JH (1986) Expression of synthetic tRNA genes under the control of a synthetic promoter. Gene 47:179–183
6. Meinnel T, Mechulam Y, Fayat G (1988) Fast purification of a functional elongator tRNAmet expressed from a synthetic gene in vivo. Nucleic Acids Res 16:8095–8096
7. Tisné C, Rigourd M, Marquet R, Ehresmann C, Dardel F (2000) NMR and biochemical characterization of recombinant human tRNA(Lys)3 expressed in Escherichia coli: identification of posttranscriptional nucleotide modifications required for efficient initiation of HIV-1 reverse transcription. RNA 6:1403–1412

8. Wallis NG, Dardel F, Blanquet S (1995) Heteronuclear NMR studies of the interactions of 15N-labeled methionine-specific transfer RNAs with methionyltRNA transformylase. Biochemistry 34:7668–7677

9. Engelke DR, Hopper AK (2006) Modified view of tRNA: stability amid sequence diversity. Mol Cell 21:144–145

10. Ponchon L, Dardel F (2007) Recombinant RNA technology: the tRNA scaffold. Nat Methods 4:571–576

11. McKenna SA, Kim I, Puglisi EV, Lindhout DA, Aitken CE, Marshall RA, Puglisi JD (2007) Purification and characterization of transcribed RNAs using gel filtration chromatography. Nat Protoc 2:3270–3277

12. Ponchon L, Beauvais G, Nonin-Lecomte S, Dardel F (2009) A generic protocol for the expression and purification of recombinant RNA in Escherichia coli using a tRNA scaffold. Nat Protoc 4:947–959

13. Neidhardt FC, Fraenkel D (1961) Metabolic regulation of RNA synthesis in bacteria. Cold Spring Harb Symp Quant Biol 26:63–74

14. Tisné C, Rigourd M, Marquet R, Ehresmann C, Dardel F (2000) NMR and biochemical characterization of recombinant human tRNA(Lys)3 expressed in Escherichia coli: identification of posttranscriptional nucleotide modifications required for efficient initiation of HIV-1 reverse transcription. RNA 6:1403–1412

Chapter 2

Selective RNase H Cleavage of Target RNAs from a tRNA Scaffold

Luc Ponchon, Geneviève Beauvais, Sylvie Nonin-Lecomte, and Frédéric Dardel

Abstract

In vivo overproduction of tRNA chimeras yields an RNA insert within a tRNA scaffold. For some applications, it may be necessary to discard the scaffold. Here we present a protocol for selective cleavage of the RNA of interest from the tRNA scaffold, using RNase H and two DNA oligonucleotides. After cleavage, we show that the RNA of interest can be isolated in a one-step purification. This method has, in particular, applications in structural investigations of RNA.

Key words: Recombinant RNA, tRNA scaffold, RNase H cleavage, RNA purification

1. Introduction

Our protocol of in vivo overproduction of tRNA chimeras yields an RNA insert within a tRNA scaffold (1). This system should have broad application in structural, biochemical, and biophysical investigations of RNA (1, 2). For some applications, it may be necessary to remove the scaffold from the target RNA. We considered several strategies: using either a dedicated ribozyme (3) or DNAzyme (4) or cleaving with RNase H using a pair of guide DNA oligonucleotides. Dual cis-acting ribozyme constructs have been used for in vitro transcribed RNA, but this approach is not compatible with the tRNA scaffold topology (5). In our hands, the method that worked best is RNase H cleavage and thus we have developed a technique for selectively cleaving the RNA of interest from the tRNA scaffold, using RNase H and two DNA oligonucleotides.

RNase H specifically cleaves the RNA strand of DNA–RNA heteroduplexes (6, 7). The strategy is therefore to use two "guide" DNA oligonucleotides complementary to the 5′ and 3′ halves of tRNA moiety of the chimera. Hence, upon incubation with RNase H, the scaffold is hydrolyzed, whereas the RNA of interest is left intact. We found that 60 pmol of *Escherichia coli* RNase H is usually sufficient to cleave 1 nmol of RNA in 2 h at 30°C (8). Commercially available RNase H can be used; however, for large-scale applications, using RNase H purified in-house is more cost-effective. The most critical step is the hybridization of the RNA with the DNA oligonucleotides. Here, as an example of the approach, we present the cleavage and the purification of the decoding site of the 16S ribosomal RNA (9). We propose a simple method to estimate the length of the RNA product by SDS-PAGE followed by a *Stains-all* staining (10).

2. Materials

Prepare all solutions using ultrapure water (prepared by purifying deionized water to attain a sensitivity of 15 MΩ cm at 25°C) and analytical grade reagents. Prepare and store all reagents at room temperature (unless indicated otherwise).

2.1. Production and Purification of RNase H

1. pET28a-(6×His)RNase H fusion protein expression vector (see Note 1).
2. Competent BL21(DE3) *E. coli* cells (Novagen).
3. Kanamycin: Prepare a stock solution of 37 mg/mL of kanamycin sulfate salt in H_2O and filter-sterilize. Store at 4°C.
4. Luria Broth (LB medium).
5. LB agar plates: Add 12 g bacto agar to 1 L LB medium before autoclaving. To prepare plates, allow medium to cool until flask or bottle can be held in hands without burning, then add 1 mL of the kanamycin stock, mix by gentle swirling, and pour or pipette approximately 30 mL into each sterile Petri dish (100 mm diameter). The final concentration of ampicillin should be 37 µg/L.
6. Isopropyl β-D-1-thiogalactopyranoside (IPTG).
7. 10% Sodium dodecyl sulfate (SDS).
8. 40% Acrylamide/bis-acrylamide solution (37:1).
9. 10% Ammonium persulfate.
10. *N,N,N,N'*-tetramethyl-ethylenediamine (TEMED).
11. SDS-PAGE running buffer: 0.025 M Tris–HCl (pH 8.3), 0.192 M glycine, and 0.1% SDS.
12. SDS loading buffer (5×): 0.3 M Tris–HCl (pH 6.8), 10% (w/v) SDS, 25% (v/v) β-mercaptoethanol, 0.1% (v/v) bromophenol blue (BPB) solution, and 45% (v/v) glycerol. Prepare 20 mL

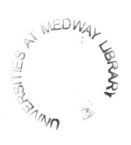

of loading buffer, leave 1 mL at 4°C for current use, and store the remaining aliquots at −20°C.

13. BPB solution: Dissolve 0.1 g BPB in 100 mL water.
14. 1 M Tris–HCl (pH 8).
15. 1 M Tris–HCl (pH 7.5).
16. Imidazole.
17. Resuspension buffer: 50 mM Tris–HCl buffer (pH 7.5) and 100 mM NaCl.
18. Elution buffer: 50 mM Tris–HCl buffer (pH 7.5), 100 mM sodium chloride, and 500 mM imidazole.
19. Storage buffer: 50 mM Tris–HCl (pH 8.0), 100 mM NaCl, and 50% glycerol.
20. Resolving gel buffer: 1.5 M Tris–HCl, pH 8.8. Add about 100 mL water to a 1-L graduated cylinder or a glass beaker. Weigh 181.7 g Tris base and transfer to the cylinder. Add water to a volume of 900 mL. Mix and adjust pH with HCl. Make up to 1 L with water. Store at 4°C.
21. Stacking gel buffer: 0.5 M Tris–HCl, pH 6.8. Weigh 60.6 g Tris base and prepare a 1 L solution as in previous step. Store at 4°C.
22. Polypropylene conical tubes, 50 mL.
23. Baffle-bottomed shake flask.
24. Temperature-controlled shaking incubator.
25. Mechanical device to disrupt *E. coli* cells (e.g., a sonicator, French press, or cell homogenizer).
26. Apparatus for gel electrophoresis.
27. Ni-NTA superflow resin (Qiagen): Pack 20 mL of the Ni-NTA superflow resin in an XK 16/40 column (GE Healthcare), following the supplier's instructions.
28. ÄKTA FPLC chromatography system (or equivalent).

2.2. RNase H Cleavage

1. Purified RNA-tRNA chimera (see Chapter 1).
2. DNA oligonucleotides (see Note 2).
3. Purified *E. coli* Ribonuclease H (from Subheading 3.1 of this protocol).
4. Hot plate.
5. ÄKTA FPLC chromatography system (or equivalent).
6. Mono-Q HR 10/10 (GE healthcare).
7. RNase-free water.
8. 1 M NaCl.
9. 1 M Tris–HCl (pH 7.4).

10. 1 M $MgCl_2$.
11. TBE Buffer (5×): 54 g Tris base, 275 g boric acid, and 4.7 g EDTA per liter of water. TBE buffer is typically stored indefinitely at room temperature.
12. Urea–acrylamide gel running buffer (0.5× TBE): Mix 100 mL of 5× TBE and 900 mL of water.
13. 5× Loading Buffer: Mix 50% (v/v) glycerol and 0.2% (w/v) xylene cyanol.
14. 40% Acrylamide/bis-acrylamide solution (19:1).
15. 1 M Potassium phosphate buffer, pH 7.0: Weigh out 107.12 g of K_2HPO_4 and 52.39 g of KH_2PO_4. Transfer to a 1-L graduated cylinder, add water to a volume of 1 L, and mix to dissolve.
16. 8 M Urea: Weigh out 480.48 g of urea. Transfer to a 1-L graduated cylinder, add water to a volume of 1 L, and mix to dissolve (see Note 3).
17. Buffer A: Weigh out 240.24 g of urea. Transfer to a 1-L graduated cylinder, add 40 mL of potassium phosphate buffer pH 7.0, add water to a volume of 1 L, and mix to dissolve.
18. Buffer B: Weigh out 240.24 g of urea and 58.44 g of NaCl. Transfer urea and NaCl to a 1-L graduated cylinder, add 40 mL of potassium phosphate buffer pH 7, add water to a volume of 1 L, and mix to dissolve.
19. Apparatus for gel electrophoresis.
20. Handheld UV lamp.

2.3. Stains-All *Staining*

1. DNA oligonucleotides (see Note 4).
2. 40% Acrylamide/bis-acrylamide solution (37:1).
3. 10% Ammonium persulfate solution.
4. *N,N,N,N'*-TEMED.
5. SDS-PAGE running buffer: 0.025 M Tris–HCl (pH 8.3), 0.192 M glycine, and 0.1% (w/v) SDS.
6. SDS loading buffer (5×): 0.3 M Tris–HCl (pH 6.8), 10% (v/v) SDS, 25% β-mercaptoethanol, 0.1% (v/v) BPB solution, and 45% (v/v) glycerol. Prepare 20 mL and leave 1 mL at 4°C for current use and store the remaining aliquots at –20°C.
7. BPB solution: Dissolve 0.1 g BPB in 100 mL water.
8. Resolving gel buffer: 1.5 M Tris–HCl, pH 8.8. Add about 100 mL water to a 1-L graduated cylinder or a glass beaker. Weigh out 181.7 g Tris base and add water to a volume of 900 mL. Mix and adjust pH with HCl. Make up to 1 L with water. Store at 4°C.
9. Stacking gel buffer: 0.5 M Tris–HCl, pH 6.8. Weigh out 60.6 g Tris base and prepare a 1 L solution as in previous step. Store at 4°C.

10. Apparatus for gel electrophoresis of protein.
11. Rinsing solution: 25% (v/v) isopropanol.
12. *Stains-all* (Sigma).
13. *Stains-all* staining buffer: Mix 30 mL of Tris–HCl (pH 8.8), 75 mL formamide, and 250 mL isopropanol, followed by addition of 0.025% (w/v) *Stains-all*. Add water to a volume of 1 L (see Note 5).
14. Lighttight containers.
15. Orbital shaker.

3. Methods

3.1. Production and Purification of RNase H

1. Transform 50 μL of competent BL21(DE3) cells with 10–100 ng of pET28a-(6×His)RNase H fusion protein expression vector, and spread 5–200 μL on an agar plate containing 37 μg/mL kanamycin. Incubate the plate overnight at 37°C.
2. Inoculate 100 mL LB medium in a 500-mL baffle-bottomed shake flask with a single colony from the transformation. Shake overnight at 220 rpm and 37°C.
3. Add 25 mL of the saturated overnight culture to 1 L fresh LB medium containing 100 μg/mL kanamycin in a baffle-bottomed shake flask.
4. Shake the flasks at 250 rpm and 37°C until the cells reach mid-log phase, OD_{600} of approximately 0.6.
5. Add IPTG to a final concentration of 1 mM. Continue shaking for 3–4 h.
6. Recover the cells by centrifugation for 15 min at $6,000 \times g$ and 4°C (see Note 6).
7. Resuspend the cells in resuspension buffer, using at least 10 mL per gram of wet cell pellet.
8. Lyse the cell suspension using a mechanical device to disrupt the *E. coli* cells (e.g., a sonicator, French press, or cell homogenizer) and centrifuge the disrupted cell suspension for at least 30 min at $15,000 \times g$.
9. Load the supernatant onto a column of Ni-NTA resin equilibrated with resuspension buffer. Wash the column with resuspension buffer and 20 mM imidazole until a stable baseline is reached. Elute the fusion protein with a linear gradient over 10 column volumes into elution buffer. The fusion protein usually elutes between 100 and 150 mM imidazole.
10. Mix 3.75 mL of resolving buffer and 3 mL of 40% acrylamide/bis-acrylamide solution (37:1), and add water to a volume of

10 mL in a 50 mL conical flask. Add 100 μL of 10% SDS, 100 μL of ammonium persulfate, and 10 μL of TEMED, and cast gel within a 7.25 × 10 cm × 1 mm gel cassette. Allow space for the stacking gel and gently overlay with ethanol or water.

11. Prepare the stacking gel by mixing 0.63 mL of stacking buffer and 0.5 mL of acrylamide mixture, and adding water to a volume of 5 mL in a 50 mL conical flask. Add 50 μL of 10% SDS, 50 μL of ammonium persulfate, and 5 μL of TEMED. Insert a ten-well gel comb immediately without introducing air bubbles.

12. Add 5 μL SDS loading buffer to a 10 μL sample of each fraction. Load the aliquots on the gel. Electrophorese at 80 V until the samples have entered the gel and then continue at 200 V.

13. Pool fractions of the eluate from the Ni-NTA column containing RNase H and then concentrate and dialyze against the storage buffer (see Note 7).

3.2. RNase H Cleavage

First, choose DNA oligonucleotides which are able to destabilize the tRNA scaffold (see Fig. 1 and Note 2).

1. Mix purified chimeric RNA and the two oligonucleotides (40 mM each, 1:1 ratio with the target RNA), incubate in boiling water (95°C) for 2 min, and then allow to cool down slowly to room temperature (25–30°C). The mix should be prepared in 250 μL maximum volume of water (see Note 8).

2. Add digestion buffer to a final concentration of 50 mM Tris–HCl (pH 7.5), 100 mM NaCl, and 10 mM $MgCl_2$. Start the cleavage reaction by adding 60 pmol of *E. coli* RNase H

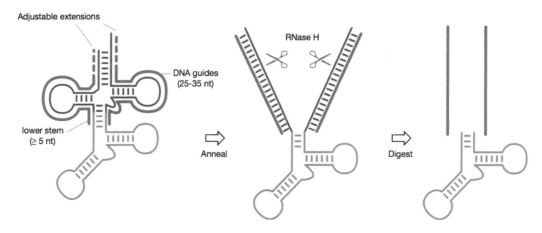

Fig. 1. The different cleavage steps carried out by RNase H. The DNA oligonucleotides are long enough to compete efficiently with the RNA–RNA interactions within the tRNA scaffold and replace them with DNA–RNA pairings after annealing. Typical lengths for these guide DNA oligonucleotides are about 30 nucleotides, but can be varied, as long as they extend at least 5 nucleotides into the lower stem of the tRNA scaffold. After cleavage, the RNA of interest is liberated from the tRNA scaffold.

per nmol of RNA. Incubate for 2 h at 30°C and then stop by addition of an equal volume of 8 M urea (see Note 9).

3. Purify preparative digests by Mono Q ion-exchange chromatography (Roche; see Note 10), under denaturing conditions: 40 mM potassium phosphate, pH 6.5, and 4 M urea (Buffer A). Wash with Buffer A until a stable baseline is reached. Elute the RNA with a 0–0.5 M NaCl gradient in Buffer B (Buffer A + 1 M NaCl) over 10 column volumes and collecting fractions of 5 mL.

4. Prepare the samples for 14% urea–acrylamide gel by mixing 20 µL of each collected fraction with 5 µL of 5× loading buffer.

5. Mix 2 mL of 5 × TBE, 4.25 mL of acrylamide mixture, and 5 g of urea, and add water to a volume of 10 mL in a 50 mL conical flask. Mix to dissolve the urea. Add 100 µL of ammonium persulfate and 10 µL of TEMED, and cast gel within a 7.25 × 10 cm × 1 mm gel cassette. Insert a ten-well gel comb immediately without introducing air bubbles.

6. Assemble the urea–acrylamide gel in the electrophoresis apparatus, fill with 0.5 × TBE running buffer, and load the samples (20 µL each). Electrophorese at 80 V until the samples have entered the gel and then continue at 200 V.

7. Following electrophoresis, pry the gel plates open with the use of a spatula. The gel will remain on one of the glass plates. Gently lift the gel from the glass plate and place it on shrink wrap (see Note 11) and place this on white paper. Reveal the RNA by UV shadowing with the handheld UV lamp placed above the gel.

8. Pool fractions identified as containing the RNA of interest. Dialyze the RNA product successively against 2 L of RNase-free water, then 2 L of 1 M NaCl (see Note 12), and finally with the buffer of your choice.

3.3. Stains-All *Staining*

1. Prepare a polyacrylamide gel for analysis of the RNA product and length marker DNA oligonucleotides, as described in Subheading 3.1, steps 10 and 11.

2. Add 5 µL SDS loading buffer to 10 µL of each DNA oligonucleotide and 10 µL of the RNA product. Load the aliquots on the gel (see Note 13). Electrophorese at 80 V until the samples have entered the gel and then continue at 200 V.

3. After electrophoresis, rinse the gel three times with 25% (v/v) isopropanol followed by washing in 30–50 mL of the same solution on a shaker for 10 min (see Note 14).

4. Replace the isopropanol by 30 mL of *Stains-all* solution. Due to the photosensitivity of *Stains-all*, gels should be incubated in

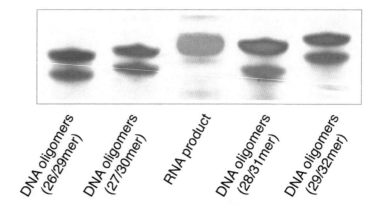

Fig. 2. The length of cleavage product of RNA is analyzed by 12% SDS-PAGE by comparison with DNA oligonucleotide markers. DNA and RNA bands were revealed by *Stains-all* staining (see Note 16). In this example, the estimated length of the RNA product was 31 mer.

a lighttight container on an orbital shaker at room temperature for at least 2 h.

5. Destain the gel with 25% (v/v) isopropanol in a lighttight container on an orbital shaker at room temperature for at least 1 h. Change the destaining solution occasionally (Fig. 2; see Note 15).

Incubation with RNase H will result in specific cleavage of the RNA strand within the DNA:RNA heteroduplexes and hence in complete cleavage of the scaffold. The RNA insert can then be recovered from the mixture and we obtained a single defined product in a quantitative manner.

4. Notes

1. The plasmid can be obtained from the Laboratory of Biological Crystallography and NMR.

2. The DNA oligonucleotides must be long enough to compete efficiently with the RNA–RNA interactions within the tRNA scaffold and replace them with DNA–RNA pairings after annealing. Typical lengths for these guide DNA oligonucleotides are about 30 nucleotides, but can be varied, as long as they extend at least 5 nucleotides into the lower stem of the tRNA scaffold. In practice, we found that they should cover at least the entire TΨC-stem and loop on one side, and the entire D-stem and loop on the other side. Previous reports of specific RNA cleavage using RNase H used modified DNA nucleotides

to improve specificity (7). In the present case, we used standard DNA oligonucleotides.

3. Urea can be dissolved faster provided the water is warmed to about 70–80°C.
4. Use DNA oligonucleotides with length comparable to that of the expected RNA product.
5. Due to the photosensitivity of *Stains-all*, the solution must be shielded from light.
6. Freeze the cell pellet at –80°C until further use (this may be for as long as several months). Perform all of the following procedures at 4°C.
7. Aliquots of RNase H can be stored at –20°C for months (final concentration of 0.25 mM).
8. After this step the RNA is no longer protected; use gloves, RNase-free solutions, and RNase-free materials.
9. Optimization of RNase H reactions: Some optimization must be made each time a new reagent is used (e.g., new plasmid preparation, new RNase H, etc.). In some cases, optimization of the RNase H reaction time is also required to maximize the yield. The critical step is the hybridization of your RNA with the DNA oligonucleotides and it is essential to use DNA oligonucleotides able to destabilize the tRNA scaffold. This step remains, however, very empirical.
10. The preferred ion exchange resin for purifying the cleavage product is MonoQ, as it provides better resolution than Source Q and hence provides better purity.
11. You can use transparent film for wrapping food or any UV transparent support preventing the adsorption of the wet gel on the white paper.
12. The dialysis against 1 M NaCl efficiently removes any remaining urea.
13. Usually denaturing urea polyacrylamide gel electrophoresis employs 8 M urea for DNA or RNA separation in a polyacrylamide gel matrix based on the molecular weight but SDS-PAGE can be used in order to obtain discreet bands.
14. The cycle of rinsing (three times) and washing should be repeated three times. This procedure ensures the removal of all SDS, which, if present, would cause the precipitation of the *Stains-all* dye.
15. Optional: Confirm the estimation of the length of the RNA product by mass spectrometry.
16. *Stains-all* allows differential staining of nucleic acids and proteins. RNA appears in pink and DNA in blue.

References

1. Ponchon L, Dardel F (2007) Recombinant RNA technology: the tRNA scaffold. Nat Methods 4:571–576
2. Nassal M (2008) Hepatitis B viruses: reverse transcription a different way. Virus Res 134:235–249
3. Soukup GA, Breaker RR (2000) Allosteric nucleic acid catalysts. Curr Opin Struct Biol 3:318–325
4. Cheong HK, Hwang E, Lee C, Choi BS, Cheong C (2004) Rapid preparation of RNA samples for NMR spectroscopy and X-ray crystallography. Nucleic Acids Res 10:e84
5. Price SR, Ito N, Oubridge C, Avis JM, Nagai K (1995) Crystallization of RNA-protein complexes. I. Methods for the large-scale preparation of RNA suitable for crystallographic studies. J Mol Biol 249:398–408
6. Donis-Keller H (1979) Site specific enzymatic cleavage of RNA. Nucleic Acids Res 7:179–192
7. Lapham J, Crothers DM (1996) RNase H cleavage for processing of *in vitro* transcribed RNA for NMR studies and RNA ligation. RNA 2:289–296
8. Ponchon L, Beauvais G, Nonin-Lecomte S, Dardel F (2009) A generic protocol for the expression and purification of recombinant RNA in Escherichia coli using a tRNA scaffold. Nat Protoc 4:947–959
9. Nonin-Lecomte S, Germain-Amiot N, Gillet R, Hallier M, Ponchon L, Dardel F, Felden B (2009) Ribosome hijacking: a role for small protein B during trans-translation. EMBO Rep 10:160–165
10. Green MR (1975) Simultaneous differential staining of nucleic acids, proteins, conjugated proteins and polar lipids by a cationic carbocyanine dye. J Histochem Cytochem 23:411–423

# Chapter 3

Preparation of Long Templates for RNA In Vitro Transcription by Recursive PCR

Jessica C. Bowman, Bahareh Azizi, Timothy K. Lenz, Poorna Roy, and Loren Dean Williams

Abstract

Preparing conventional DNA templates for in vitro RNA transcription involves PCR amplification of the DNA gene coding for the RNA of interest from plasmid or genomic DNA, subsequent amplification with primers containing a 5′ T7 promoter region, and confirmation of the amplified DNA sequence. Complications arise in applications where long, nonnative sequences are desired in the final RNA transcript. Here we describe a ligase-independent method for the preparation of long synthetic DNA templates for in vitro RNA transcription. In Recursive PCR, partially complementary DNA oligonucleotides coding for the RNA sequence of interest are annealed, extended into the full-length double-stranded DNA, and amplified in a single PCR. Long insertions, mutations, or deletions are accommodated prior to in vitro transcription by simple substitution of oligonucleotides.

Key words: In vitro transcription, RNA, DNA, Oligonucleotides, Synthetic DNA, Recursive PCR, Cloning, T7 promoter

1. Introduction

In a traditional polymerase chain reaction (PCR), an excess of oligonucleotide primers complementary to the 3′ ends of the double-stranded DNA fragment of interest (the DNA template), is combined with a small amount of DNA containing the template (1, 2). The source DNA is typically extracted from cells in the form of genomic or plasmid DNA. In the presence of deoxynucleoside triphosphates (dNTPs), Mg^{2+}, heat-stable DNA polymerase, and appropriate buffer, the template is amplified many orders of magnitude by repetitive cycling through temperatures optimal for denaturing, annealing of primers, and extension. Extension of the primers by DNA polymerase occurs in the 5′–3′ direction along the full length of the template (see Fig. 1a).

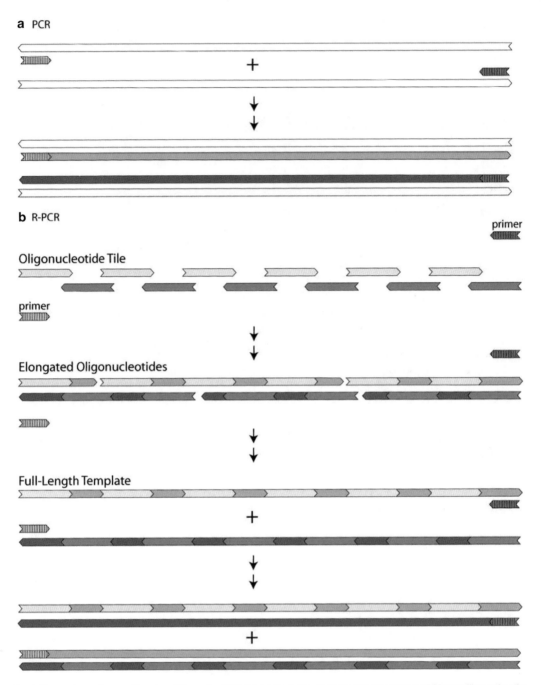

Fig. 1. Comparison of conventional and Recursive PCR. (a) A schematic diagram of a conventional PCR step illustrating the elongation of primers (*hashed arrows*) annealed to templates (*white arrows*). The direction of the chevron indicates the 5′–3′ directions. (b) A schematic diagram of an R-PCR. Initially an oligonucleotide tile is formed by synthetic oligonucleotides. The oligonucleotides are elongated and become successively longer with cycle number until some become full-length template. The added primers (*hashed arrows*) amplify the full-length template.

PCR can be used to construct long, double-stranded DNA from appropriate collections of long DNA oligonucleotides (oligos) in a process known as Recursive PCR (R-PCR). This method is named for its similarity to recursion in mathematics and computer science applications. R-PCR is also referred to as assembly PCR (3), parallel overlap assembly (4), or polymerase cycling assembly (5). R-PCR has the following advantages: (i) one-pot synthesis, (ii) a single dominant product, (iii) speed—often requires less than a day, (iv) material efficiency—chemical synthesis required for only half of the duplex DNA product (12), (v) modularity—facilitates nesting, modular synthesis, retrosynthesis, and synthesis of targeted libraries, and (vi) robustness—with no requirement for ligation.

PCR-based methods for splicing double-stranded DNA by overlap extension (6) anticipated R-PCR. The first published applications of R-PCR were the synthesis of a 522 base pair (bp) double-stranded DNA gene from ten oligos (7), and a 220 bp gene (8). Stemmer has used R-PCR for the single-step synthesis of DNA sequences up to 3 kb (3) and the approach has now achieved wide application (4, 9, 10). Genes can be obtained commercially; however R-PCR is a superior alternative to commercial genes under many circumstances. The benefits of R-PCR are greatest when fast turnaround is required, and a series of similar gene sequences is desired, whose extent of mutation, insertion, or deletion exceeds the range of a site-directed mutagenesis kit. Without R-PCR, such modification of commercially obtained genes can require de novo gene syntheses, many rounds of site-specific mutagenesis, or introduction of restriction endonuclease recognition sequences by mutagenesis followed by ligations. Modifying an R-PCR product can be as simple as swapping one or more oligos for one or more replacements, and repeating the R-PCR. Although synthesis of genes with substantial sequence modification by R-PCR adds complexity to the R-PCR oligo design process, these modifications can be quickly, reliably, and inexpensively incorporated.

In R-PCR, synthetic DNA oligos, with sequences identical to the sense and antisense strands of the target gene, are designed to form a tile. The tile contains alternating double-stranded and single-stranded regions. The 50–70mer oligos used to construct the tile are complementary on their ends giving duplex regions interleaved by single-stranded regions (see Fig. 1b). During an R-PCR, each 3′ terminus is extended, initially giving a mixture of products that coalesce to a single product as the number of PCR cycles increases (see Fig. 1b).

Here we focus on R-PCR/in vitro transcription (R-PCR/ivT)—the construction of DNA templates used for production of long RNAs by in vitro transcription. Preparation of a template for RNA in vitro transcription by R-PCR requires careful design of

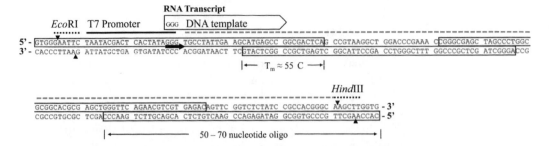

Fig. 2. Design of complementary DNA oligos for template synthesis by R-PCR. Stability nucleotides (5'-GTGG-3'), a unique restriction endonuclease recognition sequence (*Eco*RI), and the T7 promoter (*solid line*) are appended to the 5' end of the gene sense strand. A second restriction site (*Hind*III) and stability nucleotides (5'-GGTG-3') are appended to the 3' end of the gene sense strand. The resulting sequence is divided into an even number of oligos, 50–70 nucleotides in length, alternating between the sense and antisense strands. Each oligo overlaps adjacent oligos by at least 15 bp, targeting an overlap melting temperature of 55°C. Transcription following digestion with the 3' restriction endonuclease produces an RNA transcript that initiates at the tail of the arrow (shown between strands) and ends at the site of 3' endonuclease cleavage.

the synthetic DNA oligos. First, the sequence of the target RNA fragment is converted to the sense DNA sequence using DNA analysis software such as Invitrogen's Vector NTI. A T7 polymerase recognition sequence (T7 promoter) is appended at the 5' end of the sense sequence. To facilitate ligation to a vector, recognition sequences for unique restriction endonucleases, along with leading nucleotides necessary for efficient cleavage, are appended to the 5' end of the T7 promoter and the 3' end of the target sequence. The resulting DNA sequence is converted to a tile, by dividing it into partially overlapping oligos 50–70 nucleotides in length (see Fig. 2). The selected tile puts important constraints on future variants, and should therefore be chosen carefully. The nucleotides adjacent to anticipated insertions, mutations, or deletions are contained within the single-stranded regions (see Fig. 3). The oligos composing the tile, and additional 17–23mer primers for amplification of the full-length template, are obtained from a commercial vendor. The R-PCR is performed using a DNA polymerase with 3'–5' proofreading activity, equal molar concentrations of the internal oligos, and a 10-fold molar excess of amplification primers.

Subsequent preparation of the DNA template is synonymous with preparation of a native template for in vitro transcription. The amplification product is purified from secondary products and primers by preparative gel electrophoresis, ligated to a vector containing the same endonuclease recognition sequences chosen for the template, and replicated in *Escherichia coli* (*E. coli*). The purified plasmid is confirmed by sequencing analysis to contain the correct DNA template and is linearized prior to in vitro transcription.

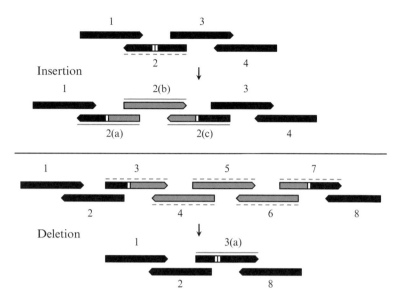

Fig. 3. Incorporating long insertions, mutations, and deletions by simple oligo substitution. Nucleotides flanking the planned modification (shown *white* in the schematic) are positioned within single-stranded regions. *Insertion*: Oligo 2 (*dashed line*) of a four-oligo template contains nucleotides flanking the planned insertion. Oligos 2(a), 2(b), and 2(c) (*solid line*) replace oligo 2 in the R-PCR to achieve the insertion (shown in *gray*). *Deletion*: Oligos 3, 4, 5, 6, 7 (*dashed line*) of an 8-oligo template contain a planned deletion (shown in *gray*). Oligo 3(a) (*solid line*) replaces oligos 3–7 in the R-PCR to achieve the deletion.

2. Materials

Prepare solutions using ultrapure water (18 MΩ cm at 25°C). Prepare and store all reagents at room temperature unless otherwise indicated.

2.1. R-PCR Components

1. DNA analysis/gene design software (see Note 1).
2. Thermocycler capable of performing a temperature gradient.
3. Nuclease-free water (see Note 2).
4. Autoclaved 1.5 mL microcentrifuge tubes (certified nuclease-free).
5. Autoclaved pipette tips (certified nuclease-free).
6. Autoclaved 0.2 mL PCR tubes (certified nuclease-free).
7. *Pfu* Polymerase (Stratagene), or an alternative DNA polymerase (see Note 3). Polymerases are usually supplied with 10× buffer. For *Pfu*: 200 mM Tris–HCl (pH 8.8 @ 25°C), 100 mM $(NH_4)_2SO_4$, 100 mM KCl, 20 mM $MgSO_4$, and 1% Triton X-100. Store at −20°C.

8. dNTP Mix: 25 mM dATP, 25 mM dCTP, 25 mM dGTP, and 25 mM dTTP. Mix 25 µL of each 100 mM stock of the four different dNTPs. Store at −20°C.

9. 2.5 µM 50–70mer oligos, commercially synthesized (see Note 4). Store at −20°C after rehydration.

10. 20 µM 17–27mer primers, commercially synthesized (see Note 4). Store at −20°C after rehydration.

2.2. Agarose Gel Electrophoresis Components

1. Horizontal agarose gel electrophoresis unit for 7×8 cm gels, and 1 and 1.5 mm thick combs with 6 and 8 wells.

2. Tris–acetate–ethylenediamine tetraacetic acid (EDTA) (TAE) Buffer (1×): 40 mM Tris–acetate and 1 mM EDTA. Use Molecular Biology Grade reagents. Can be conveniently purchased or prepared as a 40× stock: Dilute 50 mL of 40× TAE Buffer with 1,950 mL ultrapure water to prepare working concentration.

3. Agarose, LE, Analytical Grade.

4. Low-melting-temperature agarose for preparative DNA electrophoresis, such as SeaPlaque® Agarose.

5. GelStar® Nucleic Acid Gel Stain (Cambrex Bio Science Rockland, Inc.). Aliquot and store at −20°C.

6. DNA ladders for agarose gel electrophoresis: 100 bp and 1 kb DNA. Store at −20°C.

7. 1 M Tris (crystallized free base, Tris(hydroxymethyl)aminomethane): Dissolve 60.57 g in 500 mL ultrapure water. Adjust pH to 7.5 using HCl.

8. 0.5 M EDTA: Add 18.6 g to 100 mL ultrapure water and adjust pH to 8.0 using NaOH. Stir with heat until dissolved.

9. TE Buffer: 10 mM Tris, pH 7.5, 1 mM EDTA. Prepare by adding 5 mL of 1 M Tris and 1 mL of 0.5 M EDTA to 494 mL ultrapure water.

10. 6× Loading Dye, Blue: 2.5% Ficoll 400, 11 mM EDTA, 3.3 mM Tris–HCl, 0.017% SDS, and 0.015% Bromophenol Blue, pH 8.0 at 25°C. Store at −20°C.

11. Loading Dye: Add 100 µL of 6× Loading Dye, Blue, to 200 µL TE buffer. Store at −20°C.

2.3. DNA Purification Components

1. Agarose gel DNA extraction kit (see Note 5).
2. PCR and enzymatic reaction DNA purification kit (see Note 5).

2.4. Cloning Components

1. *Eco*RI and *Hind*III Restriction Endonucleases (20,000 units/mL), supplied with corresponding 10× reaction buffers, or appropriate alternatives (see Note 6).

2. pUC19 vector, or an appropriate alternative (see Note 6).

3. Phosphatase (5,000 units/mL) capable of heat inactivation at 65°C, supplied with 10× Phosphatase Buffer.
4. Quick Ligation Kit.
5. Chemically competent *E. coli* cells, such as DH5α (see Note 7).
6. Sterile inoculating loops or autoclaved toothpicks.
7. Lysogeny Broth-Ampicillin (LB-Amp) agar plates (with 50 µg ampicillin per mL agar).
8. LB medium.
9. 100 mg/mL Ampicillin.
10. Culture tubes.
11. "Mini" scale plasmid DNA preparation kit capable of purifying up to 20 µg of high-copy plasmid from 2 mL overnight *E. coli* cultures in LB, or alternative plasmid purification method.
12. "Maxi" scale plasmid DNA preparation kit capable of purifying up to 500 µg of high-copy plasmid from 100 mL overnight *E. coli* cultures in LB, or alternative plasmid purification method (for example, see Chapter 4).

3. Methods

3.1. Synthetic Oligonucleotide Design

1. Convert the sequence of the desired RNA transcript to its corresponding sense DNA sequence (see Note 8). Import the DNA sequence to the sequence editor of a DNA analysis/gene design software program (see Note 1).
2. Search the sequence for recognition sequences of common, commercially available restriction endonucleases. Take note of any that appear within the template, and eliminate these from consideration when choosing a vector and cloning site.
3. Choose a ligation vector and cloning site within the vector (see Note 9). A commonly used vector is pUC19 (see Note 10). Two commonly used restriction sites are *Eco*RI (5'-GAATTC-3') and *Hind*III (5'-AAGCTT-3') (see Note 6).
4. Using the software sequence editor, append the sense sequence of the first restriction site followed by a T7 promoter sequence (5'-TAA TAC GAC TCA CTA TAG GG-3') to the 5' end of the DNA sense template (see Note 11). Append the second restriction site to the 3' end of the DNA sense sequence.
5. Add four stability bases (e.g., GCTG or GGTG) to the 5' and 3' ends of the resulting sequence. These additional nucleotides foster stable duplex formation and are necessary at the terminal regions for efficient cleavage by many restriction endonucleases.

6. Beginning with the sense strand, divide the target sequence into an *even* number of oligos, each 50–70 nucleotides in length (see Note 12). The oligos must alternate between the sense and antisense strands. Adjacent sense and antisense oligos should overlap by at least 15 complementary nucleotides (Fig. 2). Since the first oligo is defined on the sense strand, and an even number of oligos is necessary, the last oligo is defined on the antisense strand (see Note 13). Nucleotides adjacent to any planned modifications (insertions, mutations, or deletions) by oligo substitution in the R-PCR must appear within the nonoverlapping regions (see Note 14).

7. Using the thermodynamic property analysis tool that accompanies most DNA analysis/gene design software programs, adjust the lengths of the sense and antisense oligos to achieve an estimated *overlap melting temperature* of 52–58°C (see Note 15).

8. Using DNA analysis software, check individual oligo overlap sequences for potential interfering secondary structure by searching the full target sequence for each specific overlap sequence, using a mismatch tolerance appropriate for the length of the overlap. If problematic secondary structure is found, lengthen oligos to increase specificity or shift the overlap away from secondary structure if possible. Ideally, overlapping regions are 17–20 bp in length or the length required to produce a melting temperature of 52–58°C.

9. Design standard forward and reverse amplification primers (17–27mer) complementary to the 3′ ends of the full-length DNA template (see Note 16). Here the full-length template includes the outermost stability nucleotides, the restriction sequences, and the T7 promoter. Both oligos and amplification primers can be procured lyophilized in tubes.

3.2. The R-PCR

Perform all procedures at room temperature unless otherwise specified.

1. Commercial oligos and primers are obtained in lyophilized form in tubes accompanied by a datasheet specifying the actual mass and number of moles delivered. Follow the supplier's directions for hydrating the lyophilized product to a concentration of 100 µM (strand) in nuclease-free water. After resuspension, check the final concentration with a UV spectrophotometer. Prepare 2.5 µM working stocks of each oligo, and 20 µM working stocks of each primer in nuclease-free water. Freeze the 100 µM stocks at −20°C and avoid frequent freeze/thaw cycling (see Note 17).

2. For the initial R-PCR, multiple reactions are generally prepared to facilitate PCR across a gradient of annealing temperatures, spanning a range of 45–65°C (see Note 18 and Fig. 4).

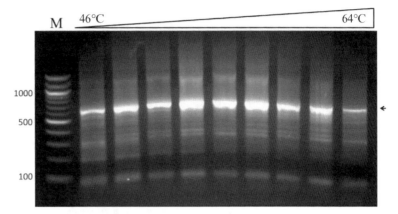

Fig. 4. Analytical gel (2% agarose) of replicate R-PCRs, showing successful synthesis of a 670 bp product amplified from 16 oligos over a range of annealing temperatures (46–64°C). Product amplification is optimal among *lane 5* (53°C), *lane 6* (55°C), and *lane 7* (58°C), centered around the design overlap melting temperature (~55°). Multiple secondary amplification products are almost always observed. Excess oligos appear near the 100 bp (smallest) marker.

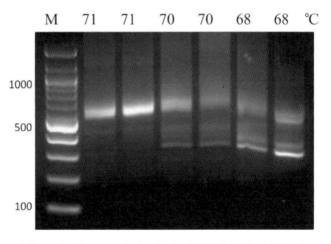

Fig. 5. Analytical gel (2% agarose) of replicate dsDNA "stitching" PCRs. Two double-stranded DNA fragments (190 and 480 bp, previously synthesized by R-PCR), containing a single 17 nucleotide overlapping region, amplified over a range of annealing temperatures: *lanes 2–3* (71°C), *lanes 4–5* (70°C), *lanes 6–7* (68°C). Lanes 2 and 3 illustrate successful amplification of the ~650 bp target.

Optimal annealing usually occurs around 55°C; however, this gradient can prove essential for optimizing amplification of templates with difficult secondary structure regions (Fig. 5). Prepare an equimolar master mix of the DNA oligos from the working stocks by combining 5.5 μL of each 2.5 μM oligo in a 1.5 mL sterile tube for every five PCRs. Assemble 50 μL reaction volumes in the order shown in Table 1 (see Notes 19 and 20).

Table 1
Components and assembly of the R-PCR

Volume	Component	Final concentration
To 50 μL total	Nuclease-free water	
5 μL	10× Polymerase reaction buffer	1×
1.25 μL	20 μM 5′ amplification primer	500 nM[a]
1.25 μL	20 μM 3′ amplification primer	500 nM[a]
0.5 μL	25 mM dNTPs (each dNTP)	250 μM
1 μL per oligo	DNA oligo master mix	50 nM each oligo[a]
1 μL	*Pfu* DNA polymerase or alternative (see Note 3)	~3 units

[a]See Note 20

Table 2
R-PCR cycling parameters

Step	Cycles	Temperature (°C)	Time (min)	Description
1	1	95	2	Initial denaturation
2	30	95	1	Cyclic denaturation
		59.5 ± 9 gradient	1	Annealing
		72	1 min per 1,000 nucleotides	Extension
3	1	72	2	Final extension
4	1	4	HOLD	

3. Program the thermocycler to cycle through the conditions shown in Table 2 (see Note 21). For the gradient annealing step, target annealing at temperatures of 53, 55, 59, 62, and 65°C (see Note 18). After thermocycling, the PCR mixture can be held at 4°C overnight or stored at −20°C.

4. Prepare an analytical agarose gel of appropriate percentage for the length of the anticipated amplification product (generally, this will be a 1.5–2% for the product size range appropriate for the R-PCR). For a 2% gel, add 1 g Agarose LE to 50 mL of 1× TAE buffer (see Note 22) in a 250 mL Erlenmeyer flask. Dissolve for 2–5 min in a microwave or heat with stirring on a hot plate. Boil until fully dissolved (less than 5 min). Prepare a horizontal gel electrophoresis apparatus by inserting the gel-casting tray sideways to seal the tray rubber against the interior

walls of the apparatus. Remove the agarose solution from heat. Before pouring, add 0.5 μL GELSTAR® Nucleic Acid Stain to the bottom of the gel-casting tray (see Note 23). Pour agarose into the casting tray as soon as it ceases to boil, to a thickness of approximately 0.5 cm. Using a pipette tip, mix the GELSTAR® into the agarose by vigorously tracing a grid of vertical and horizontal lines through the agarose. Mix well, but avoid unnecessary introduction of bubbles (see Note 24). Insert the appropriate 1 mm thick well-forming comb and allow the gel to solidify for 15–20 min.

5. Prepare a 100 bp DNA ladder and samples of each R-PCR for electrophoresis by adding 1 μL of each to 4 μL of the Loading Dye, Blue (see Note 25).

6. Check that the agarose has solidified (it should be cloudy in appearance and firm). Carefully remove the gel-casting tray containing the gel and place it in the gel apparatus in a position such that the comb is positioned nearest the black (negative) terminal of the apparatus. Submerge the gel in ~400 mL of 1× TAE buffer. Load each of the 5 μL samples prepared in the previous step to an individual well. Plug the electrodes into the power supply and run at 140 V for 20–30 min or until the dye front traverses ~70% the length of the gel.

7. Stop the power supply and remove the gel with cast from the electrophoresis apparatus.

8. Image the gel with a 302 or 312 nm UV transilluminator for dye excitation.

9. Compare amplification products with the molecular weight ladder. A bright and dominant band, approximately the same size as the calculated total length of the desired DNA template, indicates a successful R-PCR (Fig. 4). Multiple secondary amplification products (less dominant bands of varying size) are expected in R-PCR.

3.3. Purification of the DNA Template

1. Purify the desired amplification product from secondary products by preparative gel electrophoresis of the PCR product mixture. Cast a preparative (low melting) agarose gel of appropriate percentage for the length of the anticipated amplification product (1.5–2%, as for the diagnostic agarose gel). For a 2% gel, dissolve 2 g of SeaPlaque® GTG agarose in 100 mL of 1× TAE buffer in a 250 mL Erlenmeyer flask. Careful—the melting temperature of SeaPlaque® agarose is much lower than that of Agarose LE. Watch carefully while boiling to prevent boil over. Prepare a gel-casting tray as before and just before pouring, place 0.75 μL GELSTAR® in the bottom of the casting tray (see Note 23). Pour approximately 75 mL of agarose into the tray or to a thickness of 1 cm and mix in GELSTAR® as previously described. Insert the 1.5 mm side of a 6-well comb

into the agarose (see Note 26). Allow 45–60 min for the preparative gel to solidify.

2. Prepare a 100 bp molecular weight ladder by adding 1.8 µL of ladder to 18.2 µL loading dye.

3. Add 4 µL of 6× loading dye directly to each PCR, and mix well.

4. When the gel has fully solidified, submerge it in 1× TAE buffer (see Note 22). Load the molecular weight ladder–dye mix, and the full volume of each PCR–dye mix to each of the six wells. Run at 109 V for 30–45 min or until the dye front traverses ~70% the length of the gel.

5. Preheat a heating block to 55°C. Pipette 500 µL of nuclease-free water to a 1.5 mL microcentrifuge tube and place it in the heating block.

6. Image the gel with a UV transilluminator, taking care to minimize exposure time to the UV source.

7. Compare the bands on the preparative gel with the molecular weight ladder, and with the analytical gel. Secondary products that were not visible on the analytical gel may be visible on the preparative gel due to the large mass of DNA loaded. Due to a dye quenching effect, highly concentrated DNA does not stain well, and may appear as slight "parentheses" at the edges of the lane, with no definitive band visible (Fig. 6). Preparative gels

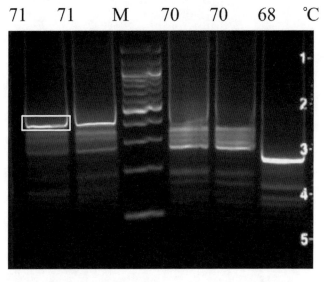

Fig. 6. Preparative gel (2% agarose) of the "stitching" PCRs shown in Fig. 5, with the second 68°C PCR omitted. The entire 50 mL volume of each PCR is loaded to a well. Due to a dye-quenching effect, the ~650 bp product band appears as "parentheses" along the sides of the well in *lanes 1* and *2*. In this preparative gel, the ~650 bp product (as seen on the analytical gel) runs between the 400 and 500 bp markers. The ~650 bp product to be excised from *lane 1* is enclosed by a box.

may also run differently relative to the molecular weight marker as compared to analytical gels. Carefully analyze and identify the location of the desired amplification product before proceeding (see Note 27).

8. Return the gel to the transilluminator and excise a minimal gel slice from each lane containing the amplification product using a razor blade. Place the gel slices in sterile 1.5 mL microcentrifuge tubes.

9. Add the volume of agarose dissolving/solubilizing buffer recommended by the gel extraction kit manufacturer to each gel slice and place the tubes in the heating block for 20 min (or until the gel slice is completely dissolved), mixing every 5 min (see Note 28).

10. Follow the gel DNA extraction kit protocol to purify the DNA from the dissolved agarose. Elute DNA in 55°C nuclease-free water. Avoid elution of DNA in a total volume greater than 30 μL.

11. Measure the UV absorbance of each eluted DNA template at 260 nm. Calculate the w/v concentration by multiplying the absorbance at 260 nm by the dilution factor (if any) and the 50 ng/μL conversion factor for dsDNA. Store at −20°C unless proceeding immediately (see Note 29).

3.4. Sequential Digest of the DNA Template and Host Vector

1. Calculate the volume of gel-purified DNA containing 200–500 ng of DNA template and transfer this volume to a sterile 1.5 mL microcentrifuge tube. Similarly, calculate the volume containing 500 ng of vector (see Note 10) and transfer that volume to a second microcentrifuge tube. Bring the total volume in each tube to 17.5 μL with nuclease-free water. Add 2 μL of 10× Restriction Enzyme Buffer and 0.5 μL of *Hind*III restriction endonuclease (or digest with an appropriate alternative). Incubate at 37°C for 1 h (see Note 30).

2. Purify the DNA from the enzyme and buffer using the PCR and enzymatic reaction DNA purification kit (see Note 31). Target an elution volume ≤17.5 μL.

3. Estimate the final elution volume using a pipette. To each tube, add nuclease-free water to a total volume of 17.5 μL. Add 2 μL of 10× *Eco*RI Buffer and 0.5 μL of *Eco*RI restriction endonuclease (or digest with an appropriate alternative). Incubate at 37°C for 1 h.

4. Preheat a heating block to 65°C. Remove tubes from the incubator. Add 24 μL nuclease-free water, 5 μL 10× Phosphatase Buffer, and 1 μL Phosphatase to the *vector sample only*. Incubate at 37°C for 1 h.

5. Remove tubes from the incubator and heat-inactivate at 65°C for 20 min.

6. Purify the digested template and vector from the phosphatase buffer using the PCR and enzymatic reaction purification kit. Elute DNA in 65°C nuclease-free water. Avoid elution of DNA in a total volume greater than 30 μL.

7. Measure the UV absorbance of each eluted DNA template at 260 nm, calculating w/v as described in Subheading 3.3. Store digested, purified template and vector at 4°C.

3.5. Ligation, Transformation, and Sequence Confirmation

1. Place two new LB-Amp plates (or LB plates with the appropriate selective antibiotic for the chosen vector) in a 37°C incubator. Add 50 ng of digested vector to each of the two sterile 1.5 mL microcentrifuge tubes. Estimate the mass required for a threefold molar excess of template insert by calculating the size of the insert as a fraction of the size of the vector and multiplying by 150. Add the calculated mass of insert to one of the two tubes containing 50 ng of vector, and bring the volume up to 10 μL (the ligation reaction). To the second of the two tubes containing 50 ng of vector, only add nuclease-free water to bring the volume up to 10 μL (background control). Add 10 μL of Quick Ligation Reaction Buffer and 1 μL of Quick T4 DNA Ligase enzyme mix to both tubes. Incubate at room temperature for 15 min (see Note 32).

2. Allow chemically competent cells to thaw on ice for 15–20 min. Transfer 5 μL of each ligation reaction to a sterile 1.5 mL microcentrifuge tube. Chill on ice for 5 min. Add 100 μL of competent cells to each 5 μL of ligation reaction. Incubate on ice for 45 min.

3. Remove the LB Amp plates from the incubator. Plate the entire 105 μL reaction (see Note 33) and incubate at 37°C for 16 h. Discard any remaining competent cells as biohazard waste.

4. Compare the number of colonies on background control plate to the ligation plate. The number of colonies on the ligation plate, relative to the number of colonies on the background control plate, dictates the recommended number of colonies to screen for plasmid containing the DNA template (see Note 34). Prepare a colony PCR master mix for screening in total reaction volumes of 10 μL. For every four colonies to be screened, combine all components for a single 50 μL PCR as listed in Table 1, omitting only the DNA oligos. Aliquot 10 μL to each of the four PCR tubes.

5. Prepare a new LB Amp plate for inoculation by sectioning into four parts. Using an inoculating loop or a sterile toothpick, touch a single colony on the ligation plate, touch the loop to one section of the prepared LB Amp plate (pre-warmed at 37°C), and then swirl the loop in one of the prepared PCR aliquots. Associate labels on the PCR tube with the plate freshly inoculated with the corresponding single colony. Incubate the

LB Amp plate(s) at 37°C for 16 h, and then store at 4°C, inverted and wrapped in parafilm.

6. Change the initial 95°C denaturing duration on the thermocycler to 5 min to facilitate cell lysis. Otherwise, cycle the PCR consistent with Table 2.

7. Prepare and load an analytical gel of the colony PCR as previously described for the R-PCR (see Subheading 3.2). Image the gel and evaluate for amplification products of similar size to the target DNA template.

8. From the LB Amp plate inoculated concurrent with preparation for the colony PCR, inoculate any colonies positive for DNA template (confirmed by analytical gel electrophoresis) into 2 mL of LB broth with 6.25 μL of 100 mg/mL ampicillin (or the appropriate selective antibiotic for the chosen vector). Culture for 16 h at 37°C with vigorous shaking.

9. Transfer 1.4 mL of each culture to a sterile 1.5 mL microcentrifuge tube. Harvest cells at $6,800 \times g$ for 3 min.

10. Prepare mini-scale plasmid purification kit buffers and purify plasmid as per the manufacturer's protocol. Elute DNA with 50 μL of 65°C nuclease-free water.

11. Measure the UV absorbance of each eluted plasmid sample. Prepare 15 μL of plasmid at a concentration of 100–300 ng/μL and send for sequencing with plasmid-specific primers flanking the cloning site (for a template ligated to the multiple cloning site (MCS) of pUC19 vector, use M13F and M13R universal primers).

12. Compare plasmid sequencing results with the full-length DNA template designed in Subheading 3.1 using DNA analysis software.

3.6. Large-Scale Replication of the Plasmid in E. coli

1. Autoclave 100 mL LB Broth in each of the two 500 mL culture flasks for step 3.

2. From the selective media plate inoculated concurrent with preparation for the colony PCR, prepare two culture tubes with 2 mL of LB broth and 6.25 μL of 100 mg/mL ampicillin (or the appropriate selective antibiotic for the chosen vector). Inoculate each with a single colony containing plasmid with the confirmed DNA template sequence from Subheading 3.5. Culture for 8 h at 37°C with vigorous shaking.

3. After 8 h, add 312 μL of 100 mg/mL ampicillin (or the appropriate selective antibiotic for the chosen vector) to each 100 mL of autoclaved LB Broth. Inoculate each with 1 mL of the starter culture. Culture for 16 h at 37°C with vigorous shaking.

4. Harvest cells at 4°C for 15 min at $6,000 \times g$. Purify plasmids per Maxi-scale plasmid purification kit as per the manufacturer's

protocol (see Note 35). Resuspend pellet in 500 μL nuclease-free water, taking care to thoroughly wash down the sides of the tube. Transfer resuspended plasmid to a sterile 1.5 mL microcentrifuge tube.

5. Measure the UV absorbance of the resuspended plasmid. Dilute and aliquot freezer stocks, if desired, but do not dilute below 150 ng/μL.

3.7. Plasmid Digestion at the 3' End of the DNA Template and Purification

1. Calculate the volume of resuspended plasmid from Subheading 3.6 containing 1 μg of plasmid DNA and transfer this volume to a 1.5 mL microcentrifuge tube. Add 2 μL of 10× Restriction Enzyme Buffer and 0.5 μL of *Hind*III restriction endonuclease (or digest with an appropriate 3' alternative). Incubate at 37°C for 2 h.
2. Heat inactivate the restriction endonuclease at 65°C for 20 min.
3. Remove tube from the heating block and allow it to cool on the bench for several minutes. Purify the DNA from the enzyme and buffer using the PCR and enzymatic reaction DNA purification kit. Elute DNA in 65°C nuclease-free water.
4. The linearized, purified plasmid containing the DNA template is now ready for in vitro RNA transcription.

4. Notes

1. Design of complementary oligos is best performed in a software program capable of showing both the sense and antisense DNA strands, calculating the melting temperature of selected regions, and recognizing common restriction sites. One example is Invitrogen's Vector NTI, though many other programs are available.
2. Nuclease-free water can be obtained from most common molecular biology supply companies, or alternately made by treating ultrapure water with diethylpyrocarbonate (DEPC). Add 0.5 mL of DEPC to 1 L ultrapure water (to 0.05%), mix well, and incubate for 2 h at 37°C. Autoclave to hydrolyze the DEPC before use.
3. While *Pfu* is routinely used by our lab for R-PCR, Freeland and coworkers (11) did not observe any full-length product when using *Pfu*, and instead reported much higher performance from *KOD* XL and *KOD* Hifi DNA polymerases which also act significantly more quickly, suggesting the potential for routine synthesis of genes up to 1 kb in under an hour. Our initial R-PCRs with Phusion® High-Fidelity DNA Polymerase and buffer (as per the manufacturer's instruction) suggest

that amplification may be superior to *Pfu* for some R-PCR applications. Alternatively, Vent DNA polymerase is reported to be effective in R-PCR (7). Xiong used *pyrobest Taq* DNA polymerase to splice double-stranded DNA fragments of intermediate length (400–500 bp), generated by R-PCR using *Pfu*, into DNA templates of multiple kb lengths (12). If using an alternative DNA polymerase, be sure to use the appropriate reaction buffer and cycling conditions.

4. Oligos are commercially available from many different companies. We order DNA oligos and primers for R-PCR at the 50 nmol synthesis scale with high-purity salt-free purification.

5. We prefer Agarose Dissolving Buffer, DNA Wash Buffer, and Zymo-Spin I Columns purchased together in the Zymoclean™ Gel DNA Recovery Kit from Zymo Research. DNA Binding Buffer, DNA Wash Buffer, and Zymo-Spin I Columns can also be purchased together in the DNA Clean and Concentrator™-5 kit from Zymo Research. Alternatives include the QIAquick® PCR Purification Kit or QIAquick® Gel Extraction Kit from Qiagen.

6. Most commercially available plasmids contain an MCS, or a region dense in common restriction sites often unique within the plasmid. Cloning into the MCS is often advantageous due to its well-defined sequence and widespread commercial availability of flanking primers. Two different restriction sites should be selected for the cloning site to ensure that the insert is ligated into the vector in the desired orientation. These sites should occur only once in the entirety of the vector sequence, and not appear in the DNA template. For convenience, endonucleases capable of double digest and heat inactivation should be selected wherever possible. The length of the plasmid relative to the length of the DNA template after ligation should be minimized. Long plasmids, relative to the size of the template to be transcribed, can reduce the efficiency of in vitro transcription. Selection of a vector 1.5–5 times the length of the DNA template is generally a good choice. If a T7 promoter is designed into the DNA template, the vector chosen for ligation should not contain its own T7 promoter region. Freeland used *Hind*III and *Bam*HI to clone their gene of interest into pUC19, but do not specify which restriction site was placed at which end of the gene (11). We have found that the double digest finder on New England Biolabs' Web site is an excellent resource for identification of compatible restriction endonucleases. If using alternate restriction enzymes, use the appropriate digestion buffers for the selected enzymes.

7. Alternatively, competent *E. coli* cells can be prepared from a fresh overnight culture. Inoculate 50 mL LB media with ~1 mL overnight culture. Incubate at 37°C for about 1 h, or until an

OD$_{550nm}$ of 0.45–0.6 is reached (no higher). Incubate on ice for 15 min, and then pellet cells for 15 min at 4°C. Resuspend pellet in 16 mL RF1 Buffer: 100 mM RbCl, 50 mM MnCl, 30 mM KOAc, 10 mM CaCl, and 15% glycerol (v/v); adjust pH to 5.8 with 0.2 M acetic acid, filter sterilize, and store at 4°C. Incubate on ice for 30 min. Pellet cells at 3,000×*g* for 15 min at 4°C. Working on ice, resuspend pellet in 4 mL RF2 Buffer: 10 mM MOPS (pH 6), 10 mM RbCl, 75 mM CaCl, and 15% glycerol (v/v); filter sterilize, and store at 4°C. Aliquot 300 μL to a prechilled, sterile 0.65 mL tube. Freeze in liquid nitrogen or a dry-ice ethanol bath. Repeat for the remaining volume. Store at −80°C.

8. This is easily done using the "Find and Replace" function of any text editor (replace all "U"s with "T"s), or by easily searchable online transcription tools.

9. Ligation of the DNA template, though time consuming, reduces transcription of undesirable secondary amplification products produced by PCR, and facilitates large-scale production of the DNA template.

10. pUC19 plasmid vector is used in this example; however alternate vectors such as the phagemid pGEM3Zf(+) have been used as well (7).

11. The specified T7 promoter is one that we have used successfully. The transcription start site is the first G residue encountered after the TATA portion of the promoter (see Fig. 2), such that this and all nucleotides after it will be incorporated into the RNA sequence by T7 RNA polymerase. Depending on the application, it may be necessary to alter the target RNA sequence to account for the presence of these initial guanosines in the transcribed RNA. There are multiple iterations of the T7 promoter published. One variation is the φ2.5 promoter, 5′-TAATACGACTCACTATT<u>A</u>GGG—3′, where the underlined adenosine is the initiating nucleotide. This promoter was shown to increase transcription efficiency and 5′ end homogeneity of the transcribed RNA (13).

12. Prodromou and Pearl recommend oligos 54–86 nucleotides long for optimal yields and minimal errors (7), while Freeland successfully utilized 40 nucleotide oligos with unoptimized 20 nucleotide overlaps, using an annealing temperature of 52°C (11).

13. When designing oligos for R-PCR, it is helpful to print a copy of the DNA sequence, showing both the sense and antisense sequence, for preliminary delineation of oligos. A simple method for delineation is to initially specify homogeneous overlaps of 15 bp and then to calculate the resulting number and length oligos required. First, calculate the number of

oligos needed for a sequence where Length T is the number of base pairs in the full-length DNA template, including stability bases, restriction sites, and T7 promoter:

$$\text{Number of oligos} = (\text{Length}_T / 40) - 0.375.$$

Round the number of oligos to the nearest *even* integer and then calculate the oligo length:

$$\text{Length of each oligo} = [(\text{Length}_T - 15)/(\text{Number of Oligos})] + 15.$$

Design initiates with the 5′ side of the sense sequence. If the length of each oligo (calculated above) is 55 bp, delineate the first 55 nucleotides of the *sense strand* by outlining or highlighting. This is preliminary oligo 1 (sense). Immediately after the last nucleotide in oligo 1, move vertically to the antisense strand. Backtrack 15 nucleotides, along the *antisense*, and delineate the 15-nucleotide overlap with oligo 1 plus the following (contiguous) 40 nucleotides of the antisense as oligo 2 (antisense). Move vertically to the sense sequence and repeat. Continue alternating sense and antisense, until preliminary oligos with complementary overlaps have been delineated for the entire DNA template. Because we are working with an even number of oligos, the last oligo delineated should (and must) be on the antisense strand.

14. When designing oligos for modifications by oligo substitution, the contiguous region to be modified must be located entirely within the nonoverlapping region of an oligo, which is roughly 20 bp in length. If the desired modification is longer, consider substitution of multiple oligos. Note that substitutions of one oligo can be made by another single oligo, three oligos, five oligos, etc. An odd number is necessary to retain the pattern of alternating sense and antisense oligos. Alternatively, it may be appropriate to extend the length of the oligo to be substituted up to 65 nucleotides. Longer oligos have a greater tendency to form interfering secondary structure, complicating synthesis and purification by the manufacturer, as well as in the R-PCR.

15. Overlapping regions of oligos should be evaluated in the same manner as amplification primers. For example, avoid overlap sequences likely to pair with an undesired overlap, seek a 3′ GC clamp, and avoid dimers and difficult secondary structure regions. DNA analysis software can be used to search for regions of nonspecific priming and secondary structure.

16. R-PCR is most efficient for DNA templates of 150–700 bp in length, with little to no secondary structure. For templates with regions of significant secondary structure or of length greater than 700 bp, we find it prudent to design additional primers for amplification of the DNA template in parts, retaining a common overlapping region. If the initial R-PCR fails to

amplify the full DNA template in a single reaction, then the oligos can be split into two separate R-PCRs, amplified individually into double-stranded DNA, and subsequently spliced into the full-length gene by dsDNA overlap extension (6, 12).

17. Careful preparation of template primer working stocks is critical. Template primers must be added to the PCR in equal molar concentrations. Take care to ensure that lyophilized primers are fully hydrated and resuspended prior to preparation of working stocks. Wu recommends resuspension of oligos in 10 mM Tris–HCl (pH 8.5) (11). For synthesis of an individual gene, a single working stock volume of 100 μL for each primer and oligo is usually more than sufficient. For more elaborate applications aliquot the 100 μM stocks in volumes anticipatory of future working stock preparation to avoid freeze/thaw cycling.

18. If this annealing temperature gradient does not produce the desired product, it may be helpful to further increase the annealing temperatures up to 71°C, particularly when the target sequence contains difficult secondary structure regions, which often interfere with R-PCR. However, in other reported cases, annealing temperature has no significant effect on R-PCR product yield. Freeland observed no perceivable difference when varying the annealing temperature from 48 to 62°C using *KOD* XL and *KOD* HiFi DNA polymerases, and consistently achieved success with a 52°C annealing temperature (11).

19. When assembling PCRs with a polymerase that exhibits 3′–5′ exonuclease activity (such as *Pfu*), the order of addition of the enzyme relative to the dNTPs is critical. Add the polymerase last to prevent possible degradation of primers and template.

20. Prodromou (7) achieved synthesis of their desired product using 0.2–0.3 pmol of each oligo in combination with 20–30 pmol of each amplification primer in a 100 μL total volume reaction with Vent DNA polymerase. They reported that the 100-fold difference proved crucial in achieving the target product. However, Freeland reports the optimal concentrations for each oligo to be 10–25 nM in a 50 μL reaction, and that the amplification primers must be at least tenfold more concentrated than the assembly oligos (11). They used 0.4 μM amplification primers, which represents a 16–40-fold excess of primer to internal oligos.

21. Alternately, Prodromou and Pearl suggest 30 cycles of 2 min at 95°C (denaturation), 2 min at 56°C (annealing), and 1 min at 72°C (extension), with a final extension at 72°C for 10 min when using Vent DNA polymerase (7). Freeman suggests additional temperature cycle options based on the performance of their preferred DNA polymerases *KOD* XL and *KOD* Hifi (11).

22. 1× TBE buffer (89 mM Tris base, 89 mM boric acid, and 2 mM EDTA at pH 8.0) may be used as a substitute for 1× TAE in agarose preparation and running buffer to improve resolution for target products below 250 bp. 10× TBE can be prepared by adding 108 g of Tris base, 55 g of boric acid, and 20 mL of 0.5 M EDTA to 1 L of ultrapure water. Dilute tenfold in ultrapure water to obtain 1× TBE. An alternate ladder with 25 bp steps, such as Bioline's Hyperladder V, can be used for molecular weight comparison when working with smaller DNA targets.

23. Optionally, add ethidium bromide to dissolved agarose or electrophoresis running buffer to a final concentration of 0.5 μg/mL.

24. If bubbles appear in the agarose upon mixing, either pierce them with a pipette tip or move them to the sides of the casting tray with the pipette to prevent interference with DNA migration.

25. A 5–10 μL total volume is appropriate for a diagnostic gel using an 8–12-well comb. A 20 μL total volume (marker) to 55 μL total volume (PCR) is appropriate for preparative gels using a 1.5 mm thick 6-well comb.

26. Note that a 1.5 mm thick 6-well comb should be selected for this gel to maximize well volume. Use of this comb may be best accommodated by adding an additional 25–50% mass of molecular weight ladder and increasing the total volume of ladder and dye loaded to the gel to 20 μL.

27. If the target band is not easily identifiable on the preparative gel, choose multiple candidate bands and excise them separately, noting the position of each excised slice on a copy of the gel image. Purify DNA from the gel slice as described in subsequent steps, and test for the presence of the target sequence by secondary PCR before proceeding with digestion and ligation (see Note 29).

28. Optionally, Prodromou used a sequential extraction with phenol, phenol/chloroform, chloroform and ether, and finally ethanol precipitation to purify the target product from the agarose (7).

29. The presence or absence of the target DNA in a given sample can be assessed by secondary PCR, which in this case is a subsequent amplification of the preparative gel-purified DNA. Assemble the secondary PCR using the same recipe as given in Table 1, replacing the DNA oligo mix with 50–100 ng of the gel-purified DNA. Use the same temperature cycling conditions used for the original PCR (e.g., if the sample was obtained from an R-PCR with a 59°C annealing temperature, use 59°C for the annealing step in the secondary PCR as well). Analyze the amplification product on an analytical agarose gel as described

(see Subheading 3.2, steps 4–9). A secondary PCR amplification product corresponding to the target DNA base pair length suggests that the original R-PCR and preparative gel DNA extraction were successful.

30. Prodromou (7) successfully digested with both *Eco*RI and *Hind*III in the same reaction; however other literature recommends the sequential digest described here for optimal cleavage. The enzyme manufacturer's literature should be consulted to determine whether a mutually compatible buffer exists for the selected pair of enzymes. If so, perform a double digest in the compatible buffer by adding 0.5 µL of both enzymes to the digestion reaction in Subheading 3.4, step 1, incubating at 37°C for 1 h, and then proceeding directly to Subheading 3.4, step 4.

31. Instead of a spin column kit, Prodromou (7) used Strataclean resin (Stratagene, Cambridge, UK) to purify the DNA from the restriction endonucleases.

32. For some DNA templates, a 15-min Quick Ligase™ reaction does not reliably yield colonies upon transformation. In such circumstance, a >16-h ligation at room temperature with T4 DNA Ligase and Buffer (New England Biolabs) is generally successful. The addition of 5–10%v/v DMSO can increase the ligation efficiency of templates with difficult secondary structure regions, but is accompanied by a decrease in transformation efficiency. Quick Ligase™ is not appropriate for extended ligations due to the presence of polyethylene glycol in the ligation buffer.

33. If using a compatible vector, optional blue/white colony screening can be performed by plating onto LB Amp plates containing X-gal (20 µg/mL) and IPTG (32 µg/mL). Colonies that appear white should have an insert ligated into the vector, while colonies that appear blue do not.

34. Freeland performed an exhaustive study on the error rates of *KOD* XL and *KOD* Hifi DNA polymerases, and formulated equations for colony screening that account for the probability of finding an insert with an exact sequence (11). These formulas are based on the length of the target product and the error rate of each polymerase.

35. DNA pelleted in isopropanol forms a glassy, translucent pellet that can be difficult to visualize. Using clear conical-bottomed centrifuge tubes and marking the tube before centrifugation may help in visualizing the pellet to ensure that it is not lost. Isopropanol pellets also do not stick to the side of centrifuge tubes well, so be very careful when drawing off the supernatant and subsequently washing the pellet.

Acknowledgments

This work was supported by the NASA Astrobiology Institute and the Georgia Institute of Technology's Center for Ribosomal Origins and Evolution.

References

1. Mullis KB, Faloona FA (1987) Specific synthesis of DNA in vitro via a polymerase-catalyzed chain reaction. Methods Enzymol 155:335–350
2. Mullis K, Faloona F, Scharf S, Saiki R, Horn G, Erlich H (1986) Specific enzymatic amplification of DNA in vitro: the polymerase chain reaction. Cold Spring Harb Symp Quant Biol 51(Pt 1):263–273
3. Stemmer WPC, Crameri A, Ha KD, Brennan TM, Heyneker HL (1995) Single-step assembly of a gene and entire plasmid from large numbers of oligodeoxyribonucleotides. Gene 164:49–53
4. Ouyang Q, Kaplan PD, Liu S, Libchaber A (1997) DNA solution of the maximal clique problem. Science 278:446–449
5. Smith HO, Hutchison CA 3rd, Pfannkoch C, Venter JC (2003) Generating a synthetic genome by whole genome assembly: phiX174 bacteriophage from synthetic oligonucleotides. Proc Natl Acad Sci U S A 100:15440–15445
6. Higuchi R, Krummel B, Saiki RK (1988) A general method of in vitro preparation and specific mutagenesis of DNA fragments: study of protein and DNA interactions. Nucleic Acids Res 16:7351–7367
7. Prodromou C, Pearl LH (1992) Recursive PCR - a novel technique for total gene synthesis. Protein Eng 5:827–829
8. Sandhu GS, Aleff RA, Kline BC (1992) Dual asymmetric PCR: one-step construction of synthetic genes. Biotechniques 12:14–16
9. Singh PK, Sarangi BK, Tuli R (1996) A facile method for the construction of synthetic genes. J Biosci 21:735–741
10. Gurevich AI, Esipov RS, Kayushin AL, Korosteleva MD (1997) Synthesis of artificial genes by PCR on a synthetic template. Bioorg Khim 23:492–496
11. Wu G, Wolf JB, Ibrahim AF, Vadasz S, Gunasinghe M, Freeland SJ (2006) Simplified gene synthesis: a one-step approach to PCR-based gene construction. J Biotechnol 124:496–503
12. Xiong AS, Yao QH, Peng RH, Li X, Fan HQ, Cheng ZM, Li Y (2004) A simple, rapid, high-fidelity and cost-effective PCR-based two-step DNA synthesis method for long gene sequences. Nucleic Acids Res 32:e98
13. Coleman TM, Wang G, Huang F (2004) Superior 5' homogeneity of RNA from ATP-initiated transcription under the T7 Φ2.5 promoter. Nucleic Acids Res 32:e14

Chapter 4

General Protocols for Preparation of Plasmid DNA Template, RNA In Vitro Transcription, and RNA Purification by Denaturing PAGE

Jo L. Linpinsel and Graeme L. Conn

Abstract

The development of methods for in vitro transcription of defined RNA sequences has been a key factor driving the tremendous advances in RNA biology over the last three decades. The numerous approaches available today to study RNA structure and function vary widely in their demands on the quality and quantity of material needed. These range for example from a few micrograms in biochemical assays, RNA structure probing or RNA folding studies using UV melting, to up to tens of milligrams or more of highly purified RNA for structural studies by nuclear magnetic resonance (NMR) or X-ray crystallography. Therefore, robust and scalable protocols, such as those described in this chapter, for production of plasmid DNA template, RNA in vitro transcription, and RNA purification, are an essential component of any RNA laboratory's experimental repertoire.

Key words: DNA plasmid preparation, RNase-free, T7 RNA polymerase, In vitro transcription, Hepatitis delta virus (HDV) ribozyme, Urea-denaturing polyacrylamide gel, Electrophoresis, RNA purification

1. Introduction

In vitro transcription of an RNA molecule requires three essential components: a polymerase enzyme, e.g., phage T7 RNA polymerase (T7 RNAP), the four ribonucleoside triphosphate building blocks, and a DNA template containing a promoter region for the polymerase directly upstream of the RNA encoding sequence (Fig. 1a). The DNA template is designed or processed before use such that the template strand ends at the desired 3′ end of the encoded RNA sequence and the polymerase "runs off" the template. Several options are available for DNA template synthesis. For short RNAs, chemically synthesized DNA oligonucleotides can be used for both strands (only the T7 RNAP promoter region needs to

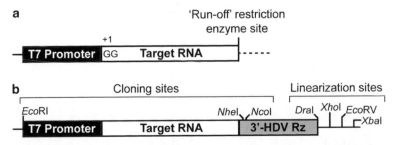

Fig. 1. Plasmid DNA construct design for RNA in vitro transcription. (**a**) The minimal requirements for a plasmid-derived transcription template: an RNA polymerase promoter, here for T7 RNA polymerase, followed directly by the target RNA sequence and ending with a restriction enzyme site to linearize the template for polymerase "run-off." (**b**) Design of an in vitro transcription construct incorporating a 3′-HDV sequence to ensure target RNA 3′-end homogeneity. Multiple linearization sites (MLS) allow adjustment of the ribozyme length to avoid close migration with the target RNA on acrylamide gels used to purify the RNA.

be double stranded; also see Chapter 5). For longer sequences, the options include total gene synthesis, recursive PCR (see Chapter 3), or standard PCR in cases where a template already exists. PCR-derived templates can be generated using a primer to incorporate the T7 RNAP promoter region and used directly for in vitro transcription. However, it can be advantageous and convenient to place each required element into a high copy number plasmid (e.g., pUC19). The only additional requirement when using a plasmid template is that it must contain a restriction enzyme site placed at the 3′ end of the RNA coding sequence to generate the "run-off" site (Fig. 1a).

T7 RNAP has become the enzyme of choice for RNA in vitro transcription (1); it is commercially available or can be produced in large quantities using recombinant constructs which add a 6×His tag for simple purification (2), and it produces large quantities of RNA in a short time. The enzyme does, however, have some limitations. First, like some other polymerases, it has the tendency to add nontemplated ("$n+1$," "$n+2$," etc.) nucleotides resulting in RNA transcripts with heterogeneous 3′-termini (3, 4). Second, the T7 RNAP promoter, typically 5′-TAATACGACGACATATA^{+1}G where the final G is the first nucleotide of the RNA transcript, imposes sequence limitations on the 5′ end. Higher yields can be obtained using two or three 5′-end G's (Fig. 1a) and minimizing the number of U nucleotides in the initial sequence but these further limit the flexibility in sequences that can be transcribed (1). In vitro transcribed RNAs will also possess a 5′-triphosphate group which is not always desirable and may require further enzymatic processing. Each of these limitations can be a problem for some downstream applications but can be overcome with *cis*-acting self-cleaving RNA sequences ("ribozymes"). We have previously generated plasmids pre-loaded with ribozyme sequences and convenient restriction enzyme sites for incorporating new target RNA sequences (5). The protocols described here include the use of a 3'-hepatitis delta virus (HDV) ribozyme sequence immediately downstream of the target RNA coding. When using this HDV-encoding plasmid, the only sequence limitation is that the final nucleotide of the target RNA should not be a cytidine because of potential base pairing with the ribozyme sequence (6). In most cases, however, the HDV ribozyme exhibits almost complete co-transcriptional cleavage from the upstream sequence yielding target RNAs with homogenous 3' ends. For some RNA constructs, where the folding of the ribozyme might be less efficient, a lower extent of initial self-cleavage may be observed. In these cases, an additional posttranscriptional annealing step can be used to enhance cleavage of the ribozyme from the RNA of interest (7).

This chapter first describes a generally applicable protocol for preparing plasmid DNA template suitable for RNA in vitro transcription. This scalable protocol will produce several milligrams of plasmid DNA from 1 L of bacterial culture. Although commercial kits are available for preparation of plasmid DNA, these use RNases during cell lysis and we have found them to produce templates of variable quality. Next, we describe a general protocol for RNA in vitro transcription that is based on conditions previously reported by Gurevich (8). We have found this to be an excellent starting point for transcribing any new RNA sequence. Although not described here, it may be necessary to test variation of some components; the most likely to affect RNA yield are the concentrations of DNA template, ribonucleoside triphosphates (rNTPs), Mg^{2+}, and the T7 RNAP. Other chapters in this book describe several variations in the in vitro transcription reaction that can also be investigated. Our plasmid construct produces RNAs fused to a 3'-HDV ribozyme (5) and a protocol is next described that can be used to enhance ribozyme cleavage (and hence target RNA yield) when this reaction is suboptimal directly in the transcription reaction. Finally, a general protocol for denaturing PAGE purification is described that complements the native chromatography and affinity approaches described elsewhere in this book (e.g., see Chapters 5, 6, and 9–11).

2. Materials

2.1. Large-Scale Plasmid DNA Template Preparation

1. Plasmid containing the target RNA sequence with an upstream promoter for T7 RNAP (5'-TAATACGACGACATATA^{+1}G; see Fig. 1).

2. Competent cells of an *Escherichia coli* strain suitable for plasmid propagation (we typically use DH5α).

3. Lysogeny Broth (LB): 10 g peptone from casein, 5 g yeast extract, and 10 g sodium chloride dissolved in water to a total volume of 1 L (see Note 1). Autoclave immediately after preparation.

4. LB-agar bacterial growth plates: 10 g peptone from casein, 5 g yeast extract, 10 g sodium chloride, and 12 g agar-agar dissolved in water to a total volume of 1 L. Divide into media bottles and autoclave. LB-agar can be stored after autoclaving; melt solid LB-agar in a microwave on low power. After autoclaving or microwaving, allow to cool to <60°C, add antibiotic corresponding to plasmid resistance at a suitable working concentration, mix by swirling, and pour plates immediately.

5. 1,000× stock solution of antibiotic corresponding to plasmid encoded resistance for selection.

6. Terrific Broth (TB): 12 g tryptone, 24 g yeast extract, 9.4 g potassium phosphate dibasic, 2.2 g potassium phosphate monobasic, and 4 mL glycerol made up to a final volume of 1 L with water. Autoclave immediately after preparation.

7. Resuspension Buffer: 25 mM Tris (pH 8.0), 10 mM EDTA, and 50 mM glucose.

8. Lysis Solution: 2% sodium dodecyl sulfate (SDS), 0.2 M NaOH. Prepare immediately before use (see Note 2).

9. Neutralization Solution: 3 M KOAc (pH 4.8).

10. 100% ethanol, 190 proof.

11. Tris–EDTA (TE) Buffer: 10 mM Tris and 1 mM EDTA (pH 8.0).

12. 7.5 M ammonium acetate.

13. Phenol:chloroform solution: Saturate phenol with TE buffer pH 8.0 and mix in a 1:1 ratio with chloroform (a small amount of TE can be left as an upper aqueous layer). Both TE-saturated phenol and phenol:chloroform solution are also available commercially.

14. Chloroform.

15. 5 M NaCl.

16. 13% Polyethylene glycol 8000 molecular weight (see Note 3).

17. Apparatus for running 1% agarose gels.

18. 70% Ethanol.

19. Preparative centrifuge with rotor for 400 mL centrifuge bottles.

2.2. RNA In Vitro Transcription

1. Plasmid DNA at a concentration of 1 μg/μL.

2. Restriction enzyme and corresponding 10× buffer provided by the supplier. For the example protocol described here, we use *Dra*I.

3. 1 M HEPES–KOH (pH 7.5), filter sterilized.
4. 1 M MgCl$_2$, filter sterilized.
5. 200 mM Spermidine: Adjust to neutral pH by addition of HCl, monitoring by spotting small aliquots onto pH test strips, then filter sterilize.
6. 1 M Dithiothreitol (DTT), filter sterilized.
7. rNTPs: 10 mM rATP, 10 mM rGTP, 10 mM CTP, and 10 mM UTP. NTPs can be purchased as mixes or individual stock solutions. If using solid NTPs, individually weigh out and dissolve in 50 mM Tris base solution (see Note 4).
8. T7 RNA Polymerase: This enzyme can be purchased commercially or prepared in-house.
9. 250 mM EDTA (pH 8.0).
10. Dialysis tubing with molecular weight cutoff appropriate for the particular RNA of interest.
11. 3 M Sodium acetate (pH 5.2).
12. 100% Ethanol, 200 proof.
13. Tris–EDTA Buffer: 10 mM Tris and 1 mM EDTA (pH 8.0).

2.3. Optimization of 3′-HDV Ribozyme Cleavage Efficiency

1. 1 M MgCl$_2$.
2. Dialysis tubing with molecular weight cutoff appropriate to the particular RNA of interest.
3. 3 M Sodium acetate (pH 5.2).
4. 100% Ethanol, 200 proof.

2.4. Analysis and Purification of RNA by Urea-Denaturing Gel Electrophoresis

1. Products of in vitro transcription resuspended in TE buffer.
2. Tris–Boric acid–EDTA Buffer (TBE, 10×): 1 M Tris, 1 M boric acid, and 10 mM EDTA.
3. Denaturing acrylamide gel solution: Acrylamide:N,N'-methylene-bis-acrylamide (19:1 ratio) and 50% w/v urea dissolved in 1× TBE (see Note 5).
4. 10% w/v ammonium persulfate: Prepare immediately before use.
5. Tetramethylethylenediamine (TEMED) (see Note 6).
6. Vertical mini-gel electrophoresis equipment for analysis of test transcription reactions, HDV annealing, etc: For example, we use the Mini-PROTEAN Tetra cell system (BioRad).
7. Large vertical gel electrophoresis apparatus: For example, we pour preparative denaturing polyacrylamide gels using 20×25 cm glass plates with 3 mm spacers and combs. This requires ~150 mL of gel solution (item 3, above) per gel and can be loaded with 2–5 mg RNA depending on the difference in migration of the target RNA and other bands on the gel.

8. Urea Loading Dye (2×): 50% urea, 0.25% bromophenol blue, and 0.25% xylene cyanol dissolved in 1× TE Buffer.
9. Handheld UV lamp (shortwave, 254 nm).
10. 0.3 M Sodium acetate (pH 5.2).
11. 100% Ethanol, 200 proof.
12. Tris–EDTA Buffer: 10 mM Tris and 1 mM EDTA (pH 8.0).
13. *Optional*: Apparatus for electroelution of RNA from gel slices, e.g., we use a "BioTrap" (Schleicher and Schuell).

3. Methods

3.1. Large-Scale RNase-Free Plasmid Preparation

The following protocol starts from a fresh transformation of competent *E. coli* cells of a strain suitable for plasmid propagation (such as DH5α). A single colony is used to produce a saturated culture in Terrific Broth from which plasmid DNA is purified. The protocol describes purification starting from a 1 L culture but can be scaled according to individual needs; at the scale described, the protocol should produce at least 1 mg purified plasmid, often much more.

1. Thaw competent *E. coli* cells on ice and transform using 50 ng of plasmid DNA (see Note 7).
2. Following heat shock and recovery on ice, add 1 mL of LB medium and incubate at 37°C for 1 h, ideally with gentle shaking sufficient to stop the cells from settling to the bottom of the tube. Plate 100 µL (see Note 8) of the transformed cells on an LB-agar plate with appropriate antibiotic and incubate for 12–16 h at 37°C.
3. Use a single colony to inoculate 5 mL of Terrific Broth containing an appropriate antibiotic and incubate at 37°C with vigorous shaking for at least 8 h (see Note 9).
4. Use the entire 5 mL starter culture to inoculate 1 L of TB with appropriate antibiotic and incubate at 37°C with vigorous shaking for 12–16 h.
5. Harvest the cells using a preparative centrifuge with sufficient r.c.f. and time to produce a compact cell pellet and completely clear supernatant, e.g., ~3,000×g at 4°C for 20 min. The cell pellets can be stored at −20°C at this point, if desired (see Note 10).
6. Resuspend the cell pellet in 10 mL of Resuspension Buffer.
7. Transfer to a 50 mL conical tube (see Note 11), add 20 mL of Lysis Buffer, and invert several times to mix. Leave for a few minutes with occasional mixing but do not exceed 5 min.

8. Add 15 mL ice-cold Solution 3 and gently invert to mix. Do *NOT* vortex. Leave on ice for 30 min.

9. Collect cell debris by centrifuging at $10,000 \times g$ for 40 min at 4°C.

10. Filter the supernatant through gauze or coarse filter paper into a 400 mL centrifuge bottle.

11. Add 110 mL ethanol and incubate on ice for at least 10 min to precipitate nucleic acids.

12. Centrifuge at $3,000 \times g$ for 10 min at 4°C. Remove the supernatant and thoroughly dry the pellet with an airstream (see Note 12). From this step on, all centrifugations are done in a swinging-bucket rotor.

13. Resuspend the pellet in 6 mL TE buffer and transfer to a 50 mL conical tube.

14. Add 3 mL of 7.5 M ammonium acetate solution, mix, and incubate for 10 min on ice to precipitate high-molecular-weight RNAs.

15. Centrifuge at $3,000 \times g$ for 10 min at 4°C.

16. Transfer the supernatant to a new 50 mL conical tube, add 20 mL of ethanol, and incubate on ice for 10 min to precipitate the plasmid DNA.

17. Centrifuge at $3,000 \times g$ at 4°C for 10 min. Pour off the ethanol and dry the pellet using an airstream (sec Note 12).

18. Dissolve the pellet in 3 mL of TE buffer and transfer to a 15 mL disposable tube.

19. Extract the DNA solution with an equal volume of phenol:chloroform (1:1). Mix by vortexing thoroughly and then centrifuge at $3,000 \times g$ for 5 min at 4°C to separate the aqueous and organic phases.

20. Remove the upper aqueous layer to a fresh tube and repeat the extraction process (step 19) one more time (see Note 13).

21. Back extract phenol from the DNA-containing aqueous phase by adding an equal volume of chloroform and vortexing as before. Centrifuge again at $3,000 \times g$ at 4°C and transfer the aqueous layer to a fresh tube.

22. Precipitate the DNA by adding two volumes of ethanol and incubating on ice for 10 min (see Note 14). Centrifuge at $3,000 \times g$ for 10 min at 4°C (see Note 15).

23. Wash the pellet with 1 mL of 70% ethanol, breaking up a large pellet. Centrifuge at $3,000 \times g$ at 4°C for 10 min.

24. Dry the pellet *thoroughly* with an airstream (see Note 12).

25. Dissolve the pellet in 330 μL TE buffer and transfer to a microcentrifuge tube (see Note 16).

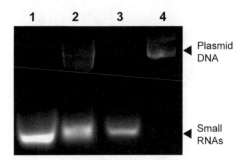

Fig. 2. RNase-free purification of plasmid DNA. (a) Agarose gel analysis of samples from the PEG 8000 precipitation step: supernatant (*Lane 1*) and resuspended pellet containing the plasmid DNA (*Lane 2*) from a first precipitation that failed to completely remove all small RNAs; supernatant from a second (repeat) PEG precipitation (*Lane 3*); and final purified plasmid DNA (*Lane 4*).

26. Add 120 μL 5 M NaCl and 750 μL 13% PEG 8000 and incubate for 30 min at room temperature to precipitate the plasmid DNA from small RNAs (see Note 3).

27. Centrifuge at $3,000 \times g$ at 4°C for 10 min. Remove the supernatant and retain for later analysis.

28. Wash the plasmid DNA pellet with 70% ethanol and allow to air-dry. Resuspend in 330 μL of TE Buffer (see Note 17).

29. Analyze the purified plasmid DNA and the supernatant retained at step 27 on a 1% agarose gel. All of the small RNAs should be removed from the plasmid sample (see Fig. 2). If not, additional PEG 8000 precipitations must be carried out on the plasmid DNA by repeating steps 26–29 (see Note 18). Once the plasmid DNA is free of small RNAs, its concentration should be determined by measuring the absorbance at 260 nm (1.0 A_{260} = 50 μg/mL double-stranded DNA).

3.2. RNA In Vitro "Run-Off" Transcription Using T7 RNA Polymerase

The following protocol is fully scalable in order to produce the desired quantity of RNA. The protocol on which these conditions are based (8) used an RNase inhibitor, pyrophosphatase, and acetylated BSA. These are omitted from the reaction conditions used here; as long as a sterile, RNase-free environment is maintained there should be no need for RNAse inhibitor, and we have found that using pyrophosphatase can produce lower quality RNA transcripts (unpublished data). For any new construct, we recommend performing at least one small-scale (50–100 μL) test transcription. Several test reactions may be needed to optimize the concentrations of some reagents (see Table 1). Reactions larger than 1 mL can be performed in multiple 1.5 mL tubes or a single larger sterile centrifuge tube; adjust volumes of reagents appropriately.

1. Digest the plasmid DNA using an appropriate restriction enzyme (see Note 19). The final concentration of DNA in the reaction should be 1 μg/μL.

Table 1
Components of the RNA in vitro transcription reaction

Component	Final concentration[a]	Volume required (μL) 100 μL reaction	1 mL reaction
1 M HEPES–KOH, pH 7.5	200 mM	20	200
1 M MgCl$_2$	28 mM	2.8	28
0.2 M Spermidine	2 mM	1	10
1 M Dithiothreitol (DTT)	40 mM	4	40
10 mM each rNTPs	6 mM (each)	60	600
Linearized plasmid DNA	30–100 μg/mL	3–10	30–100
H$_2$O	–	Up to 100	Up to 1000
T7 RNA polymerase	–	1–5	10–50

[a]These concentrations produce good yields for most RNAs but optimization of plasmid, NTPs, and/or MgCl$_2$ concentrations may be necessary with each RNA construct

2. Inactivate the restriction enzyme if this is possible, e.g., 65°C for 20 min (check the manufacturer's instructions; see Note 20).

3. Combine the reagents listed in Table 1 in the order listed (see Note 21), invert to mix, and pulse briefly in a microcentrifuge to collect the reaction at the bottom of the tube.

4. Incubate the reaction at 37°C for 3–5 h. Commonly, a white precipitate will form from the precipitation of pyrophosphate–magnesium ion complex (PPi·Mg^{2+}). This should be removed at the end of the reaction by the addition of 250 mM EDTA until the solution turns clear (see Note 22).

5. Assess the quality of the transcription reaction on an analytical 50% urea-denaturing polyacrylamide gel (see Note 23). For test transcriptions, this should confirm the presence of the target RNA product and allow determination of optimal reagent concentrations; steps 1–4 may be repeated at the final desired scale. For preparative reactions, it is necessary to dialyze the sample prior to purification.

6. Using dialysis tubing with a cutoff molecular weight of no more than half that of the target RNA, dialyze for at least 4 h against 4 L of TE buffer (see Note 24).

7. Ethanol precipitate the RNA by adding 1/10th volume of 3 M NaOAc (pH 5.2) and three volumes ethanol. Incubate on ice for at least 10 min and pellet the precipitated RNA by centrifugation at 3,000 × g for 10 min at 4°C (see Note 15).

8. Resuspend the pellet in a minimal volume of TE buffer (see Note 25).

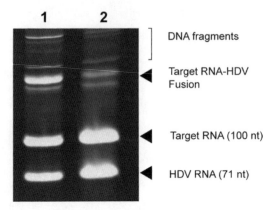

Fig. 3. Annealing to improve 3′-HDV cleavage efficiency. RNA from in vitro transcription before (*Lane 1*) and after (*Lane 2*) additional annealing step to cleave the remaining fused RNA to HDV. Typically, most target RNA-ribozyme transcripts are cleaved co-transcriptionally but with some constructs, as shown here, an additional posttranscriptional annealing step can significantly increase the fraction of free target RNA obtained.

3.3. Optional: Extra Annealing Step(s) to Enhance HDV Ribozyme Self-Cleavage

If the RNA construct is transcribed with an HDV ribozyme for 3′-end processing, it may be necessary to post-transcriptionally cleave the ribozyme from the target RNA. Although in most cases the HDV ribozyme cleaves co-transcriptionally, cleavage efficiencies vary significantly in a target RNA-dependent manner. HDV folding and cleavage can be promoted using additional "annealing" steps to achieve greater cleavage, which in turn may give higher yields of the RNA of interest (see Fig. 3). It should be noted, however, that this protocol involves heating the RNA in the presence of Mg^{2+} which can degrade the RNA. Therefore, for intermediate cases, it is necessary to balance loss of transcript due to partial HDV cleavage against loss through degradation to determine the best approach.

1. Add $MgCl_2$ to the sample to bring the concentration to 50 mM.
2. Incubate the solution at 90°C for 5 min.
3. Transfer directly to a heating block or an incubator at 55°C and incubate for at least 5 h.
4. Dialyze the sample again, ethanol precipitate, and bring up in a minimal volume TE buffer (see Note 25).

3.4. RNA Purification Using Urea-Denaturing Polyacrylamide Gel Electrophoresis

Several other chapters in this book describe various approaches for native purification of RNA using tags or FPLC chromatography (see Chapters 5, 6, and 9–11). However, as the historically most common and widely applicable approach to RNA purification away from DNA template, rNTPs, and other RNA(s) (e.g., HDV ribozyme or truncated products), a protocol such as the following for urea-denaturing polyacrylamide gel electrophoresis (urea PAGE) should be part of every RNA biologist's armory.

1. Prepare the urea gel solution and pour one or more gels. The amount of RNA to be purified that can be loaded per gel must be empirically determined as it will depend on several factors, including the gel dimensions, yield of target RNA from the transcription reaction, and relative positions of the target RNA and other bands on the gel at the optimal percentage of acrylamide.

2. Place the gel(s) into the electrophoresis apparatus. Ensure that all urea and gel fragments are cleared out from the well and flush out any air bubbles that might be present between the bottom of the gel and the lower buffer chamber. Pre-run the PAGE gel for 1 h with power settings that will be used during the RNA purification.

3. While pre-running the gel, add equal volume of 2× Loading Dye to the RNA sample and incubate at 65°C for 10 min to fully denature the RNA.

4. Again ensure that the gel well is free of urea and, directly from the heating block, load the warm RNA sample in as tight a band as possible. Run at 200 V until the marker dyes have migrated into the gel the desired distance (see Note 26).

5. Separate the gel plates and place the gel carefully between Saran Wrap. Identify and mark the target RNA by UV shadowing (shortwave, 254 nm). As quickly as possible, draw an outline of the target band on the Saran Wrap using a marker pen and turn off the UV lamp (see Note 27).

6. Excise the RNA target band using a sterile scalpel to cut across the gel above and below the band and at one end. Peel back the Saran Wrap and cut the band into small slices. Gel slices can be stored at −20°C in a 50 mL sterile disposable centrifuge tube, if desired.

7. Elute the RNA from the gel slices using one of the two possible methods: electroelution, e.g., using a "BioTrap" device (Schleicher and Schuell), or passively into buffer (also known as "crush and soak"). For electroelution, follow the manufacturer's protocols to recover the RNA and then proceed to step 11 or use the RNA directly for experiments.

8. For passive elution, place the gel slices into the barrel of a syringe, reinsert the plunger, and force the gel through into a sterile 15 mL disposable centrifuge tube. This process should shred the gel slices to maximize its surface area.

9. Add sufficient 0.3 M sodium acetate, pH 5.2, to cover the crushed gel and incubate at 4°C for at least 4 h, ideally on a roller or a similar mixing equipment. Overnight incubation is convenient and sometimes necessary.

10. Pipette the solution from around the gel and filter through a 0.2 μm filter to remove small gel fragments. (*Optional*: Additional

0.3 M sodium acetate can be added to the crushed gel to recover more RNA, if desired.)

11. Add three volumes of ethanol and incubate at −20°C for at least 30 min to precipitate the RNA. Centrifuge for 10 min at $3,000 \times g$ at 4°C in a swinging bucket rotor (see Note 15).

12. Resuspend the purified RNA in TE buffer and determine the concentration by measuring the absorbance at 260 nm (see Note 28). It is also always a good idea to check a small sample of the RNA on an analytical gel to confirm the final purity.

4. Notes

1. Although for simplicity this protocol uses LB medium for transformations, SOC medium is more commonly used in commercial kits because of the higher transformation efficiencies it can achieve. SOC medium: 2% w/v bacto-tryptone, 0.5% w/v bacto-yeast extract, 8.56 mM NaCl, 2.5 mM KCl, and 10 mM $MgCl_2$. After autoclaving the medium, add sterile filtered glucose to a final concentration of 20 mM.

2. The Lysis Solution should be prepared directly before use to be effective. For convenience, 10% SDS and 5 M NaOH stocks can be stored at room temperature and mixed at the appropriate ratio before use.

3. The precipitation of contaminating RNAs is most efficient when the PEG 8000 solution is prepared fresh.

4. To prepare rNTPs for in vitro transcription, place 60–100 mg of each powder into individual tubes and add 1.5 mL 50 mM Tris base (no pH adjustment) to each. Zero a spectrophotometer with 1 mL of TE Buffer in a quartz cuvette. Add 1 μL of the first dissolved rNTP and measure its absorbance at the appropriate wavelength: ATP at 259 nm ($\varepsilon = 15{,}400$ M^{-1} cm^{-1}); GTP at 254 nm ($\varepsilon = 11{,}100$ M^{-1} cm^{-1}); CTP at 272 nm ($\varepsilon = 7{,}300$ M^{-1} cm^{-1}); and UTP at 261 nm ($\varepsilon = 9{,}700$ M^{-1} cm^{-1}). Repeat with each rNTP stock solution in turn and use the Beer–Lambert Law to determine the concentration, c (in molar, M):

$$A = \varepsilon \times c \times l,$$

where A is the measured absorbance, ε is the extinction coefficient (at the given wavelength), and l is the cell path length (cm). Using the measured concentrations calculate the volume of each rNTP required to mix to yield a 10 mM solution of each rNTP (the total volume will be determined by the most dilute rNTP). Save any remaining individual samples at −20°C for later rNTP preparations but avoid repeated freeze–thaw cycles. After mixing, bring to the appropriate volume with 50 mM Tris base (again, do not adjust the pH). Sterile filter this solution and aliquot into 1.5 mL tubes for storage at −20°C.

5. Acrylamide can be purchased in either powder or premixed forms. Acrylamide is a neurotoxin that is easily absorbed through the skin and is more dangerous when handled in powder form. For this reason, we typically purchase premixed solutions of 30 or 40% acrylamide:bis-acrylamide (19:1). The final acrylamide percentage required depends on the size of the RNA of interest, e.g., for a 100 nt RNA, samples are run on an 8% gel. When preparing the gel solutions, it is necessary to warm the solution in order to fully dissolve the urea. Let the solution cool before pouring the gel.

6. TEMED is used to catalyze the polymerization of polyacrylamide gels. Because of this, it should always be added last and the gel should be poured directly after its addition.

7. The volume and quantity of DNA can be varied but it is important for transformation efficiency that the volume added does not exceed 10% of the volume of the competent cells.

8. *Optional*: The remaining cells in LB can be also plated as follows: pellet by spinning in a microfuge for 2 min at 3,000 × g, decant the supernatant leaving no more than 200 μL, gently resuspend the cells by flicking the tube, and then spread them on a second LB-agar plate with antibiotic. If transformation efficiency is low for some reason this second plate should still yield some colonies.

9. Typically, the 8-h starter culture is grown over the course of a day and used to inoculate the 1 L culture for growth overnight. This allows the plasmid prep to be started immediately the following morning, if desired.

10. It is more convenient (and considerate of colleagues in the lab!) to store cell pellets in disposable 50 mL tubes rather than centrifuge bottles. After cell harvesting, pour off the cleared medium setting aside about 20–30 mL for later use. Scrape off and transfer as much of the cell pellet as possible, e.g., using a disposable pipette, to a clean 50 mL tube. Use the set aside medium to resuspend the remaining cells in the centrifuge bottle and then combine this with the cell paste in the 50 mL tube. Alternatively, the entire cell pellet can be directly resuspended in 20–30 mL of medium and then transferred to a 50 mL tube (this may be the best option in some cases, e.g., where a swinging bucket rotor is used resulting in a thin and more loosely packed pellet in the centrifuge tube).

Centrifuge the cells in the 50 mL disposable tube, pour off the medium, and store at −20 or −80°C.

11. The protocol is designed for the next two steps to be done in one 50 mL tube. If the resuspended cell volume is greater than 15 mL, split the solution evenly into two separate tubes to perform subsequent steps.

12. It is critical to ensure that the pellet is thoroughly dried. If it is not, we have found the subsequent precipitation steps to be inefficient.

13. Commonly there will be a white precipitate of protein between the organic and aqueous layers. It is important to avoid transferring this when removing the upper aqueous layer.

14. Depending on the yield of the plasmid preparation, more ethanol might be required to precipitate the plasmid. If no pellet is seen in this step following centrifugation, bring up to three volumes of ethanol and centrifuge again.

15. The centrifugation speed may need to be increased to ensure complete recovery if using a fixed angle rotor. This centrifugation step can be performed at a speed up to the limit of the disposable tube being used.

16. The PEG precipitation is designed to be performed in a microcentrifuge tube. If the pellet will not completely dissolve in 330 μL of TE buffer, dilute further and split the sample into multiple aliquots of 330 μL.

17. It is convenient to resuspend the plasmid in 330 μL as this allows additional PEG 8000 precipitations to be carried out directly if they are needed.

18. It is important to compare samples from the PEG 8000 precipitation pellet and the final purified plasmid. Only small RNAs should be observed in the pelleted material and no plasmid. In final plasmid sample there should be a single band of appropriate size relative to markers for the plasmid with no small RNAs present. If small RNAs remain, the PEG 8000 precipitation steps should be repeated.

19. Follow the manufacturer's protocol for the specific restriction enzyme used in this step. If lower units-to-DNA ratios are used, the reaction time may be extended (e.g., overnight). It is critical for the in vitro transcription that the plasmid be completely linearized and this should be checked on an agarose gel. Incomplete digestion may lead to extended templates (without the "run-off" site) that may produce spurious products and rapidly deplete the rNTPs.

20. Denaturing the restriction enzyme is often (but not always) important to produce the best quality RNA in vitro transcript. If the enzyme used cannot be heat inactivated, two options are

available: (1) the enzyme can be removed via phenol/chloroform extraction or (2) a small-scale test transcription (50–100 μL) can be performed without inactivation or extraction.

21. The order of addition of transcription reaction components (Table 1) is important to prevent spermidine from precipitating the linearized plasmid. Also note that all solutions being used in the reaction have been filter sterilized through a 0.2 μM filter to minimize RNase contamination.

22. Most commonly, 250 μL of 250 mM EDTA added to a 1 mL in vitro transcription will redissolve the precipitate. After adding the EDTA, invert tube and wait for 30–60 s to make sure that the solution is clear. If not, add additional EDTA in 50 μL aliquots and repeat until no precipitate is visible.

23. For the analytical gel, 1 μL of the reaction, 4 μL water, and 5 μL 2× urea loading dye are mixed, heated to 65°C for 10 min, and then loaded on the gel. Make sure to thoroughly clear out the wells immediately before loading.

24. The molecular weight of RNA can be roughly calculated as 330 multiplied by the number of nucleotides.

25. The pellet should be resuspended in the smallest possible volume of buffer to minimize the sample size for loading onto the preparative gel and ensure tight, well-resolved RNA band(s). The precise amount that can be loaded will depend on specific gel dimensions; for our gel system, 2–5 mg RNA in 0.5–2 mL typically produces good results. Remember, the sample volume doubles with addition of loading dye.

26. From the analytical gel run previously, you will know where to expect the RNA of interest band relative to the dyes.

27. The time that the RNA is exposed to UV light should be kept to a minimum as it can damage the nucleic acid.

28. An absorbance of 1.0 at 260 nm is generally considered to be equivalent to 40 μg/mL for single-stranded RNA. However, this can vary significantly for structured RNAs. For more accurate determination of RNA concentration, an extinction coefficient can be calculated from the base composition using the "nearest neighbor method." Several Web sites offer calculators requiring the user enter only the RNA sequence. Alternatively, extinction coefficients can be empirically determined via complete digestion of a small sample of the RNA to individual nucleotides (e.g., using nuclease P1) and calculation of the free nucleotide concentration and thus the starting RNA concentration (9). The nucleotide pool concentration is calculated from a weighted average of the accurately known nucleotide extinction coefficients and the digested sample absorbance using the Beer–Lambert Law (see Note 4).

Acknowledgments

This work was supported in part by laboratory start-up funds from the Department of Biochemistry and the University Research Council of Emory University (grant 2010050). Research in the Conn Laboratory is also supported by the NIH (R01-AI088025). We thank Dr. Christine Dunham for critical comments on the manuscript during its preparation.

References

1. Milligan JF, Uhlenbeck OC (1989) Synthesis of small RNAs using T7 RNA-polymerase. Methods Enzymol 180:51–62
2. Ichetovkin IE, Abramochkin G, Shrader TE (1997) Substrate recognition by the leucyl/phenylalanyl-tRNA-protein transferase. J Biol Chem 272:33009–33014
3. Kholod N, Vassilenko K, Shlyapnikov M, Ksenzenko V, Kisselev L (1998) Preparation of active tRNA gene transcripts devoid of 3′-extended products and dimers. Nucleic Acids Res 26:2500–2501
4. Schürer H, Lang K, Schuster J, Mörl M (2002) A universal method to produce in vitro transcripts with homogeneous 3′ ends. Nucleic Acids Res 30:e56
5. Walker SC, Avis JM, Conn GL (2003) General plasmids for producing RNA in vitro transcripts with homogeneous ends. Nucleic Acids Res 31:e82
6. Obayashi E, Oubridge C, Pomeranz Krummel D, Nagai K (2007) Crystallization of RNA-protein complexes. Methods Mol Biol 363:259–276
7. Searles MA, Lu D, Klug A (2000) The role of the central zinc fingers of transcription factor IIIA in binding to 5 S RNA. J Mol Biol 301:47–60
8. Gurevich VV (1996) Use of bacteriophage RNA polymerase in RNA synthesis. Methods Enzymol 275:382–397
9. Sutton DH, Conn GL, Brown T, Lane AN (1997) The dependence of DNase I activity on the conformation of oligodeoxynucleotides. Biochem J 321:481–486

Chapter 5

Preparation of Short RNA by In Vitro Transcription

Cheng Lu and Pingwei Li

Abstract

Short RNA oligomers are required in many biochemical and biophysical studies. In vitro transcription using T7 RNA polymerase can produce a large amount of specific RNA sufficient for structural studies in a more economical way than chemical synthesis. Here, we provided protocols optimized for the synthesis of very short RNA of 10–20 nucleotides in length by in vitro transcription. These RNA oligomers can be purified conveniently by gel filtration chromatography. We also described how to study RNA and protein binding by gel filtration chromatography.

Key words: In vitro transcription, T7 RNA polymerase, Short RNA, RNA purification, Gel filtration chromatography, Protein–RNA binding studies

1. Introduction

Since bacteriophage T7 RNA polymerase (T7 RNAP) was first cloned and expressed from *E. coli* cells in 1984 (1), it has been widely used in vitro to produce milligram quantities of RNA polymers ranging from less than 100 nucleotides (nt) to as long as 30,000 nt (2, 3). Viral RNA with 5′ triphosphate stimulates the secretion of type I interferons via the cytosolic RNA sensor RIG-I (4, 5). Short oligonucleotides with 5′ triphosphate can be synthesized conveniently by in vitro transcription using T7 RNAP for structural and functional studies (6). The protocols provided here describe the in vitro synthesis and purification of very short RNA of 10–20 nt in length. Generally, in vitro transcription using T7 RNAP requires a linear DNA template containing T7 promoter, ribonucleoside triphosphates (rNTPs), a buffer containing dithiothreitol (DTT), magnesium ion (Mg^{2+}), and T7 RNAP.

Although T7 RNAP is commercially available, it can be expressed in *E. coli* and purified in the laboratory for large-scale RNA synthesis. T7 RNAP specifically recognizes the T7 promoter

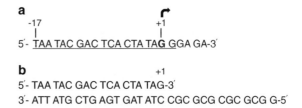

Fig. 1. (a) Consensus sequence of class III promoter of bacteriophage T7 RNA polymerase. The transcription start (position +1) is indicated by the *arrow*. (b) Double-stranded DNA template designed for the transcription of a 14 nucleotide GC-rich RNA.

(class III) consensus sequence as shown in Fig. 1a. The sequence is strictly conserved and variations in the transcribed region of nucleotides +1 to +6 affect the transcription efficiency. Nucleotides at positions +1 and +2 are especially important and significantly influence the transcription yields, whereas nucleotides +3 to +6 have smaller effects (2). The transcription must initiate with a G at +1 position, while replacing of the second base by either A or C results in only half relative yield. No RNA can be synthesized if U is at either of the first two positions (7).

The DNA template for in vitro transcription can be generated in several different ways (8). To synthesize very short RNA, we used chemically synthesized DNA oligonucleotides as templates. Two complementary oligonucleotides containing the T7 promoter sequence and the template sequence are annealed to make a double-stranded (ds) DNA template (see Note 1). After the in vitro transcription reaction, the quality and yield of the products were analyzed by denaturing polyacrylamide gel electrophoresis (PAGE) and gel filtration chromatography. Instead of purifying the RNA by conventional denaturing PAGE technique, the short RNA can be purified conveniently by gel filtration chromatography. The purified RNA products are of high quality and can be used in many biochemical and biophysical studies. In addition, we also describe how to use gel filtration chromatography to study the interactions between RNA and RNA-binding proteins.

2. Materials

RNase-free water is used to make all the solutions unless otherwise indicated.

2.1. In Vitro Transcription

1. RNase-free water (DEPC-treated water or commercially available Ultrapure water).
2. Recombinant T7 RNAP (4 mg/ml): This enzyme is commercially available but we recommend obtaining a clone and expressing your own (see Note 2).

3. Chemically synthesized promoter and template DNA oligo-nucleotides (see Note 1).
4. rNTPs: rATP, rCTP, rGTP, and rUTP. Prepare stock solutions of each rNTP at 480 mM in RNase-free water, adjust pH to about 7.0 with NaOH. The working rNTP mixture solution containing each NTP at 120 mM is prepared by mixing equal amount of each of the stock solution. Store at –20°C.
5. 10× Transcription reaction buffer: 0.4 M Tris buffer at pH 8.0 with 0.2 M $MgCl_2$ and 20 mM spermidine. Store at 4°C.
6. 1 M Dithiothreitol (DTT). Store at –20°C.
7. Inorganic pyrophosphatase (IPP, 100 U/ml). Store at –20°C.

2.2. Analysis of the In Vitro Transcribed RNA by Denaturing PAGE

1. Mini-PROTEAN 3 (Bio-Rad) or an equivalent electrophoresis system. Gel size 75 × 100 × 1 mm.
2. 10× TBE electrophoresis buffer: 0.89 M Tris, 0.89 M boric acid, and 10 mM EDTA. Store at 4°C.
3. 20% Acrylamide solution: 1× TBE, 19% acrylamide, 1% bisacrylamide, and 7 M urea. Commercially available acrylamide mix (19:1) with 7 M urea can also be used.
4. 10% Ammonium persulfate.
5. N,N,N',N'-Tetramethylenediamine (TEMED).
6. Denaturing gel sample-loading buffer: 7.0 M urea in 1× TBE plus 0.05% bromophenol blue and 0.05% xylene cyanol. Store at 4°C.
7. Ethidium bromide (10 mg/ml). Store at 4°C in dark bottles (or cover with aluminum foil).

2.3. Analysis, Purification, and Protein–RNA Binding Studies by Gel Filtration Chromatography

1. ÄKTA FPLC System with Superdex200 10/300 GL (analytical grade) and Superdex75 16/60 (preparative grade) columns (GE Healthcare).
2. FPLC running buffer: 20 mM Tris-HCl, 150 mM NaCl at pH 7.5. Filter sterilize and store at room temperature or 4°C.
3. Centrifugal concentrator units with 10 kDa molecular weight cut-off (e.g., Millipore Amicon Ultra).

3. Methods

3.1. In Vitro Transcription

The following protocol has been optimized for short RNA transcription using T7 RNAP. If a large amount of RNA is required, the reaction can be scaled up accordingly.

1. Dissolve the two chemically synthesized promoter and template DNA oligonucleotides in RNase-free water at 100 μM each. Mix the two strands at 1:1 molar ratio and anneal by first heating the mixture in a boiling water bath (about 300 ml water in a 1,000 ml beaker) and then gradually cooling down the beaker to room temperature for 30 min. The resulting 50 μM dsDNA template is stored at −20°C.

2. At room temperature (see Note 3) combine 10 μl of 10× transcription reaction buffer, 1 μl of 1 M DTT, 1 μl of 120 mM rNTP mix, 1 μl (0.1 U) of IPP, 4 μl of 50 μM dsDNA template, 4 μl of 4 mg/ml T7 RNAP, and 79 μl of RNase-free water. This will make a reaction solution with a final volume of 100 μl.

3. Incubate at 37°C for 3 h in a water bath. The purpose of this small-scale experiment is to test whether the specific RNA can be synthesized in vitro or not (see Note 4).

4. Analyze the transcription product from the small-scale experiment by denaturing PAGE (follow protocol in Subheading 3.2). Results for the analysis of an in vitro transcribed 14 nt RNA are shown in Fig. 2.

5. Analyze the transcription product by gel filtration chromatography. Load 100 μl of the sample on a Superdex200 10/300 GL column and elute with FPLC running buffer at 0.5 ml/min. Results for the analysis of the in vitro transcribed 14 nt RNA are shown in Fig. 3.

6. If a white pyrophosphate precipitate appears in the reaction solution after incubation (see Note 5), remove the precipitate by centrifugation at $14,000 \times g$ for about 5 min immediately after the transcription reaction.

If the yield and purity of the products are satisfactory, the reaction can be scaled up to 1–10 ml reactions according to the protocol in step 2. If the yield of the product is too low, the sequence of the RNA should be modified. The quality of the RNA from the large-scale transcription should also be checked by denaturing PAGE and gel filtration chromatography before purification.

3.2. Analysis of RNA by Denaturing PAGE

1. Mix an equal volume of the RNA sample with denaturing gel sample-loading buffer and then heat the sample in a 95°C water bath for 5 min.

2. Assemble the glass plates for the gel (75×100 mm with 1 mm spacers).

3. Add 100 μl of 10% ammonium persulfate and 10 μl of TEMED to 10 ml of the 20% acrylamide solution.

5 Preparation of Short RNA by In Vitro Transcription

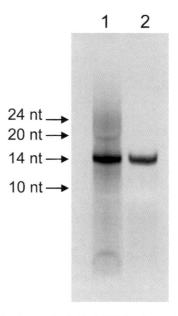

Fig. 2. Analysis of in vitro transcribed 14 nt RNA by denaturing polyacrylamide gel electrophoresis. The transcription product before purification was shown in *lane 1*. The RNA purified by gel filtration chromatography was shown in *lane 2*.

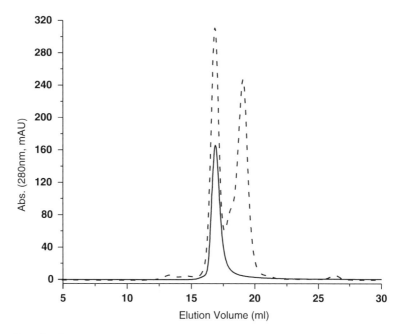

Fig. 3. Gel filtration chromatography analysis of in vitro transcribed 14 nt RNA before and after purification. The *solid curve* represents the purified 14 nt RNA, while the *dotted curve* represents the in vitro transcription product before purification. The samples were analyzed using a Superdex200 10/300 GL column.

4. Pour the gel mixture between the plates and insert the comb immediately.
5. It takes about 5–10 min for the gel to polymerize. Remove the comb as soon as the gel has set (see Note 6). Flush the sample wells with 1× TBE buffer immediately after removal of the comb.
6. Set up the electrophoresis apparatus. Add 1× TBE electrophoresis buffer to the top and bottom chambers of the electrophoresis cell.
7. Right before loading the sample, rinse the sample wells thoroughly with 1× TBE buffer to dissolve any urea in the sample wells (see Note 7).
8. Load the samples carefully into the wells (see Note 8).
9. Run the gel at constant voltage of 300 V until the bromophenol blue and xylene cyanol have migrated to appropriate positions (see Note 9).
10. Stain the gel in 1× TBE buffer containing 500 ng/ml ethidium bromide for 10–20 min.
11. Visualize and document the gel(s) using an imaging system (e.g., we use a Bio-Rad Gel Doc XR system). Results for the analysis of the 14 nt RNA before and after gel filtration purification are shown in Fig. 2.

3.3. RNA Purification by Gel Filtration Chromatography

1. Concentrate the RNA prepared by in vitro transcription to 1–2 ml using the 10 kDa cutoff centrifugal concentrators (see Note 10).
2. Load the concentrated sample onto a Superdex75 10/60 column.
3. Elute the column with FPLC running buffer at a flow rate of 1.0 ml/min. Peaks for the RNA of 10–20 nt in length appear at elution volumes of 70–80 ml on a Superdex75 16/60 column.
4. Collect 1 ml fractions for each of the RNA peaks and analyze by denaturing PAGE.
5. Combine the fractions containing the expected RNA product. Measure the sample concentration by ultraviolet (UV) absorption at $\lambda = 260$ nm.
6. Analyze the quality of the purified RNA by denaturing PAGE and gel filtration chromatography.
7. Concentrate the RNA to required concentration using the 10 kDa cutoff centrifugal concentrators.

8. Flash-freeze the sample in liquid nitrogen and store at −20°C (see Note 11).

9. If dsRNA is needed, anneal the two ssRNA samples with complementary sequences (or one ssRNA designed to be self-complementary) by heating the samples in a boiling water bath and then gradually cooling down to room temperature for over 30 min.

3.4. RNA–Protein Binding Studies by Gel Filtration Chromatography

Gel filtration chromatography can be used to study the binding interactions between RNA and proteins. It can provide useful information about the stoichiometry between the protein and the RNA. We have used gel filtration chromatography to study the binding interactions between the C-terminal domains of human RIG-I and MDA5 and various forms of RNA (6, 9, 10).

1. Prepare the RNA and the protein in the FPLC running buffer at concentrations of 50–200 µM. The concentrations of the protein and RNA should be at least a few folds higher than the estimated binding affinity (K_D) between the RNA and the protein.

2. Mix the RNA and the protein at specific molar ratios according to the estimated stoichiometry (see Note 12). At the same time, prepare the RNA and protein individually in separate samples using an equal volume of buffer to replace the binding partner.

3. Inject 100 µl of each sample (see Note 13) over a Superdex200 (10/300 GL) column and elute with FPLC running buffer at 0.5 ml/min.

4. Export the chromatograms of the RNA alone, the protein alone, and the RNA/protein mixture as spreadsheet files and plot in overlay using graphing software such Excel, Origin, Kaleidagraph, or Unicorn.

   A peak in the mixture chromatogram with an elution volume (corresponding to RNA/protein complex) shifted away from either the protein or the RNA alone indicates formation of a complex (Fig. 4). In contrast, if peaks in the mixture chromatogram overlap with peaks of the protein and RNA in isolation, this indicates that there is no binding or the binding affinity is too low. The formation of the RNA/protein complex can be observed for binding affinities as low as 5 µM. This technique can be used to purify protein and RNA complexes at preparative scale for structural studies. Either Superdex75 16/60 or Superdex200 16/60 columns can be used for the purifications, depending on the size of the complexes.

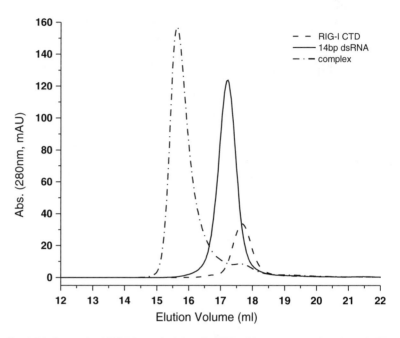

Fig. 4. Binding study of RIG-I C-terminal domain (CTD) with a 14 bp 5′ triphosphate dsRNA by gel filtration chromatography using a Superdex200 10/300 GL column.

4. Notes

1. To design the template DNA oligonucleotides, the T7 promoter sequence should be added upstream of the sequence to be transcribed. Two complementary strands should be annealed to make a dsDNA template. However, only part of the DNA template, the −17 to +1 region of the promoter sequence, needs to be double-stranded to bind the RNA polymerase and initiate the transcription (11). Therefore it is more economical to synthesize one short and one long oligonucleotide, generating a template with the coding region (i.e., from +1 on) single-stranded. For example, the short promoter DNA oligonucleotide can be synthesized as 5′-TAA TAC GAC TCA CTA TAG. This can be used with multiple templates. A template DNA oligonucleotide may be synthesized with the sequence 5′-G GCG CGC GCG CGC CTA TAG TGA GTC GTA TTA. By annealing these two DNA strands, we obtain the DNA template shown in Fig. 1b. In vitro transcription using this template results in the formation of a 14 nt RNA product with the palindrome sequence 5′-GGC GCG CGC GCG CC. Annealing of this self-complementary RNA generates a 14 bp dsRNA used in our protein–RNA binding and structural studies (6). When designing the RNA sequences, one should always keep in mind that the base composition of +1 and +2 is critical for efficient transcription. The RNA sequence must start with a G (+1),

while the second base may be a G for the best yield. Either C or A at the +2 position results in reduced yield of the RNA product.

2. Starting from a single colony, our enzyme was expressed in *E. coli* strain BL21(DE3) at 15°C overnight and purified by nickel-affinity chromatography followed by gel filtration chromatography. The enzyme was concentrated to about 4 mg/ml in 20 mM Tris-HCl, 150 mM NaCl pH 7.5 buffer plus 20% glycerol and 5 mM DTT. Aliquots of the enzyme were flash frozen in liquid nitrogen and stored at −80°C. Avoid repeated freeze and thaw of the enzyme.

3. The transcription reaction should be set up at room temperature, because spermidine in the reaction buffer tends to precipitate the template DNA at low temperature (12).

4. The yield of RNA is somewhat sequence dependent and is also affected by other factors. When a new DNA template is used for the first time, a small transcription test (100 µl scale) should be performed. The yield of the RNA may be improved by adjusting the concentrations of the ribonucleotides and T7 RNAP or the incubation time. If satisfactory yield and quality can be achieved in the test, large-scale transcription reaction can be performed from 1 ml up to 10 ml. A 1 ml transcription reaction can produce up to 200 µg of short RNA.

5. During transcription reactions, inorganic pyrophosphate is released when rNTP is incorporated into the growing chain. Therefore IPP is needed to catalyze the hydrolysis of pyrophosphate to phosphate. In transcription reactions without pyrophosphatase or when pyrophosphatase activity is low, a white pyrophosphate–Mg^{2+} precipitate may form. This can be removed by centrifugation before purification (7).

6. Have everything ready before pouring the gel because the solution will polymerize quickly. Keep the remainder of the gel solution to check for polymerization. Remove the comb immediately after the gel has completely polymerized (no more than 15 min). Otherwise, the wells may become blocked, preventing samples from being loaded to the bottom of the wells.

7. It is critical to rinse the sample wells right before loading, as urea will diffuse into the wells. A syringe with a bent needle can be used to flush the wells.

8. 200–300 ng RNA will be sufficient to show clear bands on the gel. A loading volume of 3–5 µl will give tight bands, but up to 15 µl sample can be loaded. The samples should be loaded evenly on the bottom of the wells. Long, thin gel-loading pipette tips should be used.

9. On a 20% polyacrylamide gel, bromophenol blue migrates with RNA of 8 nt in length, while xylene cyanol migrates with

RNA of 28 nt. It takes about 1 h for bromophenol blue to reach the bottom of the gel.

10. Millipore centrifugal filters of molecular weight cutoff of 10 kDa were used to concentrate the RNA. Although the molecular weight of the very short RNA is much less than 10 kDa, they will not pass through the filters since RNA are elongated molecules. Analyze the flow through when necessary.

11. RNA is less stable than DNA. The 5′ triphosphate group is especially easily degraded. The RNA samples must always be stored frozen and thawed on ice. Store samples in aliquots of 100–200 μl and avoid repeated freeze–thaw of the samples.

12. If stoichiometry between the RNA and its binding partner is not known, a titration can be performed by fixing the concentration of one binding partner while increasing that of the other.

13. Care must be taken when loading the 100 μl sample onto the FPLC to maintain the reproducibility of the results and to avoid introduction of air bubbles into the column. If a 100 μl sample loop is used, prepare 200 μl of sample and inject only 150 μl into the sample loop, leaving 50 μl in the loading syringe.

References

1. Davanloo P, Rosenberg AH, Dunn JJ, Studier FW (1984) Cloning and expression of the gene for bacteriophage T7 RNA polymerase. Proc Natl Acad Sci USA 81: 2035–2039
2. Milligan JF, Uhlenbeck OC (1989) Synthesis of small RNAs using T7 RNA polymerase. Methods Enzymol 180:51–62
3. Pokrovskaya ID, Gurevich VV (1994) In vitro transcription: preparative RNA yields in analytical scale reactions. Anal Biochem 220: 420–423
4. Hornung V, Ellegast J, Kim S, Brzózka K, Jung A, Kato H, Poeck H, Akira S, Conzelmann KK, Schlee M, Endres S, Hartmann G (2006) 5′-triphosphate RNA is the ligand for RIG-I. Science 314:994–997
5. Pichlmair A, Schulz O, Tan CP, Näslund TI, Liljeström P, Weber F, Reis e Sousa C (2006) RIG-I-mediated antiviral responses to single-stranded RNA bearing 5′-phosphates. Science 314:997–1001
6. Lu C, Xu H, Ranjith-Kumar CT, Brooks MT, Hou TY, Hu F, Herr AB, Strong RK, Kao CC, Li P (2010) The structural basis of 5′ triphosphate double-stranded RNA recognition by RIG-I C-terminal domain. Structure 18: 1032–1043
7. Gruegelsiepe H, Schön A, Kirsebom LA, Hartmann RK (2005) Enzymatic RNA synthesis using bacteriophage T7 RNA polymerase. In: Hartmann RK, Bindereif A, Schön A, Westhof E (eds) Handbook of RNA biochemistry. WILEY-VCH Verlag GmbH & Co. KGaA, Germany, pp 3–21
8. Beckert B, Masquida B (2011) Synthesis of RNA by in vitro transcription. Methods Mol Biol 703:29–41
9. Lu C, Ranjith-Kumar CT, Hao L, Kao CC, Li P (2011) Crystal structure of RIG-I C-terminal domain bound to blunt-ended double-strand RNA without 5′ triphosphate. Nucleic Acids Res 39:1565–1575
10. Li X, Lu C, Stewart M, Xu H, Strong RK, Igumenova T, Li P (2009) Structural basis of double-stranded RNA recognition by the RIG-I like receptor MDA5. Arch Biochem Biophys 488:23–33
11. Milligan JF, Groebe DR, Witherell GW, Uhlenbeck OC (1987) Oligoribo-nucleotide synthesis using T7 RNA polymerase and synthetic DNA template. Nucleic Acids Res 15:8783–8798
12. Clarke PA (1999) Labeling and purification of RNA synthesized by in vitro transcription. Methods Mol Biol 118:1–10

Chapter 6

Native RNA Purification by Gel Filtration Chromatography

Evan P. Booy, Hui Meng, and Sean A. McKenna

Abstract

In vitro transcription of RNA from DNA templates by T7 RNA polymerase allows for the generation of large quantities of RNA suitable for many downstream applications. The resulting RNA can be purified by a number of methodologies. Herein, we describe the native isolation of RNA molecules by FPLC purification using Superdex 75 or 200 gel filtration columns. This approach can be extended to purify biologically interesting RNA complexes such as RNA–protein complexes that have been generated from either synthetic or in vitro transcribed RNAs and recombinant proteins.

Key words: Native RNA purification, Non-denaturing, Gel filtration, Size exclusion, T7 RNA polymerase, In vitro transcription, Fast-performance liquid chromatography

1. Introduction

Advances in the chemical synthesis of nucleic acids by the phosphoramidite process have led to the automated production of both DNA and RNA molecules and have yielded valuable material for molecular biology, biochemistry, and biophysics (1). DNA oligonucleotides of up to 200 residues in length are readily and efficiently synthesized. Currently, RNA molecules as long as 50 nucleotides are routinely synthesized; however, due to complications in protecting the 2′-hydroxyl group of the ribose sugar, large-scale synthesis of longer RNAs has remained prohibitively expensive and technically difficult (2). Due to the high cost of chemical synthesis, the preferred method employed to generate large quantities of RNA is in vitro transcription from a linearized plasmid template using T7 RNA polymerase (3). The T7 RNA polymerase is a commercially available enzyme or alternatively the recombinant protein can be expressed and purified from *Escherichia coli* in-house (4). This procedure generates milligram quantities of RNA within a relatively short time frame (~3 h); however the resulting RNA requires extensive purification. Contaminants include the T7 RNA polymerase, plasmid template, excess nucleotide triphosphates (NTPs), as well as aborted/terminated transcripts and hydrolyzed RNA (5).

Fast-performance liquid chromatography (FPLC) provides a large-scale and rapid means of isolating transcribed RNA (6). Gel filtration columns, which separate molecules on the basis of their hydrodynamic volume, are employed to separate the various molecules in the transcription reaction. This technique is based upon a varying rate of migration of molecules in solution as they pass through a column packed with beads composed of cross-linked dextran and agarose (7). Smaller molecules that are able to penetrate every pore within the matrix are exposed to a larger column volume and elute later than large molecules that do not enter the matrix. This non-denaturing approach allows for the isolation of monomeric RNA and avoids precipitation steps which can lead both to RNA aggregation and misfolding. A further advantage over PAGE-based RNA purification is that this technique avoids the problem of acrylamide contamination of the purified RNA, as these contaminants can present a hindrance for downstream functionality in high-resolution structural studies or biophysical techniques (8). While this method is unable to provide nucleotide resolution to isolate transcribed RNA with homogenous 3′ ends, the inclusion of an appropriate ribozyme in the construct design can mitigate this problem (9, 10). Following transcription and ribozyme cleavage, the ribozyme is efficiently separated from the transcript of interest on the gel filtration column. The resulting RNA can be concentrated using centrifugal ultrafiltration devices of an appropriate molecular weight cutoff (MWCO) to yield RNA of high concentration and purity for many downstream applications.

2. Materials

All solutions should be prepared using ultrapure water (Milli-Q or equivalent) and should be filtered through a 0.22 μm membrane. Wear gloves when handling all materials and instruments to prevent RNAse contamination. Chemicals and reagents should be of molecular biology grade, RNAse-free, and should be stored, handled, and disposed of according to the manufacturer's instructions and institutional policy.

2.1. Plasmid Design, Cloning, Purification, and Linearization

1. DH5α, TOP10, or other appropriate strains of chemically competent *E. coli*.
2. pUC119 or other appropriate vectors containing an antibiotic resistance gene and multiple cloning site.

3. *Bsa*I, *Hin*dIII, and *Eco*RI restriction endonucleases or other appropriate enzymes for your RNA-encoding plasmid (see Subheading 3.1).

4. 50× Tris–acetate–EDTA (TAE) Buffer: Prepare by adding 242 g Tris, 57.1 mL glacial acetic acid, and 100 mL of 0.5 M EDTA solution (see Note 1) to 700 mL water. Adjust pH to 8.5 and bring to 1 L.

5. Agarose Gel: Dissolve 1.5 g agarose in 100 mL 1× TAE Buffer, heat in a microwave until boiling and agarose has completely dissolved (see Note 2). Allow to cool for 5–10 min and then add ethidium bromide to a final concentration of 0.5 μg/mL (see Note 3).

6. T4 DNA Ligase.

7. Plasmid Mini-prep Kit.

8. Plasmid Maxi-prep Kit.

9. Phenol:chloroform:isoamyl alcohol (24:24:1) buffered solution.

10. 95% Ethanol.

11. 3 M Sodium acetate, pH 5.2.

12. Lysogeny broth (LB) medium.

13. SOC medium.

14. LB-agar.

15. 37°C Incubator/shaker.

16. Temperature-adjustable water bath.

17. Agarose gel electrophoresis equipment.

2.2. In Vitro Transcription and Polyacrylamide Gel Electrophoresis

1. T7 RNA polymerase (see Note 4).

2. NTP stocks: Prepare 100 mM stock of each NTP in water with the pH adjusted to 7.0 (see Note 5). Prepare a working stock of 50 mM by combining each NTP at a concentration of 12.5 mM. Store NTPs in working volumes at −20°C and avoid repeated freeze/thaw cycles.

3. 10× Transcription Buffer: 400 mM Tris–HCl (pH 8.1) (see Note 6), 10 mM spermidine, 0.01% Triton X-100, and 100 mM DTT in HPLC water (see Note 7).

4. 1 M $MgCl_2$ stock: Dissolve $MgCl_2$ at a concentration of 1 M in HPLC water.

5. 10× Tris–Borate–EDTA (TBE) Buffer: Prepare by combining 108 g of Tris, 55 g of boric acid, and 40 mL of 0.5 M EDTA (pH 8.0). Bring to 1 L (see Note 8).

6. TBE/urea denaturing polyacrylamide gels: 10% gels can be cast by combining 1.5 mL of 10× TBE Buffer, 3.75 mL of 40% acrylamide/bis-acrylamide (29:1), 7.2 g of urea, 5 mL of

water, 150 μL of 10% ammonium persulfate (APS), and 10 μL of TEMED (see Note 9).

7. 2× Denaturing TBE Gel Load Dye: Prepare by combining 24 g of urea, 10 mL of 10× TBE Buffer, 2 mL of 0.5 M EDTA, 25 μg of bromophenol blue, and 25 μg of xylene cyanol. Bring to 50 mL with water.

8. 0.1% Toluidine Blue Gel Stain: Prepare by dissolving 1 g Toluidine Blue in 800 mL of water. Add 10 mL glacial acetic acid, bring to 1 L, and pass through a 0.22 μm filter.

9. Vertical gel electrophoresis system with accessories and power supply (see Note 10).

10. Temperature-adjustable water bath.

11. Rocking platform.

2.3. Desalting and FPLC Gel Filtration Chromatography

1. Disposable gravity flow desalting columns, e.g., 10DG desalting column (Bio-Rad) or PD-10 desalting columns (GE Healthcare).

2. RNA Buffer: 10 mM sodium phosphate pH 6.6 and 100 mM NaCl (see Note 11).

3. FPLC system and fraction collector (see Note 12).

4. HiLoad Superdex 75 P 26/60 (GE Life Sciences).

5. HiLoad Superdex 200 PR 26/60 (GE Life Sciences).

2.4. Purity Assessment, Concentration, and Storage

1. Centrifugal concentrators of appropriate MWCO, e.g., Vivaspin 20 (Sartorius Mechatronics) or Amicon Ultra 15 (Millipore Corporation) (see Note 13).

2. Native TBE Gel: Combine 3.75 mL of 40% acrylamide/bis-acrylamide (29:1), 1.5 mL of 10× TBE Buffer, 150 μL of 10% APS, 10 μL of TEMED, and 9.6 mL of water.

3. Toluidine Blue Gel Stain (see Subheading 2.2, item 8).

3. Methods

3.1. Template Design, Amplification, and Linearization

While an in-depth discussion of the theory and technique governing plasmid design for in vitro transcription is beyond the scope of this chapter, general methodology and design parameters are presented here. Other chapters in this volume (e.g., see Chapter 4) and detailed reviews, widely available in the literature (8, 11), should be consulted if further information is necessary. Briefly, plasmids for in vitro transcription should contain the following in the 5′ to 3′ direction: a restriction endonuclease cutting site (*Eco*RI is appropriate for the pUC119 vector), the T7 RNA polymerase promoter (see Note 14), the specific nucleotide sequence to be transcribed followed by a 3′ linearization site (*Bsa*I allows for upstream cutting to maintain inclusion of only the sequence of interest at the 3′ end), and finally a 3′ restriction endonuclease cutting site for cloning (*Hin*dIII is appropriate for the pUC119 vector). The sequence of interest to be inserted can be purchased as a double-stranded DNA oligonucleotide or a synthetic gene contained within a plasmid or can be generated by PCR (see Note 15).

1. Digest the DNA sequence to be inserted as well as the cloning plasmid with the appropriate restriction endonucleases.

2. Ligate the DNA sequence and vector with T4 DNA ligase and use to transform chemically competent DH5α *E. coli* or other suitable strain.

3. Screen for successful transformants by plasmid purification, digestion with restriction endonucleases, and agarose gel electrophoresis (see Note 16).

4. Use the validated plasmid to transform the competent DH5α *E. coli* and inoculate a 5 mL LB culture with a single colony from a freshly streaked plate containing the appropriate resistance marker (ampicillin is suitable for pUC119). Incubate for 8 h at 37 °C in a shaking incubator.

5. Inoculate 150 mL of LB containing the appropriate antibiotic in a 1 L flask with 100 μL of the starter culture. Grow for 16 h at 37 °C in a shaking incubator.

6. Isolate the plasmid using a DNA Maxi-Prep kit according to the manufacturer's instructions. Resuspend the purified plasmid in HPLC water (see Note 17).

7. Linearize the plasmid template with the appropriate restriction endonuclease (see Note 18). Assess complete plasmid linearization by performing agarose gel electrophoresis.

8. Following linearization, purify the plasmid by phenol extraction (see Note 19). Add an equal volume of phenol/chloroform to the restriction digest reaction and mix by vortexing. Centrifuge at $3,000 \times g$ for 5 min to separate the phases and carefully pipette off the upper (aqueous) phase and transfer to a new tube.

9. Add 1/10 volume of 3 M sodium acetate (pH 5.2) and mix by pipetting. Precipitate the plasmid DNA by addition of a threefold excess volume of cold 95% ethanol. Pellet the precipitated plasmid by centrifugation at $35,000 \times g$ for 15 min at 4 °C.

10. Discard the supernatant and add three volumes of cold 70% ethanol to wash the pellet (see Note 20).

11. Resuspend the pellet in an appropriate volume of HPLC water. Check plasmid concentration by measuring the absorbance at 260 nm with a spectrophotometer and dilute to a final concentration of 500 μg/mL.

3.2. In Vitro Transcription

50 μL trial transcriptions are recommended to assess optimal reaction conditions. The parameters that are variable are the concentration of T7 RNA polymerase as well as the $MgCl_2$ concentration within the reaction.

1. Combine the following in 1.5 mL microfuge tubes: 5 μL 10× transcription buffer, 5 μL linearized template DNA (500 μg/mL), 8 μL 50 mM NTPs, 2–10 μL 100 mM $MgCl_2$ (1 or 2 μL increments), and 0.5–2 μL T7 RNA polymerase (0.5 μL increments). Bring the final reaction volumes to 50 μL with HPLC water (see Note 21).
2. Incubate trial transcriptions for ~1 h at 37°C (see Note 22).
3. Combine 10 μL of each transcription reaction with 10 μL of 2× Denaturing TBE Gel Load dye. Heat at 95°C for 5 min and load the entire volume on a 10% TBE/urea polyacrylamide gel (see Note 23). Run gel in 1× TBE buffer at 100 V until the bromophenol blue dye has migrated to the bottom of the gel (see Note 24).
4. Following electrophoresis, immerse the gel in Toluidine Blue staining solution for 10 min. Destain with deionized water, changing the water frequently until background staining is minimal.
5. Proceed with large-scale transcriptions using the conditions identified to produce the highest yield of the RNA of interest with minimal nonspecific products. Small-scale transcriptions can be scaled up to any desired volume. Often a 10 mL transcription reaction will yield sufficient RNA (1–5 mg) for multiple experiments. For structural/biophysical studies requiring abundant quantities of RNA this can be scaled up further depending upon the yield of a 10 mL transcription. Large-scale transcriptions generally produce maximal product following a 3-h incubation at 37°C.
6. Following large-scale transcription, the accumulated pyrophosphate precipitate should be cleared by centrifugation at $3,000 \times g$ for 5 min. Transfer the supernatant to a new 50 mL tube.
7. The transcription reaction should then be quenched by the addition of EDTA to a final concentration of 50 mM to chelate the Mg^{2+} and inactivate the T7 RNA polymerase.
8. To remove the T7 RNA polymerase, add an equal volume of phenol/chloroform to the reaction and mix by vortexing. Centrifuge at 25°C for 10 min at $3,000 \times g$. Carefully remove the upper aqueous phase by pipetting and transfer to a new tube.

3.3. Desalting/Buffer Exchange of the Transcribed RNA

Desalting of the transcription reaction serves to eliminate a large portion of the unused NTPs as well as any phenol carried over from the phenol/chloroform extraction. This is a critical step as residual phenol can be damaging to the Superdex columns. Desalting using a gravity flow column is preferred over desalting with centrifugal ultrafiltration devices as concentration of the RNA at this stage can lead to aggregation.

1. Equilibrate a 10-DG desalting column with 20 mL RNA buffer.
2. Apply 3 mL of the phenol-extracted sample to the column and allow the column to empty completely.
3. Add 1 mL of RNA buffer to the column and allow it to flow through.
4. Elute the RNA transcripts from the column by applying 5 mL RNA buffer and collect the entire flow-through.
5. For sample volumes >3 mL, apply 25 mL of RNA buffer to the column and repeat the process again with an additional 3 mL of sample. For high-volume transcriptions multiple desalting columns can be run in parallel. The columns can be washed and stored in deionized water for future reuse.
6. Once the entirety of the sample has been desalted, store the RNA at 4°C or proceed directly with purification of the RNA by FPLC.

3.4. Gel Filtration by FPLC

Following desalting, the sample is ready to be loaded onto the gel filtration column. This step will separate the RNA transcript from the plasmid template as well as any abortive transcripts, hydrolyzed or aggregated RNA, remaining free NTPs, and other small molecule contaminants. Generally, smaller RNAs (<100 nucleotides) are separated efficiently on a HiLoad Superdex 75 P 26/60 (see Note 25). For longer RNAs, better resolution may be obtained by using a HiLoad Superdex 200 PR 26/60; however, separation largely depends on the native conformation of the RNA of interest and optimal conditions will need to be determined empirically. We use the ÄKTA Purifier 10 system connected to a Frac-950 fraction collector under the control of the UNICORN software suite.

1. Filter the RNA sample as well as all buffers through a 0.22 μm filter prior to injecting onto the gel filtration column.
2. Equilibrate the column by running 1–2 column volumes of RNA buffer at a flow rate of 1–2.5 mL/min (see Note 26).
3. Inject the sample into the FPLC at a flow rate of 1 mL/min. Generally, resolution decreases with increasing sample volume and therefore sample volume is recommended not to surpass 15 mL for the HiLoad 26/60 columns.
4. Following injection, elute the RNA transcript by loading the column with RNA buffer at a flow rate of 1–2.5 mL/min. Absorbance at 260 nm (peak absorbance wavelength of nucleic

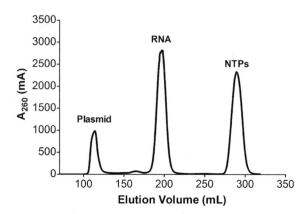

Fig. 1. Elution Profile of a monomeric viral RNA. A 100-nucleotide fragment of adenoviral noncoding RNA was in vitro transcribed in a 10 mL transcription volume. The RNA was separated from contaminating plasmid and free NTPs on a Superdex 200 26/60 gel filtration column.

acids) and 280 nm (peak absorbance wavelength of protein) should be monitored to detect eluted nucleic acids and achieve an approximate assessment of purity and yield. Collect fractions (5 mL) to allow for isolation and pooling of the RNA of interest.

5. Analyze fractions on a denaturing TBE gel. It is recommended that when developing a protocol every fraction that gives significant absorbance measurements should be analyzed. Once a protocol has been established, desired fractions can be chosen based on a signature chromatogram.

6. Pool desired fractions containing the RNA transcript.

Typical elution profiles are presented in Figs. 1 and 2. The plasmid template as well as any aggregated RNA will elute near the void volume of the column, around 110 mL for the Superdex 26/60 columns. RNA multimers, if present, will elute shortly before the monomeric RNA peak and can usually be separated with minimal loss of the monomeric RNA. Smaller fractions can be collected if there is overlap of the eluted RNAs. Flexible/natively disordered RNAs may elute in a broad and poorly defined peak, and native gel electrophoresis will be necessary to identify fractions containing the RNA/conformation of interest. Degraded/aborted transcripts will elute in a broad peak followed by excess NTPs. If a ribozyme is used to generate homogenous 3′ ends, additional peaks will be present corresponding to uncleaved full-length transcripts, the free ribozyme as well as the RNA of interest. To avoid overlapping elution of the ribozyme and free RNA, modifications to the ribozyme such as the addition of extra nucleotides at the 3′ end or change of ribozyme of choice may be necessary (12, 13).

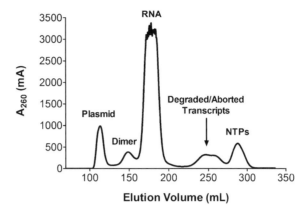

Fig. 2. Elution profile of a transcription reaction containing multimeric RNA and small RNA contaminants. A 159-nucleotide fragment of adenoviral noncoding RNA was transcribed in a 10 mL transcription volume. The RNA was purified on a Superdex 200 26/60 gel filtration column. Labeled peaks correspond to the plasmid template, dimerized RNA, monomeric RNA, as well as small contaminating RNAs arising from aborted and/or degraded transcripts.

3.5. Purity Assessment, Concentration, and Storage

1. To assess the purity of the separated RNA transcript, analyze 20 µL of the pooled fractions by native gel electrophoresis using a 10% native TBE gel. Gels should be run for 2–3 h at 75 V in 0.5× TBE at 4°C.

2. Stain the gel with Toluidine Blue staining solution to visualize the RNA in the pooled fractions (see Note 27).

3. Assess the concentration of the purified RNA by measuring the absorbance at 260 nm. Accurate concentration measurements will require the appropriate extinction coefficient. Information on calculation of RNA extinction coefficients is available elsewhere (14).

4. Concentrate the purified RNA by applying the sample to a centrifugal ultrafiltration device of appropriate MWCO (see Note 28).

5. The purified RNA can be kept at 4°C for several weeks without any observable degradation; however, for longer term storage, the RNA can be aliquoted and stored at −20°C (see Note 29).

4. Notes

1. To prepare 0.5 M EDTA, add 186.1 g EDTA to 800 mL water. Place on a stir plate and add ~20 g NaOH pellets while stirring. Continue to stir and bring pH to 8.0 by adding NaOH dropwise from a 10 M stock. Bring final volume to 1 L.

2. It is important at this stage not to overheat the agarose as the solution will tend to boil over when heated at high power. Once the agarose solution begins to boil remove it from the microwave using insulated gloves and swirl to mix. Replace in the microwave and bring to a second boil. Continue this process until all of the agarose is fully in solution.

3. Ethidium bromide is a potential mutagen and should be handled only with nitrile gloves. Once the gel has been prepared with ethidium bromide the gel also should only be handled with gloves. As an alternative to ethidium bromide, the SYBR Safe DNA gel stain is available from Invitrogen Corporation and provides comparable sensitivity.

4. The T7 RNA polymerase can be produced in-house using established protocols and standard nickel-affinity protein purification techniques (3, 4).

5. Adjust pH with sodium hydroxide being careful not to allow the pH to rise above 7.0. Neutral pH is essential for optimal performance of the NTP stocks.

6. The transcription reaction is highly dependent upon an accurate pH of the transcription buffer. Adjust the pH of a 1 M stock of Tris–HCl at 37°C.

7. The 10× transcription buffer can be stored at −20°C without DTT. DTT should be added fresh from a 1 M stock prior to use. Any remaining 1× buffer containing DTT should be discarded and not be reused.

8. After long-term storage a precipitate will often form in the 10× TBE buffer. To prevent this, the buffer should be passed through a 0.22 μm filter prior to storage.

9. To facilitate the dissolving of the urea, combine the urea, 10× TBE Buffer, and acrylamide/bis-acrylamide and incubate in a 37°C water bath for 5–10 min. Once fully dissolved add the 10% APS and TEMED and immediately pour the gel.

10. A popular model is the Bio-Rad Mini-PROTEAN tetra-cell; however, any standard vertical electrophoresis system is appropriate.

11. This buffer can be used as a starting point; however, as the separation by gel filtration is not buffer dependent any number of buffer conditions can be used and modified to suit the downstream applications of the RNA being purified.

12. Our lab uses the ÄKTA Purifier 10 with Frac-950 fraction collector produced by GE Healthcare; however any alternative FPLC system employing suitable gel filtration columns may be used.

13. In general, an MWCO of no greater than half the molecular weight of the RNA of interest should be used to avoid any sample loss due to flow-through.

14. The standard T7 promoter consists of the sequence 5′-TAATAC GACTCACTATAGG-3′. Use of this promoter sequence will result in the inclusion of two guanosine residues at the 5′ end of the transcribed RNA. An alternative T7 promoter sequence 5′-TAATACGACTCACTATTAG-3′ will result in the inclusion of an adenosine followed by a guanosine residue at the start of the RNA sequence. Alteration of the first two nucleotides beyond these options results in significantly reduced efficiency of transcription (11). Should these nucleotides present a problem, the inclusion of a ribozyme 5′ to the RNA of interest may be useful (12).

15. Ordering of a synthetic gene designed according to the above specifications eliminates all cloning steps; other methods are cheaper alternatives but will add to the experimental time frame.

16. While observing the correct banding pattern by agarose gel electrophoresis is often indicative of successful ligation, it is always advised to confirm the cloned vector by sequencing.

17. HPLC water is used as it is a relatively inexpensive source of RNAse-free water.

18. Complete linearization is essential for efficient transcription from the plasmid template. Circular plasmids will result in high amounts of long, heterogeneous RNA contaminants and will severely reduce yield of the transcript of interest. Plasmid linearization can be carried out overnight at 37°C to ensure complete digestion. Generally 1 U of a restriction enzyme should be sufficient to efficiently cut 2 μg of plasmid.

19. Phenol is highly toxic and should only be worked with under a fume hood and while wearing nitrile gloves.

20. Gentle pipetting can help avoid dislodging the pellet at this stage. If the pellet becomes dislodged centrifuge a second time for 5–10 min to pellet the precipitated DNA.

21. T7 RNA polymerase should be the final component added to the reaction. Mix the reaction well by gently pipetting up and down with a 200 μL pipette set to ~30 μL.

22. The production of pyrophosphate in the transcription reaction may result in the presence of a white precipitate.

23. Gel concentrations from 6 to 15% can be used depending on the length of the RNA being analyzed. Typically a 10% gel is suitable for RNAs of 50–100 nucleotides. For shorter and longer RNAs the acrylamide concentration should be adjusted accordingly.

24. Bromophenol blue will migrate close to the length of a 25 nucleotide RNA on a 10% denaturing gel. To eliminate obscuring of the bands upon staining, bromophenol blue can be eliminated from the load dye when analyzing smaller RNAs.

The fluorescent dye SYBR Green II can be used to visualize RNA at low concentrations and will not be affected by the presence of loading dye.

25. Due to their extended structure, RNA molecules will typically behave as much as three- to six-fold larger on a gel filtration column than a protein with a similar molecular weight (6).

26. Flow rates within this range are generally suitable; however, the pressure over the column must be monitored to ensure that the maximum column pressure recommended by the manufacturer is not exceeded.

27. RNA transcripts that form a defined secondary structure should run as a discreet band whereas unstructured RNAs may exhibit a degree of smearing on a native gel.

28. Following concentration, a small amount of the RNA should be analyzed again on a native TBE gel to ensure that aggregation has not occurred.

29. RNAs stored at −20°C may form aggregates upon thawing. This can be determined by native gel electrophoresis. Heating of the RNA to 95°C for 5 min followed by rapid cooling on ice for 5–10 min and then equilibration to room temperature may return the RNA to its native and monomeric state. Should aggregates persist the RNA can be repurified on the gel filtration column.

Acknowledgments

The work was supported by a Natural Sciences and Engineering Research Council of Canada Discovery Grant and a Manitoba Health Research Council Establishment Grant.

References

1. Caruthers MH (2011) A brief review of DNA and RNA chemical synthesis. Biochem Soc Trans 39:575–580
2. Somoza A (2008) Protecting groups for RNA synthesis: an increasing need for selective preparative methods. Chem Soc Rev 37:2668–2675
3. Milligan JF, Groebe DR, Witherell GW, Uhlenbeck OC (1987) Oligoribonucleotide synthesis using T7 RNA polymerase and synthetic DNA templates. Nucleic Acids Res 15:8783–8798
4. Davanloo P, Rosenberg AH, Dunn JJ, Studier FW (1984) Cloning and expression of the gene for bacteriophage T7 RNA polymerase. Proc Natl Acad Sci U S A 81:2035–2039
5. McKenna SA, Kim I, Puglisi EV, Lindhout DA, Aitken CE, Marshall RA, Puglisi JD (2007) Purification and characterization of transcribed RNAs using gel filtration chromatography. Nat Protoc 2:3270–3277
6. Kim I, McKenna SA, Viani Puglisi E, Puglisi JD (2007) Rapid purification of RNAs using fast performance liquid chromatography (FPLC). RNA 13:289–294
7. O'Fagain C, Cummins PM, O'Connor BF (2011) Gel-filtration chromatography. Methods Mol Biol 681:25–33
8. Lukavsky PJ, Puglisi JD (2004) Large-scale preparation and purification of polyacrylamide-free RNA oligonucleotides. RNA 10:889–893

9. Schurer H, Lang K, Schuster J, Morl M (2002) A universal method to produce in vitro transcripts with homogeneous 3′ ends. Nucleic Acids Res 30:e56
10. Walker SC, Avis JM, Conn GL (2003) General plasmids for producing RNA in vitro transcripts with homogeneous ends. Nucleic Acids Res 31:e82
11. Beckert B, Masquida B (2011) Synthesis of RNA by in vitro transcription. Methods Mol Biol 703:29–41
12. Ferre-D'Amare AR, Doudna JA (1996) Use of cis- and trans-ribozymes to remove 5′ and 3′ heterogeneities from milligrams of in vitro transcribed RNA. Nucleic Acids Res 24: 977–978
13. Ferre-D'Amare AR, Scott WG (2010) Small self-cleaving ribozymes. Cold Spring Harb Perspect Biol 2:a003574
14. Puglisi JD, Tinoco I Jr (1989) Absorbance melting curves of RNA. Methods Enzymol 180:304–325

Chapter 7

Cis-Acting Ribozymes for the Production of RNA In Vitro Transcripts with Defined 5′ and 3′ Ends

Johanna M. Avis, Graeme L. Conn, and Scott C. Walker

Abstract

The use of in vitro transcribed RNA is often limited by sequence constraints at the 5′-end and the problem of transcript heterogeneity which can occur at both the 5′- and 3′-ends. This chapter describes the use of *cis*-acting ribozymes, 5′-end hammerhead (HH) and 3′-end hepatitis delta virus (HDV), for direct transcriptional processing to yield target RNAs with precisely defined ends. The method is focused on the use of the pRZ and p2RZ plasmids that are designed to simplify the production of such dual ribozyme templates. These plasmids each bear a 3′-HDV modified with a unique restriction site that allows the ribozyme to remain on the plasmid and, therefore, be omitted from the cloning procedure. The additional steps required to design a unique hammerhead ribozyme tailored to the 5′-end of each target RNA are detailed. In most cases, a transcriptional template bearing a 5′-HH ribozyme and a 3′-HDV ribozyme can be achieved by cloning a single PCR product into either the pRZ or p2RZ vector. Protocols for optimization of transcription yields from these templates and the isolation of the homogeneous target RNA are also described.

Key words: In vitro transcription, T7 RNA polymerase, RNA, Ribozyme, Hammerhead, HDV

1. Introduction

The use of the bacteriophage T7 RNA polymerase (T7 RNAP) for RNA in vitro transcription is widespread (1, 2). However, the RNA produced in a typical in vitro transcription reaction may not be ideal for every intended use. The enzyme prefers to initiate from certain sequences (constraining the 5′-end) and is also prone to nontemplated errors at both the 5′-end and 3′-end of the RNA transcript (1, 3, 4). In many applications the exact nucleotide identity and chemical nature of the 5′-end or 3′-end can be essential for function; examples are tRNA aminoacylation, RNA end-labeling, RNA ligation, and crystallization. When producing RNA for a specific purpose it is important to consider the limitations of in vitro transcribed RNA and whether any additional steps or post-processing will be required to yield a functional RNA.

1.1. The Limitations of In Vitro Transcription

T7 RNAP utilizes two promoters, class II (TAATACGACTCACTATTA$_{(+1)}$) and the more widely utilized class III (TAATACGACTCACTATAG$_{(+1)}$). In each case the purine (A/G) shown at the +1 position is strongly preferred to promote efficient transcription initiation (5). In practice, a guanine is usually also included at the +2 position to further improve the yield of RNA. Thus, to ensure high yields the T7 RNAP system places a sequence requirement on the 5′-end of the RNA transcripts produced from each promoter (5′-AGNN… or 5′-GGNN…). When other sequences are used at the 5′-end, transcription initiation is poor and yields can be significantly lower, although tolerable for some purposes. In many applications, such as RNA–protein binding or in vitro transcription/translation, the sequence preferences at the 5′-end of an RNA will not interfere with its function and are easily accommodated in favor of RNA yield. However, for more demanding applications the nucleotide identity and the exact chemical nature of the 5′-end can be essential for function and must be considered.

1.1.1. Sequence Preference at the 5′-End

1.1.2. The 5′-End Triphosphate

An in vitro transcribed RNA will carry a 5′-triphosphate derived from the initiating nucleotide triphosphate (NTP) in the transcription mix. A 5′-triphosphate is not suitable for end-labeling or RNA ligation and must first be removed to yield a 5′-hydroxyl using alkaline phosphatase (AP). The 5′-hydroxyl is then converted to a 5′-monophosphate using ATP (or γ-^{32}P-ATP) and polynucleotide kinase (PNK). The 5′-monophosphate generated is suitable for ligation to the 3′-hydroxyl of another RNA species. As described in Chapter 13, it is also possible to directly prepare in vitro transcribed RNA with a 5′-hydroxyl (or 5′-monophosphate) by using an excess of the initiating nucleoside (or nucleotide monophosphate) in the transcription mix (6, 7). However, yields are generally lower and some fraction of 5′-triphosphate products will remain due to the nucleotide triphosphate present in the transcription mix. Additionally, these methods do not address the potential for nontemplated errors that can occur at the 5′-end.

1.1.3. Transcript Heterogeneity at the 5′- and 3′-Ends

Possibly the most significant problem with in vitro transcribed RNAs is the potential for nontemplated nucleotides to be inserted at the 3′-end of a transcript resulting in a heterogeneous population of RNA transcripts. This "run-over" heterogeneity at the 3′-end can be reduced, although rarely eliminated, by using DNA templates bearing a 2′-methoxy on the last two nucleotides of the template strand (8, 9). It is less common to find sequence heterogeneity at the 5′-end, although with some initiating sequences this can also be a significant problem (3, 4). Heterogeneity at the 5′-end has been shown to be less prevalent when the class II promoter is used (10). Collectively these unintended transcripts are usually referred to as $n+1$ or $n+2$ (etc.) species and can pose a significant problem when the RNA requires a defined 5′-end or 3′-end for its proposed use.

1.2. Processing RNA Transcripts to Yield Defined Ends

When entirely homogeneous populations are required it is usually necessary to employ some form of processing of the RNA by initiating precise cleavage to yield a defined 5′-end or 3′-end. Direct transcriptional processing can be achieved through the use of *cis*-acting ribozymes that are engineered into the DNA template prior to transcription (see below and Fig. 1). There are also a number of post-processing techniques that use an external factor to induce a precise cleavage, see Chapters 8 and 9. These techniques differ in their application as well as the exact chemical nature of the products formed. Post-processing by oligonucleotide-directed RNase H (11, 12) or by tRNA-structure directed RNase P (13) will result in the formation of a 5′-phosphate and a 3′-hydroxyl. Alternatively, post-processing via a template-directed DNAzyme (14) or by

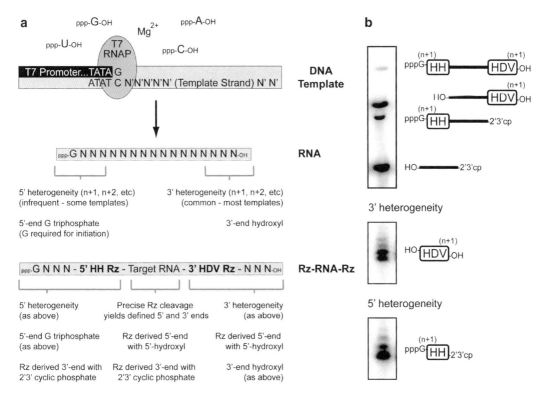

Fig. 1. In vitro transcription of RNA using T7 RNA polymerase. (**a**) The transcript is shown with the 5′-G-triphosphate and 3′-hydroxyl typically produced under standard transcription conditions. A dual ribozyme transcript (5′-HH/3′-HDV) is also shown for comparison. (**b**) Transcription of a target RNA flanked by 5′-HH and 3′-HDV ribozymes. Precise ribozyme cleavage yields a target RNA with a defined 5′-end and 3′-end (*upper gel panel*—4% PAGE). The matured HH and HDV ribozymes demonstrate the problem of 5′-end and 3′-end heterogeneity associated with most RNA in vitro transcripts (*lower gel panels*—8% PAGE).

trans-acting ribozymes (15, 16) will result in a 5′-hydroxyl and a 2′3′-cyclic phosphate. The activity of a DNAzyme or RNase H can be relatively easily directed to either the 5′-end or 3′-end of a target RNA by adjusting the sequence of the DNAzyme or the guide oligonucleotide, respectively. On the other hand *trans*-acting ribozymes (including RNase P) are usually employed only at the 3′-end and directed by a specific sequence tag that must be incorporated into the transcript itself. The *trans*-acting forms of the Hepatitis delta virus (HDV) ribozyme or the Varkud satellite (VS) ribozyme require only short sequence tags unlike the tRNA structure required by RNase P. In each case the post-processing technique chosen must be carefully optimized and one technique may be more successful than another with any particular target RNA.

1.3. Using Cis-Acting Ribozymes to Produce Defined 5′- and 3′- Ends

Direct transcriptional processing is often the best approach when high yields of an entirely homogeneous RNA transcript are required. The hammerhead ribozyme (HH Rz) can be used at either the 5′-end or 3′-end of a transcript (see Fig. 2a). When used at the 5′-end the HH Rz does not place any sequence requirements upon the target RNA. Both the 5′ and 3′ versions of the HH Rz form a stem structure with the target sequence and require a unique HH Rz to be tailored to each target RNA (see Fig. 2a). The hepatitis delta virus ribozyme (HDV Rz) does not form any structure with the target RNA and is ideal for cleaving at the 3′-end with no sequence requirements on the target RNA (see Fig. 2b). Thus the use of a 5′-HH Rz and a 3′-HDV Rz is a common approach for the production of homogeneous RNA transcripts.

It is important to consider the chemical products of ribozyme cleavage as both the HH Rz and HDV Rz yield a 5′-hydroxyl and a 2′3′-cyclic phosphate (see Fig. 2c). The 5′-hydroxyl on a ribozyme-derived 5′-end is generally more useful than its 5′-triphosphate counterpart. Direct phosphorylation of a ribozyme-derived 5′-hydroxyl is usually highly efficient since the reaction is no longer reliant upon the successful removal of the 5′-triphosphate by alkaline phosphatase. However, the 2′3-cyclic phosphate on a ribozyme-derived 3′-end is generally less useful than its 3′-hydroxyl counterpart. It is important to be aware that RNA ligation or 3′-end radiolabeling (via ligation of (5′-^{32}P)-cytidine-3′,5′-bisphosphate) is not possible without first removing the 2′3′-cyclic phosphate using the phosphatase activity of the T4 PNK enzyme (17, 18). It should also be noted that an RNA with a 2′3-cyclic phosphate carries additional charge and will migrate approx 1 nt faster during electrophoresis than its 3′-hydroxyl counterpart.

1.4. Cassettes to Assist the Production of 3′-HDV Rz and 5′-HH Rz/3′-HDV Rz Templates

The vectors described in this chapter have been designed to aid in the preparation of transcripts bearing a 3′-HDV Rz or both 5′-HH Rz and 3′-HDV Rz (19). The pRZ and p2RZ vectors each bear a modified HDV Rz with a unique restriction site, adjacent to the cleavage site (see Fig. 3). These engineered restriction sites allow

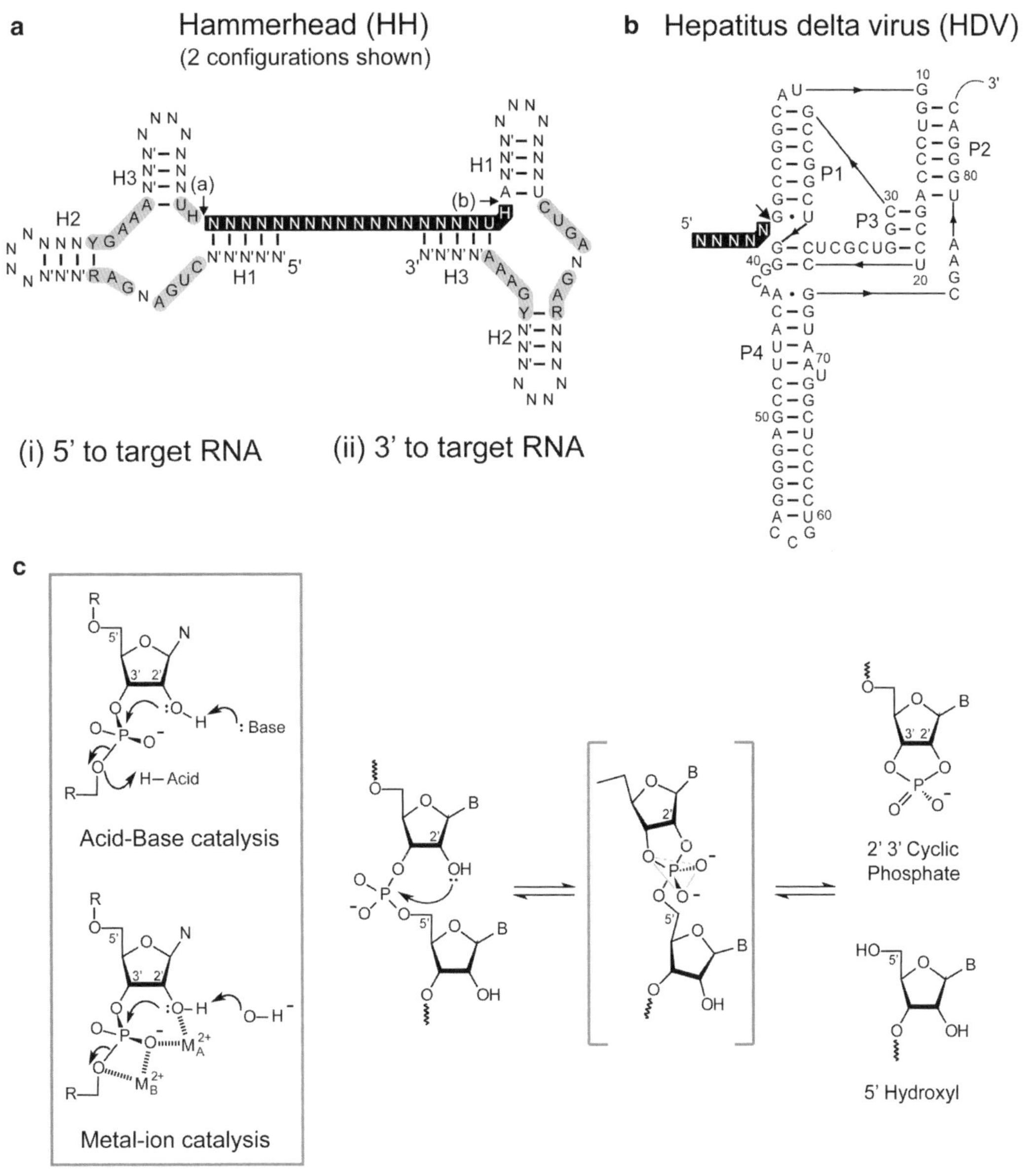

Fig. 2. Ribozyme RNA secondary structures and chemistry. (a) The hammerhead (HH) ribozyme is shown in both 5' and 3' configurations; the cleavage sites are marked with an *arrow*. The required consensus nucleotides are shown with a *grey background* and the target sequence is shown with a *black background*. N = any nucleotide, N' = nucleotide complementary to N, R = purine, Y = pyrimidine, H = any nucleotide except G. (b) The Hepatitus delta virus (HDV) ribozyme is shown at the 3'-end of a target RNA. The target sequence is shown with a *black background* and the cleavage site is marked with an *arrow*. (c) RNA cleavage proceeds via an internal transesterification reaction involving the adjacent 2'hydroxyl. The reaction is favored when the 5'phosphate and the 2'-hydroxyl are correctly aligned to resemble the trigonal bipyramidal transition state (*shown in brackets*). The reaction can be catalyzed in multiple ways (*boxed*) including general acid–base catalysis or by involving inner sphere coordinated metal ions (*dashed lines*) to activate the nucleophile/stabilize the leaving group. Some ribozymes (hammerhead, hairpin, and VS ribozymes) are also able to catalyze the reverse (ligation) reaction.

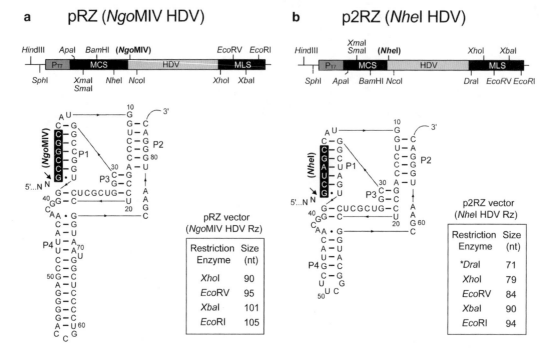

Fig. 3. Plasmids for the production of RNA transcripts with homogeneous ends. (**a**) pRZ bearing the HDV ribozyme modified with a unique *Ngo*MIV restriction site (*black background*). (**b**) p2RZ bearing the HDV ribozyme with a shortened P4 stem and a unique *Nhe*I restriction site (*black background*). Both plasmids have the bacteriophage T7 RNAP promoter (P_{T7}) (class III), multiple cloning sites (MCS) to facilitate cloning, and multiple linearization sites (MLS) to control the size of the HDV Rz and aid in the purification of similarly sized target sequences. *The *Dra*I restriction site in p2RZ is not unique to the vector.

the HDV Rz to remain on the vector and reduce the number of steps required for the construction of in vitro transcription templates bearing a 3′-HDV Rz. The two different HDV ribozymes allow for a choice in the restriction site as well as the size of the HDV ribozyme. Additionally, multiple linearization sites (MLS) allow further adjustments to the size of the HDV and aid in the separation of the ribozyme from similarly sized target RNAs. The linearization sites produce either 5′-overhangs or blunt ends to reduce the potential for extraneous transcription that is often associated with incomplete termination at 3′-overhangs (20).

When dual ribozymes are required, a 5′-HH Ribozyme will still need to be tailored to suit each target RNA. The uniquely designed HH Rz sequence is added to the target sequence by PCR. The pRZ and p2RZ vectors have multiple cloning sites (MCS) to facilitate the introduction of target sequences bearing a 5′-HH Rz. This strategy allows the T7 promoter to remain on the vector and also allows transcription to be initiated from a high yield initiating sequence. The undesired sequence derived from the MLS region will be subsequently removed through the cleavage of the 5′-HH Rz.

2. Materials

2.1. Design of Hammerhead Rz Sequences

1. Computer with an RNA secondary structure prediction program or access to Web-based servers for RNA folding prediction is required. Downloadable programs and links to Web-based RNA folding servers can be found at the following addresses:

P.C.	RNAstructure (http://rna.urmc.rochester.edu/rnastructure.html)
	RNAdraw (http://www.rnadraw.com).
Mac	Mulfold (http://iubio.bio.indiana.edu/soft/molbio/mac/).

2.2. PCR Amplification of Target Sequence and Cloning Target Sequence into pRZ Vectors

1. Destination vector(s) for the target RNA-encoding sequences. The pRZ plasmids described in this chapter are available from Addgene (http://www.addgene.org), a nonprofit plasmid repository:

Addgene ID# 27663	pRZ vector (*Ngo*MIV HDV)	(19)
Addgene ID# 27664	p2RZ vector (*Nhe*I HDV)	(Described here)
Addgene ID# 27667	pVAiHDV4 vector (*Nhe*I HDV)	(19)

2. Template DNA for PCR, either genomic DNA or plasmid-borne sequence. Adjust concentration to 50 μg/ml.
3. DNA oligonucleotides. See Subheading 3.2 for detailed description of DNA sequence design. Dissolve in water to a final concentration of 100 pmol/μl.
4. DNA polymerase, supplied with commercial buffer.
5. Agarose gel electrophoresis equipment.
6. DNA purification kit (for recovery of DNA from a PCR reaction or an agarose gel slice).
7. Restriction enzymes appropriate to the cloning strategy, supplied with commercial buffer.
8. T4 DNA ligase, supplied with commercial buffer.
9. Competent DH5α or XL1-Blue *E. coli* cells and reagents for bacterial transformation and culture according to your standard lab protocol, e.g., LB medium and LB-agar plates with 100 μg/ml ampicillin.
10. DNA plasmid mini-prep kit.
11. Access to an automated DNA sequencing facility.

2.3. Transcription of RNA

1. Sequence-verified plasmid encoding the target RNA produced in Subheading 3.2. Plasmid DNA produced from the DNA mini-prep kit can be used for test transcriptions and reaction optimization. For preparation of large quantities of plasmid DNA suitable for RNA in vitro transcription, follow the protocols of Chapter 4.

2. Restriction enzyme for plasmid linearization within the MLS (Fig. 3) for run-off transcription, supplied with commercial buffer.

3. Phenol/chloroform/isoamylalcohol (25:24:1).

4. Chloroform.

5. 3M Sodium Acetate (pH 5.2).

6. Ethanol, absolute.

7. RNA Transcription Buffer (10×): 800 mM K-Hepes (pH 7.5), 10 mM spermidine, 200 mM DTT, and 0.1% Triton-X100.

8. T7 RNAP, approximately 1 mg/ml (~400,000 U/mg).

9. Ribonucleotide triphosphates (rNTPs): 100 mM ATP, 100 mM GTP, 100 mM CTP, 100 mM UTP. Combine equal volumes to yield a 25 mM stock of rNTPs (25 mM each rNTP).

10. Yeast inorganic pyrophosphatase (YIP) (Sigma # I1891).

11. Optional: Ribonuclease inhibitor (RNasin or SuperaseIn—Ambion).

12. Optional: Radiolabeled ribonucleotide triphosphate (α-^{32}P-rNTP).

Specific activity	Supplied concentration
6,000 Ci/mmol	40 µCi/µl (6.7 µM)
3,000 Ci/mmol	10 µCi/µl (3.3 µM)
800 Ci/mmol	10 µCi/µl (12.5 µM)

13. Formamide loading dye: 95% (v/v) deionized formamide, 2% (v/v) 0.5 M ethylenediaminetetraacetic acid (EDTA; pH 8.0), 0.1% (w/v) sodium dodecyl sulfate (SDS), 0.02% (w/v) xylene cyanol, and 0.02% (w/v) bromophenol blue (optional). SDS can be prepared as a 10% (w/v) stock solution and added to the formamide and other reagents.

14. Analytical scale polyacrylamide gel electrophoresis equipment (~0.4 mm spacers and combs).

15. Methylene blue stain.

16. Phosphorstorage screen and phosphorimager (if using α-^{32}P-rNTP).

2.4. Purification of Target RNA

1. Preparative polyacylamide gel electrophoresis equipment (1.5–3.0 mm spacers and combs).
2. Autoradiography intensifying screen.
3. Shortwave (254 nm) handheld UV lamp.
4. Gel Elution Buffer: 300 mM sodium acetate (pH 5.2), 5 mM EDTA, and 0.1% SDS.

3. Methods

3.1. Guidelines for Designing 5′-Hammerhead Ribozymes

The sequence shown in Fig. 4a is the suggested staring point for the design of 5′-HH ribozymes. The three nucleotides directly upstream of the target RNA are the optimal sequence (GUC) for achieving high cleavage efficiency (21). The target RNA forms part of helix 1 (H1) and a unique complementary sequence must be designed for each target RNA. The 10 base pair stem is suggested to compete with structure formation within the target RNA (see Note 1). Both the length and the sequence identity of helix 2 (H2) and helix 3 (H3) can be adjusted in the variable regions (N and N′) although the 4 base pair stems are usually sufficient for folding and cleavage. Closing the stem loops of H2 and H3 with thermodynamically stable tetraloops is also recommended to promote the desired folding, e.g., GNRA or UNCG (where R is any nucleotide and R is G or A).

After designing a 5′-HH Rz, it is helpful to predict the folding of the sequence in silico. Secondary structure prediction programs based upon the Mfold algorithm (22) such as RNAstructure/Mulfold or the Vienna algorithm (23) such as RNAdraw are freely available (Subheading 2.1). To identify potential folding problems it is useful to initially test the folding of the isolated HH Rz before examining potential competing structures within the context of the target RNA. Ultimately, the only true test of function is to produce the template and assess the ribozyme cleavage by performing in vitro transcription under various conditions (Subheading 3.3).

If poor ribozyme performance cannot be tackled by adjusting the transcription conditions then the ribozyme design can be adjusted and this new template must be produced. Further manipulation of the existing templates can be aided by including additional restriction sites within the initial HH Rz design. The first HH Rz example shown in Fig. 4b has a *Kpn*I site (GGTACC) within the 3′-half of H3 and the other example has an *Nhe*I site (GCTAGC) within the stem loop of H3.

3.2. Cloning the Target Sequence

Once a 5′-HH Rz has been designed to suit a target RNA it can be fused to the target sequence using PCR (see Fig. 4). Previously, we have used a two-stage PCR protocol to introduce the HH Rz using

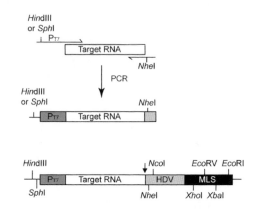
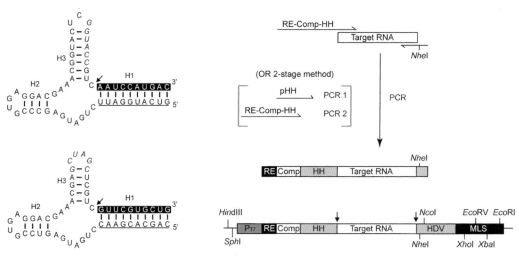

Fig. 4. Example designs and strategy for generating constructs for RNA in vitro transcription with cis-acting ribozymes. (**a**) A HH ribozyme is shown in the correct configuration for cleavage at the 5'-end of a target RNA. The 5' region of the ribozyme is unique to each target sequence and must be designed to complement the target and allow for helix 1 (H1) formation. The sequence of helix 2 (H2) and helix 3 (H3) can be adjusted to favor ribozyme folding in the context of a given target sequence. (**b**) Examples of unique 5'-HH ribozymes are shown that have been used successfully in the lab. (**c**) Strategy for the construction of 3'-HDV transcription cassettes. (**d**) Strategy for the construction of 5-HH/3' HDV transcription cassettes. PCR is used to introduce the 5'-HH Rz which must be specifically designed for each target RNA. A restriction enzyme (RE) chosen from the vector's multiple cloning sites (MCS) is added to facilitate cloning. In some cases two sequential PCR reactions may be needed to introduce the HH Rz.

two sequential PCR steps (19). However, when the small HH Rz design shown in Fig. 4a is used, a single oligo (~80 nt) can be used in one PCR step. Oligos of this length can now be more reliably synthesized and this approach has been used with a high success

Table 1
PCR reaction components

Component	Volume	(Stock)	(Final)
10× Buffer	30 µl	10×	1×
dNTPs	30 µl	2 mM	0.2 mM
DNA template	3 µl	50 ng/µl	0.5 ng/µl
DNA polymerase	3 µl	2.5 U/µl	0.025 U/µl
Forward oligo	3 µl	100 pmol/µl	1 pmol/µl
Reverse oligo	3 µl	100 pmol/µl	1 pmol/µl
Water	228 µl	–	–

rate (see Note 2). The forward oligo is designed as follows: flanking sequence to aid in restriction site cleavage (~10 nt), restriction site (6 nt), complementary region (10 nt), HH Rz core (35 nt), and 20 nt of complementarity to direct the PCR reaction to the 5′-end of the target RNA. The reverse oligo is designed with 20 nt of complementarity to direct the PCR reaction to the 3′-end of the target RNA and either the *Nhe*I or *Ngo*MIV restriction site (+10 nt to aid in cleavage) is added to allow cloning adjacent to the HDV Rz of the desired destination vector.

1. Set up the PCR reaction according to Table 1.
2. Split the PCR mix into four thin-walled PCR tubes (4 × 75 µl) and perform the following protocol on a thermal cycler (PCR machine): 94°C for 1 min, then 25 cycles of 94°C for 45 s, 50°C for 45 s, and 72°C for 1 min per kilobase of expected product, and 72°C for 4 min (see Note 3).
3. Examine the products of the PCR reaction on an agarose gel with appropriate size markers loaded in an adjacent lane.
4. Remove the polymerase and dNTPs by purifying the PCR reaction using a silica-based PCR cleanup kit.
5. Digest the PCR fragment with the appropriate restriction enzymes and gel purify the digested fragment from an agarose gel.
6. Using T4 DNA ligase, insert the purified RNA-encoding fragment into the chosen pRZ or p2RZ plasmid which has been similarly digested at the appropriate restriction sites and purified.
7. Transform competent bacterial host cells (e.g., *E. coli* DH5α or XL1-Blue cells) using the ligation reaction and plate onto LB-Agar plates with 100 µg/ml ampicillin.

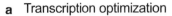
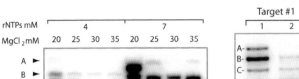
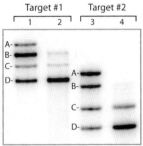
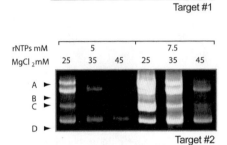
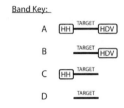

Fig. 5. The influence of rNTP and Mg^{2+} concentrations on overall transcription and ribozyme cleavage. (**a**) Two different targets are shown to illustrate that the optimum transcription conditions can be different for each template. 5% PAGE analysis with autoradiography of internally radiolabeled transcripts (*upper panel*) or staining with ethidium bromide (*lower panel*). (**b**) Ribozyme cleavage can be enhanced by thermal cycling to allow the RNAs to unfold/refold and promote the cleavage of each of the flanking ribozymes. Two internally labeled transcripts are visualized by 5% PAGE immediately after transcription at 5 mM rNTPs and 20 mM $MgCl_2$ (lanes 1 and 3) and following adjustment to 40 mM $MgCl_2$ and three rounds of thermal cycling (lanes 2 and 4).

8. Prepare small-scale (2–5 ml) cultures using individual colonies and isolate plasmid DNA using a mini-prep kit.
9. Verify the presence and correct sequence of the PCR insert by appropriate restriction enzyme digests and automated DNA sequencing.

3.3. RNA In Vitro Transcription Optimization

The availability of rNTPs and free magnesium ion (Mg^{2+}) will affect both the transcription yield of RNA and the likelihood of correct ribozyme folding and cleavage. The best conditions are often different from one target RNA to the next (see Fig. 5a), making it necessary to experimentally identify optimal transcription conditions by varying the rNTPs:Mg^{2+} ratio in a series of small-scale (50 μl) transcription trials (see Note 4). Also, to ensure that the identified optimal conditions can be scaled up in a reproducible manner it is important to use YIP in the reaction (see Note 5). In some cases the level of overall transcription can be relatively good, although the yield of target RNA can be limited by incomplete ribozyme cleavage. It is often possible to improve the yield of target RNA by employing a brief heat denaturing step allowing the ribozymes to refold and leading to enhanced cleavage (see Fig. 5b).

Table 2
RNA in vitro transcription reaction components

Component	Volume	(Stock)	(Final)
10× Buffer	5 μl	10×	1×
rNTPs	10 μl	25 mM	5 mM
$MgCl_2$	(Y) μl	100 mM	15–35 mM
DNA template	5 μl	500 ng/μl	50 ng/μl
T7 RNAP	2.5 μl	1 mg/ml	50 μg/ml
YIP	0.1 μl	1 U/μl	2 U/ml
α-^{32}P-NTP[a]	0.9 μl	10 μCi/μl	Trace
RNase inhibitor[a]	2.5 μl	20 U/μl	1 U/μl
RNase-free water	24-(Y) μl	–	–

[a]*Optional*: If omitted use water to maintain the reaction volume

1. Linearize the transcription template by digesting the plasmid DNA at an appropriate restriction enzyme site (MLS region).

2. Purify the digested DNA by extraction with phenol/chloroform/isoamylalcohol (25:24:1) followed by a chloroform extraction.

3. Precipitate the DNA by adding 0.1 volumes of 3 M Sodium acetate (pH5.2) followed by 2.5 volumes of ethanol and centrifuging at maximum speed in a microcentrifuge.

4. Resuspend the DNA pellet in nuclease-free water and adjust the final concentration to 500 ng/μl.

5. Set up the transcription reaction(s) according to Table 2 and incubate at 37°C for 2–4 h.

6. *Optional*: To test if thermal cycling is effective in promoting further ribozyme cleavage, remove an aliquot (20 μl) and transfer to a thin-walled PCR tube. Perform at least three cycles of the following program in a thermocycler: 72°C for 1 min, 65°C for 5 min, and 37°C for 10 min (see Note 6).

7. Add an equal volume of formamide loading dye to each sample.

8. Load 2–5 μl from each transcription onto an analytical urea-denaturing polyacrylamide gel using an appropriate percentage gel to resolve RNA transcripts of the expected size.

9. Run the gel and visualize the transcription products using a phosphor screen (if α-^{32}P-NTP was included in the transcription reaction) or by staining the gel with methylene blue.

3.4. Purification of the Target RNA

Once optimal reaction conditions are established, the target RNA should be transcribed on the desired scale (an example 1 ml transcription is used here) and purified away from the ribozymes and uncleaved intermediate species.

1. Set up a 1 ml transcription using the optimal transcription conditions previously established in Subheading 3.3.
2. Add an equal volume of formamide loading dye to the transcription.
3. Load onto a pre-warmed preparative polyacrylamide gel and run the gel an appropriate distance to fully separate the RNA products (see Note 7).
4. Split the gel plates and transfer the gel between Saran Wrap. Identify the correct band by locating the UV shadow against the intensifying screen and quickly mark its position by drawing on the Saran Wrap with a marker pen (see Note 8).
5. Excise the gel slice by first cutting through the Saran Wrap using a new blade and then removing the strip of Saran Wrap with two sterile pipette tips. Slice the gel band into approx 1 mm strips and then cut across the strips to form 1 mm cubes.
6. Transfer the gel cubes to a fresh tube and add approximately two volumes of gel extraction buffer. Elute the RNA by end-over-end rotation. A few hours at room temperature is usually sufficient, or this can be performed in the cold room overnight.
7. Recover the RNA by precipitation with ethanol (2.5 volumes) or isopropanol (1 volume).

4. Notes

1. In a stubborn case where the target RNA had extensive structure at the 5′-end, the complementarity of the 5′-hammerhead ribozyme within helix 1 was extended from the suggested 10 base pairs to 18 base pairs. Only a modest increase in HH Rz cleavage was observed and more complete cleavage was achieved with thermal cycling.
2. Longer oligonucleotides often benefit from additional purification which can be purchased at the time of synthesis. A fast and cost-effective alternative is to bind and wash the oligo using a small amount of DEAE resin. The entire procedure can be monitored by UV spectroscopy and results in the removal of contaminants absorbing in the 220–240 nm range. This approach has been successful many times when the initial PCR reaction has failed.

3. If necessary, further optimization of the PCR can be carried out using a gradient PCR machine.

4. The optimum for most transcripts is typically in the range 0.75–1.75 for total rNTPs:Mg^{2+}. A useful starting point is to fix the rNTPs at 5 mM each (20 mM total) and vary the concentration of $MgCl_2$: 15 mM (ratio = 0.75), 20 mM (1.0), 25 mM (1.25), 30 mM (1.5), and 35 mM (1.75).

5. YIP is used to remove the pyrophosphate (PP_i) released during polymerization. Pyrophosphate is prone to precipitation and will co-precipitate magnesium and rNTPs which can directly affect the result of the transcription trials.

6. Heating RNA in the presence of magnesium ions is often not recommended as this can result in hydrolysis of the RNA. However, the results will differ with each RNA target and in many cases brief heat cycling has been successful in increasing ribozyme cleavage and overall yields of the target RNA. If hydrolysis is particularly evident then alternative heat cycles can be tested or chemical denaturants can be tried. The unmodified HDV Rz retains activity in urea (up to 5 M) and formamide (up to 10 M) (24).

7. In some instances, when loading large-scale transcriptions, the RNA has precipitated at the gel surface. This behavior was not observed when the same RNA was produced without ribozyme cleavage. The problem was overcome by first dialyzing the RNA against a suitable buffer, e.g., 1× TE or TBE, prior to loading onto the gel.

8. The exposure to shortwave UV (254 nm) should be kept as brief as possible to avoid cross-linking and degradation of the RNA.

References

1. Milligan JF, Uhlenbeck OC. Synthesis of small RNAs using T7 RNA polymerase. Methods Enzymol. 1989;180:51–62.
2. Pokrovskaya ID, Gurevich VV. In vitro transcription: preparative RNA yields in analytical scale reactions. Anal Biochem. 1994;220:420–3.
3. Helm M, Brule H, Giege R, Florentz C. More mistakes by T7 RNA polymerase at the 5′ ends of in vitro-transcribed RNAs. RNA. 1999;5:618–21.
4. Pleiss JA, Derrick ML, Uhlenbeck OC. T7 RNA polymerase produces 5′ end heterogeneity during in vitro transcription from certain templates. RNA. 1998;4:1313–7.
5. Lee SS, Kang C. Two base pairs at −9 and −8 distinguish between the bacteriophage T7 and SP6 promoters. J Biol Chem. 1993;268: 19299–304.
6. Huang F. Efficient incorporation of CoA, NAD and FAD into RNA by in vitro transcription. Nucleic Acids Res. 2003;31:e8.
7. Sampson JR, Uhlenbeck OC. Biochemical and physical characterization of an unmodified yeast phenylalanine transfer RNA transcribed in vitro. Proc Natl Acad Sci USA. 1988;85: 1033–7.
8. Kao C, Zheng M, Rudisser S. A simple and efficient method to reduce nontemplated nucleotide addition at the 3 terminus of RNAs transcribed by T7 RNA polymerase. RNA. 1999;5:1268–72.
9. Sherlin LD, Bullock TL, Nissan TA, Perona JJ, Lariviere FJ, Uhlenbeck OC, Scaringe SA. Chemical and enzymatic synthesis of tRNAs for high-throughput crystallization. RNA. 2001;7: 1671–8.

10. Coleman TM, Wang G, Huang F. Superior 5′ homogeneity of RNA from ATP-initiated transcription under the T7 phi 2.5 promoter. Nucleic Acids Res. 2004;32:e14.
11. Inoue H, Hayase Y, Iwai S, Ohtsuka E. Sequence-dependent hydrolysis of RNA using modified oligonucleotide splints and RNase H. FEBS Lett. 1987;215:327–30.
12. Lapham J, Crothers DM. RNase H cleavage for processing of in vitro transcribed RNA for NMR studies and RNA ligation. RNA. 1996;2:289–96.
13. Ziehler WA, Engelke DR. Synthesis of small RNA transcripts with discrete 5′ and 3′ ends. Biotechniques. 1996;20:622–4.
14. Santoro SW, Joyce GF. A general purpose RNA-cleaving DNA enzyme. Proc Natl Acad Sci USA. 1997;94:4262–6.
15. Perrotta AT, Been MD. Cleavage of oligoribonucleotides by a ribozyme derived from the hepatitis delta virus RNA sequence. Biochemistry. 1992;31:16–21.
16. Ferre-D'Amare AR, Doudna JA. Use of cis- and trans-ribozymes to remove 5′ and 3′ heterogeneities from milligrams of in vitro transcribed RNA. Nucleic Acids Res. 1996;24:977–8.
17. Cameron V, Uhlenbeck OC. 3′-Phosphatase activity in T4 polynucleotide kinase. Biochemistry. 1977;16:5120–6.
18. Povirk LF, Steighner RJ. High ionic strength promotes selective 3′-phosphatase activity of T4 polynucleotide kinase. Biotechniques. 1990;9:562.
19. Walker SC, Avis JM, Conn GL. General plasmids for producing RNA in vitro transcripts with homogeneous ends. Nucleic Acids Res. 2003;31:e82.
20. Schenborn ET, Mierendorf Jr RC. A novel transcription property of SP6 and T7 RNA polymerases: dependence on template structure. Nucleic Acids Res. 1985;13:6223–36.
21. Birikh KR, Heaton PA, Eckstein F. The structure, function and application of the hammerhead ribozyme. Eur J Biochem. 1997;245:1–16.
22. Zuker M. Mfold web server for nucleic acid folding and hybridization prediction. Nucleic Acids Res. 2003;31:3406–15.
23. Hofacker IL (2004) RNA secondary structure analysis using the Vienna RNA package. Curr Protoc Bioinformatics Chapter 12, Unit 12 2
24. Rosenstein SP, Been MD. Self-cleavage of hepatitis delta virus genomic strand RNA is enhanced under partially denaturing conditions. Biochemistry. 1990;29:8011–6.

Chapter 8

Trans-Acting Antigenomic HDV Ribozyme for Production of In Vitro Transcripts with Homogenous 3′ Ends

Milena Szafraniec, Leszek Blaszczyk, Jan Wrzesinski, and Jerzy Ciesiolka

Abstract

During in vitro run-off transcription with T7 RNA polymerase, transcripts with heterogenous 3′ ends are commonly synthesized. Here, we describe an efficient procedure for correct processing of transcript 3′ ends with the use of antigenomic HDV ribozyme. The procedure involves the extension of nascent transcripts with seven nucleotides complementary to the ribozyme's recognition site and, subsequently, the removal of those nucleotides with the HDV ribozyme acting in trans. Sufficient reaction rates and final cleavage extents of approx. 90% can be obtained with just twofold excess of the ribozyme. The highest concentration of RNA substrate suggested for practical applications turns out to be 3 μM. The procedure is an alternative to the use of ribozymes as *cis*-cleaving autocatalytic cassettes attached to transcript 3′ ends.

Key words: Transcription in vitro, T7 RNA polymerase, RNA heterogeneity, 3′ homogeneity, Ribozyme cleavage

1. Introduction

It has been observed that during in vitro run-off transcription T7 RNA polymerase often attaches one or two nontemplate encoded nucleotides to the 3′ end of the nascent RNA transcript (1, 2). Homogenous transcripts with a predefined length are, however, indispensable in many applications such as X-ray crystallographic studies, NMR spectroscopy, and ligation reactions (3, 4). To produce RNA in vitro transcripts with homogenous 3′ ends several approaches have been developed. A commonly used procedure is a careful purification of transcription products by denaturing polyacrylamide gel electrophoresis or HPLC but for relatively long RNAs this procedure works very inefficiently. Another approach employs ribozymes acting in cis that excise full-length RNAs from flanking regions ((5–9); also see Chapter 7). Ribozymes acting in trans, the hepatitis delta virus (HDV) ribozyme (10, 11), the *Neurospora* Varkud satellite VS ribozyme (6), or the catalytic RNA subunit of a bacterial RNase P (9), can also be used for correct processing of transcript's 3′ ends.

Here, we describe the use of antigenomic HDV ribozyme acting in trans for the purpose of correct processing of the 3′ ends of RNA in vitro transcripts. The ribozyme can be transcribed from a template consisting of chemically synthesized oligodeoxyribonucleotides (see Fig. 1); thus it is easily available for practical applications. The general scheme of the proposed procedure is shown in Fig. 2. In the first step, a transcription template is generated, which encodes the RNA sequence of interest extended with additional seven nucleotides GGGUCGG complementary to the HDV ribozyme recognition site (RRS). Following RNA transcription, these extra nucleotides are cleaved off with the *trans*-acting ribozyme in a reaction induced by magnesium ions. The ribozyme does not require any particular sequence upstream of the cleavage site, and therefore it can be applied to any RNA. To ensure high cleavage efficiency of RNA intermediates, the additional 7-nucleotide-long stretch should be accessible for ribozyme hybridization. Thus, any possibility of extensive pairing of that stretch with other regions of the transcript should be avoided while constructing the transcription template (12). Our procedure is an effective and simple alternative to the use of 3′ *cis*-cleaving autocatalytic cassettes. In those cases, improper folding of ribozymes within the context of full-length molecules is likely to be responsible for the often observed low cleavage efficiency. Moreover, when isotopically labeled RNA transcripts are needed for NMR studies, the use of *trans*-acting ribozymes spares the expensive nucleotide precursors, which otherwise would be incorporated in the *cis*-acting ribozyme sequence and discarded upon cleavage.

2. Materials

Prepare all reagents using ultrapure water of 18.2 MΩ cm resistance at 25°C and analytical grade chemicals. Make up all the reagents at room temperature and sterilize them by autoclaving (solutions of KCl, $MgCl_2$, EDTA, Tris, sodium acetate) or filtering (solution of DTT and all buffers made in small quantities). For filtering, use sterile disposable plastic syringes and 0.22 μm filters. Store all the reagents at –20°C, unless marked otherwise.

2.1. Construction of DNA Template Encoding trans-Acting HDV Ribozyme

1. HDV template oligodeoxyribonucleotides: RA, 5′-*TAATACG ACTCACTATA* GGGCATCTCCACC-3′; RW, 5′-GAAAAGT GGCTCTCCCTTAGCCATCC GAGTGCTCGGATGCCCA GGTCGGACCGCGAGGAGGTGGAGATGCCC-3′ (the T7

RA oligomer	5' *TAATACGACTCACTAT*<u>AGGGCATCTCCACC</u> 3'
RW oligomer	3' CCCGTAGAGGTGGAG GAGCG CCAGGCTGGACCC GTAGGC TCGTGAGCCTACCGATTCCCTCTCGGTG AAAAG 5'

↓ synthesis of DNA template

HDV template	5' *TAATACGACTCACTAT*AGGGCATCTCCACCTCCTCGCGGTCCGACCTGGGCATCCGCAGCACTCGGATGGCTAAGGGAGAGCCACTTTTC 3' 3' *ATTATGCTGAGTGATA*TCCCGTAGAGGTGGAGGAGCGCCAGGCTGGACCCGTAGGCTCGTGAGCCTACCGATTCCCTCTCGGTGAAAAG 5'

↓ *in vitro* transcription

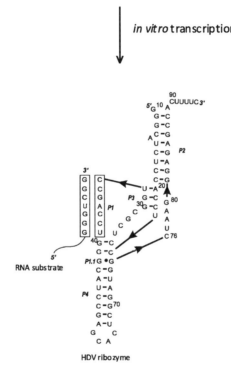

Fig. 1. Preparation of *trans*-acting antigenomic HDV ribozyme. Numbering of nucleotides corresponds to the wild-type RNA sequence. In the ribozyme structure, base-paired segments are denoted P1 to P4. The RNA substrate that is to be made homogenous at its 3' end is also shown in the figure. Regions which are base-paired in the ribozyme–substrate complex are *boxed*.

RNA polymerase promoter is marked in italics; complementary sequences are underlined). DNA oligomers can be purchased from any commercial supplier and a synthesis on the 0.2 μmol scale is typically sufficient for these protocols.

2. Tris–EDTA (TE) buffer: 10 mM Tris–HCl pH 8.0, 1 mM EDTA. Prepare 0.1 M solution of EDTA by dissolving 0.292 g EDTA in 10 mL of water. Weigh 12.114 mg Tris and add about 7 mL of water. Adjust pH with concentrated HCl, continuously mixing the solution on a magnetic stirrer. Add 100 μL of previously prepared 0.1 M EDTA and fill the solution with water up to 10 mL (see Notes 1 and 2).

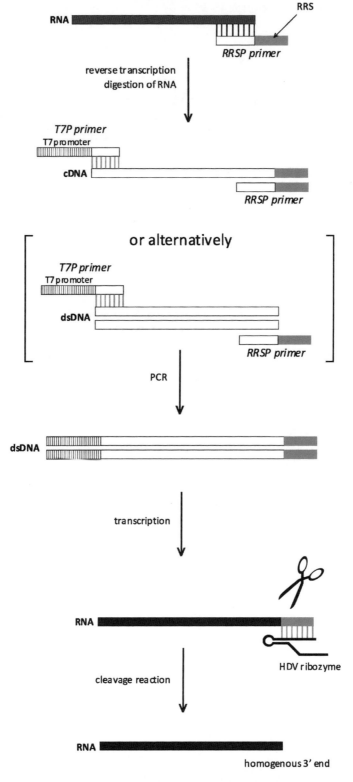

Fig. 2. Scheme presenting the procedure for obtaining RNA in vitro transcripts with homogenous 3′ ends. The abbreviation RRS denotes the 7-nucleotide-long stretches that correspond to the HDV ribozyme's recognition site. An alternative way of obtaining the dsDNA template encoding RRS is shown in *parenthesis*.

3. Taq polymerase, 1 U/μL.
4. Taq polymerase buffer (10×): 750 mM Tris–HCl pH 8.8, 200 mM $(NH_4)_2SO_4$, 0.1% (v/v) Tween 20. This buffer is usually supplied with commercial Taq polymerase.
5. 25 mM $MgCl_2$. This may be supplied with the Taq polymerase.
6. 10 mM each deoxyribonucleotide (dNTP) mixture.
7. 3 M Sodium acetate, pH 5.5. Dissolve 2.461 g sodium acetate in 7 mL of water. Adjust pH to 5.5 using concentrated acetic acid and fill with water up to 10 mL.
8. 96% Ethanol.

2.2. In Vitro Transcription

1. T7 RNA polymerase, 200 U/μL (see Note 3).
2. Transcription buffer (5×): 200 mM Tris–HCl pH 7.9, 30 mM $MgCl_2$, 50 mM DTT, 50 mM NaCl, and 10 mM spermidine.
3. 25 mM each ribonucleotide (NTP) mixture.
4. 100 mM DTT.

2.3. Purification of Nucleic Acids by Polyacrylamide Gel Electrophoresis

1. Tris–borate–EDTA (TBE) buffer (10×): 1 M Tris, 1 M boric acid, 10 mM EDTA, pH 8.3. To prepare 10× TBE, weigh 121.14 g Tris, 61.83 g boric acid, and 3.72 g EDTA and dissolve in 1 L of water. Store at room temperature. For electrophoresis use diluted 1× TBE buffer.
2. 8% Polyacrylamide/8.3 M urea gel mixture: 8% (w/v) acrylamide:N,N′-methylenebisacrylamide (29:1), 100 mM Tris, 100 mM boric acid, 1 mM EDTA, and 8.3 M urea. Prepare a 40% acrylamide:N,N′-methylenebisacrylamide (29:1) solution by weighing 193.33 g acrylamide and 6.67 g N,N′-methylenebisacrylamide and filling with water up to 500 mL (see Note 4). Mix the solution using a magnetic stirrer. Store in a dark bottle at 4°C. Weigh 420 g urea, dissolve it in 200 mL of the previously prepared 40% acrylamide:N,N′-methylenebisacrylamide solution, and fill with water up to 800 mL. Add a spatula of resin beads AG 501-X8 (Bio-Rad) and mix for 1 h on a magnetic stirrer (see Note 5). Having all the urea dissolved, filter the mixture using water pump and paper filter. Add 100 mL of 10× TBE buffer and fill up with water to 1,000 mL. Store at room temperature.
3. Polyacrylamide gel polymerization catalysts: N,N,N′,N′-tetramethyl-ethylenediamine (TEMED) and 10% (w/v) ammonium persulfate (APS). Store at 4°C.
4. Gel electrophoresis system with 20×20 cm plates and 1 mm thick spacers, e.g., PROTEAN II Vertical Electrophoresis Cells (Bio-Rad) or a homemade apparatus of a similar size.
5. XC loading buffer (2×): 8 M urea, 0.05% (w/v) xylene cyanol, and 10 mM EDTA. Store at 4°C.

6. BB loading buffer (2×): 8 M urea, 0.05% (w/v) bromophenol blue, and 10 mM EDTA. Store at 4°C.
7. 0.3 M Sodium acetate, pH 5.5.
8. Thermomixer, e.g., Thermomixer Comfort (Eppendorf).
9. Glycogen, 30 mg/mL.
10. 96% Ethanol.
11. TLC plate with a fluorescent indicator with a 254 nm excitation wavelength and a UV lamp with 254 nm light output.

2.4. Reverse Transcription

1. RRSP primer with the 7-nucleotide-long stretch 5′-CCGACCC-3′ at its 5′ end followed by at least 15 nucleotides complementary to the 3′ end of the RNA of interest (see Fig. 2).
2. 500 mM Tris–HCl pH 8.0. Weigh 0.606 g Tris, dissolve in about 7 mL of water, and adjust pH with concentrated HCl. Fill with water up to 10 mL.
3. 10 mM each deoxyribonucleotide (dNTP) mixture.
4. 500 mM KCl.
5. 100 mM $MgCl_2$.
6. 100 mM DTT.
7. M-MuLV reverse transcriptase, 200 U/µL.
8. RNase A, 50 U/µL.

2.5. Amplification of cDNA

1. RRSP primer (see Subheading 2.4).
2. T7P primer containing T7 RNA polymerase promoter 5′-TAATACGACTCACTATA-3′ and at least 12 nucleotide-long sequence complementary to the 5′ end of your RNA (see Fig. 2).
3. 100 mM Tris–HCl pH 8.3. Weigh 0.121 g Tris, dissolve in about 7 mL of water, adjust pH with concentrated HCl, and fill with water up to 10 mL.
4. 10 mM each deoxyribonucleotide (dNTP) mixture.
5. 500 mM KCl.
6. 100 mM $MgCl_2$.
7. Taq polymerase 1 U/µL.
8. Phenol saturated with TE buffer. Mix 0.5 mL of phenol with the same volume of TE buffer. Vortex firmly and centrifuge for about 0.5 min at 2,000 × g to separate phenol and aqueous layers. Use the lower layer of the mixture. Store at 4°C.
9. Chloroform–isoamyl alcohol mixture (24:1, v/v). Store at 4°C.
10. 3 M Sodium acetate pH 5.5.
11. 96% Ethanol.
12. TE buffer (see Subheading 2.1).

2.6. Ribozyme Cleavage Reaction

1. Reaction buffer (10×): 500 mM Tris–HCl pH 7.5, and 1 mM EDTA.
2. 100 mM $MgCl_2$.

3. Methods

3.1. Preparation of trans-Acting HDV Ribozyme

3.1.1. Construction of a dsDNA Template

1. A double-stranded DNA template encoding the HDV ribozyme is created from two overlapping oligodeoxyribonucleotides that cover the catalytically active ribozyme sequence. Additionally, one of these oligomers is equipped with T7 RNA polymerase promoter at its 5′ end (see Fig. 1 and Subheading 2.1). Prepare 100 pmol/μL solutions of RA and RW oligomers in TE buffer. Assemble the PCR reaction in 300 μL total volume, by mixing: 222.5 μL of nuclease-free water, 5 μL of each oligomer, 30 μL of 10× Taq polymerase buffer, 24 μL of 25 mM $MgCl_2$, 6 μL of 10 mM each dNTP mixture, and 7.5 μL of Taq polymerase. The reaction mixture should be kept on ice during the whole procedure of its assembly. Gently vortex and briefly centrifuge the mixture, and then divide it into three portions of 100 μL in thin-wall PCR tubes.

2. Perform a PCR reaction on a thermocycler as follows. Step 1, initial denaturation: 2 min at 94°C. Step 2, eight cycles of denaturation, annealing, and elongation: 30 s at 94°C, 30 s at 46°C, and 2 min at 72°C. Step 3, final elongation: 5 min at 72°C.

3. Precipitate the obtained DNA by adding 30 μL of 3 M sodium acetate pH 5.5 and 990 μL of ethanol to the combined 300 μL reaction mixture. Incubate overnight at −20°C (see Note 6).

4. Centrifuge the sample for 20 min at 4°C and $17,000 \times g$. Remove the supernatant and dry the pellet in an open tube for 5 min at 37°C. When dry, dissolve the pellet in 100 μL of TE buffer.

5. Measure the concentration of DNA using UV spectrophotometer (see Note 7). The conversion factor for dsDNA is 0.05 μg/μL per optical density unit (1 OD) at 260 nm. Store the template at −20°C.

3.1.2. In Vitro Transcription and Transcript Purification

1. Combine in vitro transcription reaction components at room temperature, by mixing in order 4 μL of 5× transcription buffer, 2 μL of 100 mM DTT, 0.8 μL of 25 mM each NTP mixture, 2 μg of the dsDNA template (obtained as described in Subheading 3.1.1), 2 μL of T7 RNA polymerase, and water to a final volume of 20 μL. Incubate the mixture for 4 h at 37°C (see Note 8).

2. Purify the obtained RNA by polyacrylamide gel electrophoresis in denaturing conditions. Prepare an 8% denaturing polyacrylamide gel using TBE buffer, with 20 μL of TEMED and 350 μL of APS per 50 mL of gel mixture (see Note 9). Perform pre-electrophoresis of the gel for about 0.5 h at 400–600 V and 10–15 mA. Add 20 μL of BB loading buffer to the transcription reaction mixture, mix it, and load into one well of the gel (see Note 10). To observe the progress of the electrophoresis, put 20 μL of XC loading buffer into another well. Continue electrophoresis at 800–1,000 V and 20–25 mA (see Note 11), until XC marker dye migrates about 6 cm below the well bottom.

3. After finishing electrophoresis, remove one of the glass plates and cover the gel with a plastic wrap. Transfer the gel, plastic wrap-side-down, on top of a TLC plate with fluorescent indicator. Visualize your product by UV shadowing, applying 254 nm UV lamp, and excise proper bands using sterile surgical blades (see Note 12).

4. In order to recover RNA from the gel, put the excised gel piece into a 1.5 mL tube and cover it with 150 μL of 0.3 M sodium acetate pH 5.5 (see Note 13). Perform the elution using a thermomixer at 25°C and 650 rpm or at room temperature shaking the tube occasionally. After 1.5 h harvest the RNA solution over the gel, put it into a new tube, flood the gel with a new portion of sodium acetate solution, and repeat the procedure. Combine the supernatants (250–300 μl) in one tube and precipitate the RNA by adding 1.5 μL of glycogen and 3 volumes of ethanol. Vortex the mixture and keep it at −20°C overnight (see Note 6).

5. Centrifuge the sample for 20 min at 4°C and 17,000×g, remove supernatant, dry the pellet for 5 min at 37°C, and dissolve it in 50 μL of sterile water.

6. Measure the concentration of the obtained RNA using a UV spectrophotometer. The conversion factor for RNA is 0.04 μg/μL per 1 OD at 260 nm. Taking into consideration that the molecular weight of a single nucleotide is on average 330 Da, estimate the concentration of RNA in picomoles per microliter. Store the RNA at −20°C.

3.2. Generating the RNA of Interest Susceptible to Ribozyme Cleavage

The scheme of the procedure to obtain RNA molecules that are susceptible to ribozyme cleavage is outlined in Fig. 2. In the first step, a cDNA is obtained *via* reverse transcription reaction using RRSP primer and the RNA which is to be made homogenous at its 3′ end as a template. Subsequently, RNase A enzyme is added to digest the RNA (Subheading 3.2.1). The cDNA is then amplified by PCR with T7P and RRSP primers as described in Subheading 3.2.2. Alternatively, if a dsDNA template is available for the RNA of interest, one can omit reverse transcription and generate the extended template directly from this dsDNA (see Fig. 2). To do that, re-amplify your template by PCR, using T7P and RRSP primers. Perform PCR as described in Subheading 3.2.2. Then conduct in vitro transcription using the extended template and purify the transcript as described in Subheading 3.1.2.

3.2.1. Reverse Transcription of RNA with a Primer Containing the HDV RRS Sequence

1. Perform a reverse transcription reaction using the RNA which is to be made homogenous at its 3′ end in order to generate a cDNA encoding RRS. Use RRSP primer with a region complementary to the 3′ end of the RNA of interest (see Fig. 2 and Subheading 2.4). Mix 15 pmol of RNA with 45 pmol of the primer (see Note 14) and dissolve them in deionized water to a final volume of 35 µL. Perform denaturation and renaturation of RNA molecules by incubating the mixture for 2 min at 100°C, for 10 min at 0°C, and, finally, for 10 min at 37°C. Next, add 7 µL of 10 mM each dNTP mixture, 7 µL of 500 mM Tris–HCl pH 8.0, 7 µL of 500 mM KCl, 2.8 µL of 100 mM $MgCl_2$, 7 µL of 100 mM DTT, and 0.7 µL of 200 U/µL M-MuLV reverse transcriptase. Fill the mixture with water up to 70 µL. Conduct the reaction for 1.5 h at 42°C.

2. Cleave the template RNA with 5 µL of RNase A for 30 min at 35°C (see Note 15).

3.2.2. Amplification of cDNA and RNA Transcription

1. Amplify the obtained cDNA by PCR, using RRSP primer and T7P primer (see Fig. 2 and Subheading 2.5). To do this, use equimolar amounts of T7P and RRSP oligomers (the final concentration of the primers should be 1 µM), half of the cDNA obtained in Subheading 3.2.1 (ca. 35 µL), 30 µL of 100 mM Tris–HCl pH 8.3, 6 µL of 100 mM $MgCl_2$, 30 µL of 500 mM KCl, 6 µL of 10 mM each dNTP mixture, and 7.5 µL of Taq DNA polymerase in a final volume of 300 µL.

2. Perform the reaction in three 100 µL PCR tubes applying the following conditions. Step 1, initial denaturation: 2 min at 94°C. Step 2, 20 cycles of denaturation, annealing, and elongation: 30 s at 94°C, 30 s at 42°C, and 2 min at 72°C.

3. Extract the obtained dsDNA as follows. Recombine the three 100 µL samples in PCR tubes into a single microfuge tube, add an equal volume (300 µL) of TE buffer-saturated phenol, and shake intensively for 3 min at room temperature. Next, carefully remove the aqueous phase from over the phenol and put it into a new microfuge tube. Add 300 µL of a chloroform–isoamyl alcohol mixture and shake as before. After again removing the upper aqueous phase, precipitate the dsDNA by adding 1/10 volume of 3 M sodium acetate pH 5.5 and three

volumes of ethanol. Perform the precipitation overnight at −20°C (see Note 6).

4. Centrifuge the sample for 20 min at 4°C and 17,000×g. Remove the supernatant and dry the pellet in an open tube for 5 min at 37°C. When dry, dissolve the pellet in 60 µL of TE buffer. Store the dsDNA at −20°C.

5. Using the obtained dsDNA as a template perform in vitro transcription, and subsequently, purify the transcript by polyacrylamide gel electrophoresis in denaturing conditions as described in Subheading 3.1.2.

3.3. Cleavage Reaction

The cleavage reaction should be performed with excess of HDV ribozyme, which allows it to be conducted in a relatively short time (see Note 16). Several ribozyme-to-substrate ratios have been tested (11) and the results are shown in Fig. 3a. It turns out that a decrease in the ribozyme excess from 100-fold to just twofold is almost irrelevant to the final cleavage extent. As a sufficient reaction rate and the final cleavage extent of approx. 90% can be obtained with just double excess of the ribozyme (11), we suggest applying such conditions for practical usage. Different concentrations of ribozyme and substrate at a constant 2:1 ratio have also been examined ((11); see also Fig. 3b). Considering the results, we recommend to use a 6 µM concentration of ribozyme and 3 µM of RNA substrate. At higher concentrations of the ribozyme and the substrate the reaction becomes less specific and some side products appear.

1. To perform the cleavage reaction with the ribozyme and substrate concentrations of 6 µM and 3 µM, respectively, mix 120 pmol of HDV ribozyme with 60 pmol of substrate RNA, add 2 µL of reaction buffer, and fill with water up to 18 µL. Subject the mixture to a denaturation–renaturation procedure at 100°C for 2 min, then at 0°C for 10 min, and at 37°C for 10 min.

2. Initiate the reaction by adding 2 µL of 100 mM $MgCl_2$ solution and proceed at 37°C for 10 min.

3. Quench the reaction by adding 20 µL of BB loading buffer.

4. Purify the cleaved RNA using an 8% denaturing polyacrylamide gel and perform elution as described in Subheading 3.1.2.

4. Notes

1. Use graduated cylinder instead of a plastic tube or a beaker scale, as it is more accurate.

2. TE buffer is also commercially available.

a Ribozyme / substrate ratio

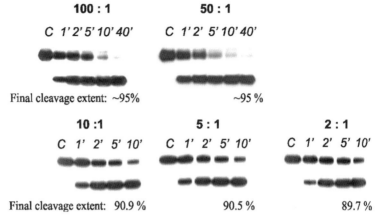

b Various ribozyme and substrate concentration at their constant 2 : 1 ratio

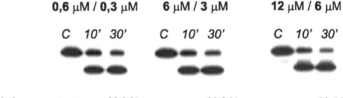

Fig. 3. Cleavage reaction of (5'-^{32}P)-end-labeled tRNA^{Phe}/7 nucleotide intermediate with *trans*-acting antigenomic HDV ribozyme. (**a**) Dependence of the cleavage reaction on different ribozyme-to-substrate ratios. The reactions were carried out in the buffer Tris–HCl pH 7.5 in the presence of 10 mM MgCl$_2$, the products were separated on 12% polyacrylamide gels and visualized by autoradiography. (**b**) Dependence of the cleavage reaction on various ribozyme and substrate concentrations at their constant 2:1 ratio (reproduced from ref. 11 with permission from Oxford University Press).

3. Alternatively, for in vitro transcription reagents of AmpliScribe™ High Yield Transcription Kit (Epicentre Biotechnologies) can be used, in accordance with the manufacturer's protocol.

4. Acrylamide is highly toxic. Wear a mask when weighing it. Prepare acrylamide solution inside a fume hood and avoid spreading acrylamide in laboratory. It is worth noting that premixed solutions at various ratios are also commercially available. These are more costly but much safer to use.

5. Dissolving urea in water is highly endothermic, so it is advisable to use a heated magnetic stirrer to raise its solubility.

6. Precipitation of DNA or RNA with ethanol can also be performed for 1 h on dry ice. However, in such conditions precipitation of salt buffers sometimes occurs.

7. We recommend using a NanoDrop spectrophotometer, as it allows measuring the concentration of a nucleic acid solution

in very small volumes, and additionally, the sample purity can be estimated. Using a NanoDrop, you should obtain a peak with maximum at 260 nm and the 260/280 absorption ratio should be in the range of 1.8 and 2.0.

8. Yield of the transcription reaction can be raised by previous purification of the oligomers used for the synthesis of the DNA template by polyacrylamide gel electrophoresis in denaturing conditions. Perform purification as described in Subheadings 2.3 and 3.1.2.

9. If the gel mixture polymerizes too fast, you can reduce the amount of TEMED.

10. Before loading the sample, wash the well thoroughly with TBE buffer to remove any gel fragments or urea from it.

11. Check the temperature of the plates. It should not exceed 50°C, because at higher temperatures the plates may crack.

12. Use protective glass goggles, as UV light is extremely harmful for the eyes.

13. You may briefly centrifuge the tube to make the gel pieces go to its bottom.

14. 1 OD = 33 µg of DNA/mL. Taking the average molecular weight of a nucleotide as 330 Da, 1 OD of a 20-nucleotide-long oligomer corresponds to $(0.033~\mu g/\mu L)/(20 \times 0.00033~\mu g/pmol) = 5~pmol/\mu L$ of oligomer.

15. Prepare RNase A free of DNase activity by boiling commercial RNase A at 100°C for 10 min.

16. The *trans*-acting HDV ribozyme is able to work in several rounds, so it could also be used in sub-stoichiometric amounts. However, to achieve satisfactory cleavage extents, the reaction time has to be considerably extended. This in turn might increase nonspecific degradation of RNA and is thus not recommended in practical applications.

Acknowledgements

This work was supported by Wroclaw Research Center EIT+ under the project "Biotechnologies and advanced medical technologies—BioMed" (POIG 01.01.02-02-003/08-00) financed from the "European Regional Development Fund (Operational Programme Innovative Economy, 1.1.2)" and earlier by grants from the Ministry of Science and Higher Education.

References

1. Milligan JF, Groebe JF, Witherell DR, Uhlenbeck OC (1987) Oligoribonucleotide synthesis using T7 RNA polymerase and synthetic DNA templates. Nucleic Acids Res 15:8783–8798
2. Cazenave C, Uhlenbeck OC (1994) RNA template-directed RNA synthesis by T7 RNA polymerase. Biochemistry 91:6972–6976
3. Price SR, Ito N, Outbridge C, Avis JM, Nagai K (1995) Crystallization of RNA-protein complexes. I. Methods for the large-scale preparation of RNA suitable for crystallographic studies. J Mol Biol 249:398–408
4. Sherlin LD, Bullock TL, Nissan TA, Perona JJ, Lariviere FJ, Uhlenbeck OC, Scaringe SA (2001) Chemical and enzymatic synthesis of tRNAs for high-throughput crystallization. RNA 7:1671–1678
5. Grosshans CA, Cech TR (1991) A hammerhead ribozyme allows synthesis of a new form of the *Tetrahymena* ribozyme homogenous in length with a 3′ end blocked for transesterification. Nucleic Acids Res 19:3875–3880
6. Ferre-D'Amare AR, Doudna JA (1996) Use of *cis*- and *trans*-ribozymes to remove 5′ and 3′ heterogeneities from milligrams of *in vitro* transcribed RNA. Nucleic Acids Res 24:977–978
7. Schürer H, Lang K, Schuster J, Mörl M (2002) A universal method to produce *in vitro* transcripts with homogenous 3′ ends. Nucleic Acids Res 30:e56
8. Walker SC, Avis JM, Conn GL (2003) General plasmids for producing RNA *in vitro* transcripts with homogenous ends. Nucleic Acids Res 31:e82
9. Mörl M, Lizano E, Willkomm DK, Hartmann RK (2005) Production of RNAs with homogenous 5′ and 3′ ends. In: Hartmann RK, Bindereif A, Schon A, Westhof E (eds) Handbook of RNA biochemistry. Wiley-VCH GmbH & Co, KGaA, Weinheim, pp 22–35
10. Wrzesinski J, Łęgiewicz M, Smolska B, Ciesiołka J (2001) Catalytic cleavage of *cis*-and *trans*-acting antigenomic *delta* ribozymes in the presence of various divalent metal ions. Nucleic Acids Res 29:4482–4492
11. Wichłacz A, Łęgiewicz M, Ciesiołka J (2004) Generating *in vitro* transcripts with homogenous 3′ ends using *trans*-acting antigenomic delta ribozyme. Nucleic Acids Res 32:e39
12. Świątkowska A, Dutkiewicz M, Ciesiołka J (2007) Structural features of target RNA molecules greatly modulate the cleavage efficiency of trans-acting delta ribozymes. Biochemistry 46:5523–5533

Chapter 9

Rapid Preparation of RNA Samples Using DNA-Affinity Chromatography and DNAzyme Methods

Hae-Kap Cheong, Eunha Hwang, and Chaejoon Cheong

Abstract

Milligram quantities of RNA are commonly synthesized by in vitro transcription from a DNA template with T7 RNA polymerase. However, the run-off transcription method results in heterogeneity at the RNA 3′-terminus. RNA purification requires single-nucleotide resolution to separate the transcript of the correct length from the aborted or add-on transcripts that are usually present in comparable amounts. Here, we describe an RNA preparation method that uses a *trans*-acting DNAzyme and sequence-specific affinity column chromatography. This purification method is simple, fast, and suited for high throughput.

Key words: RNA, DNAzyme, Affinity chromatography, RNA purification, In vitro transcription

1. Introduction

Structural and functional studies of RNA often require milligram quantities of pure material. For example, to obtain useful structural information using X-ray crystallography and NMR spectroscopy, milligram quantities of RNA oligonucleotides are efficiently prepared by in vitro transcription from DNA templates using T7 RNA polymerase (1). Large-scale chemical synthesis of RNA is still technically difficult and expensive. However, the resulting RNA transcripts are not chemically pure. T7 RNA polymerase produces short, abortive, and add-on transcripts that are usually present in amounts comparable to those transcripts of the correct length. Denaturing polyacrylamide gel electrophoresis (PAGE) followed by size-exclusion chromatography is commonly used to purify the desired RNA (2). Although PAGE purification of RNA provides nucleotide resolution, it is time-consuming and leads to acrylamide oligomer impurities associated with the RNA (3).

For high-throughput RNA preparation, several different methods and protocols to overcome the disadvantages of PAGE purification have been proposed (3–9). A method to reduce non-templated nucleotide addition by T7 RNA polymerase using modified DNA templates has been suggested (4). To obtain medium-sized (20–50 nts) RNAs with a homogeneous length, *trans*-cleavage with a hammerhead ribozyme and ion-exchange chromatography are used (5, 6). Chromatographic purification after RNA transcription facilitates large-scale preparation. Size-exclusion chromatography is one of the methods that can resolve small abortive products and the correct RNA transcript under native conditions (3, 7). RNA purification tags have been developed to immobilize and affinity-capture RNA transcripts. A recently developed procedure uses RNA–protein interactions to immobilize and a *cis*-acting ribozyme to elute the desired RNA (8).

In this chapter, we describe a high-throughput method of preparing RNA samples using DNA-affinity chromatography and DNAzymes to liberate the RNA product. DNAzymes, also known as deoxyribozymes or DNA enzymes, are single strands of DNA with catalytic activity that were discovered by in vitro selection (10). The best-studied DNAzymes are the 10:23 and 8:17 DNAzymes, which catalyze the cleavage of RNA substrates. DNAzymes have a small catalytic core that anneals to RNA targets by hybridizing the two flanking arms of 7–13 nucleotides. Upon the addition of Mg^{2+} or other divalent ions, the DNAzyme specifically cleaves the RNA at the designated site. To simplify and increase the speed of the purification steps, immobilized DNA oligonucleotides were used to affinity-capture the tagged RNA transcripts. The affinity tag is removed by sequence-specific cleavage using a *trans*-acting DNAzyme. The arm lengths of the DNAzyme are each optimized at ~13 nt to maximize the turnover number under the reaction conditions. The procedure used for high-throughput RNA sample preparation is illustrated in Fig. 1.

2. Materials

Prepare all solutions using ultrapure water (RNase-free or DEPC-treated water) and biochemical grade (RNase-free) reagents. The sequence of the oligonucleotides used to prepare an RNA sample is illustrated in Fig. 2.

2.1. In Vitro Transcription

1. DNA templates: Synthetic oligonucleotide or linearized plasmid.
2. T7 RNA polymerase: Clones of T7 RNA polymerase are available and we recommend that you obtain a clone and purify

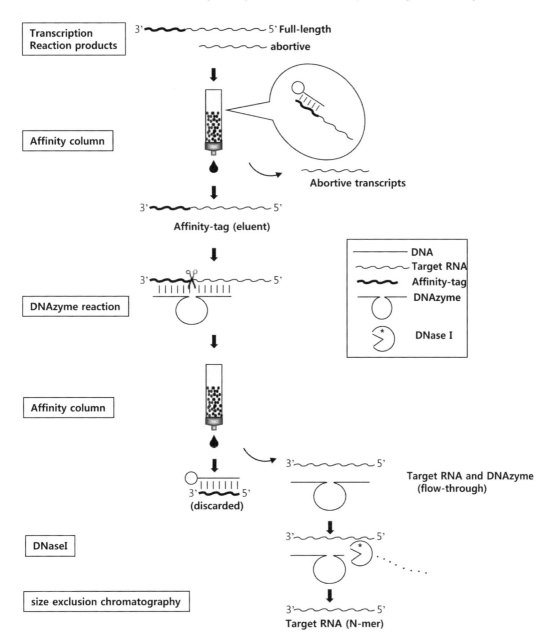

Fig. 1. Overview schematic of the steps involved in preparing RNA samples in a high-throughput manner using DNA affinity column and DNAzyme methods.

your own enzyme. T7 RNA polymerase is also commercially available from several suppliers.

3. 5× NTPs: 20 mM each of ATP, GTP, CTP, and UTP. Adjust to pH 8.1 with 1 M NaOH. Store at −20°C.

4. 1× Transcription Buffer: 40 mM Tris–HCl, pH 8.1, 1 mM spermidine, 0.01% Triton X-100, 5 mM DTT, and 28 mM $MgCl_2$. Make a 10× stock and store at −20°C.

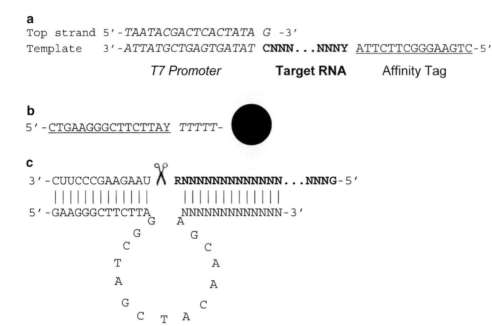

Fig. 2. The sequence of the oligonucleotides used to prepare an RNA sample. (**a**) DNA templates for in vitro transcription. (**b**) DNA affinity support that is chemically synthesized on the Oligo Affinity Support. (**c**) 10–23 DNAzyme used in this study. The DNAzyme cuts the substrate RNA after the unpaired purine residue.

5. 5× Polyethylene glycol: 400 mg/mL PEG8000 in water.
6. 0.5 M EDTA, pH 8.0.
7. Ethanol, reagent grade.
8. 3 M Sodium acetate, pH 5.2.

2.2. DNA-Affinity Chromatography

1. DNA oligonucleotide column on an Oligo Affinity Support (Glen Research) (see Note 1).
2. Binding Buffer: 250 mM NaCl and 20 mM sodium phosphate, pH 7.0 (see Note 2).
3. Elution Buffer: 20 mM sodium phosphate, pH 7.0 (see Note 2).
4. Empty column: I.D. 10 mm and length 10 cm.
5. UV spectrometer to measure oligonucleotide concentrations. 1 optical density (OD) at 260 nm corresponds to a concentration of ~50 μg/mL for oligonucleotides.

2.3. DNAzyme Reaction

1. DNAzyme oligonucleotide (see Note 3).
2. 2× DNAzyme Reaction Buffer: 300 mM NaCl and 80 mM Tris–HCl, pH 7.5.
3. 1 M $MgCl_2$.

4. RNase-free DNase I.
5. 10 kDa molecular weight cutoff (MWCO) spin concentrator.
6. Fast protein liquid chromatography (FPLC) system.
7. Superdex-75 column (GE Healthcare).
8. Denaturing polyacrylamide gel: 15% acrylamide/bis-acrylamide (29:1) solution in 1× TBE buffer (89 mM Tris–borate and 2 mM EDTA) and 7 M urea denaturing gel.
9. 0.1% Toluidine blue.

3. Methods

3.1. In Vitro Transcription

More detailed descriptions of the in vitro transcription procedure are given in other Chapters in this book (see Chapters 4 and 5). A brief protocol suitable for generating samples for the following DNAzyme purification approach is given below. For a 10 mL transcription reaction:

1. Mix the transcription reaction reagents in the following order:
   (a) 1 mL of 10× Transcription Buffer.
   (b) 2 mL of 5× NTPs.
   (c) 2 mL of 5× polyethylene glycol.
   (d) 100 μL of DNA template (~1 nmole).
   (e) Water to achieve a final volume of 10 mL.
   (f) 100 μL of T7 RNA polymerase (~30,000 unit/mL final concentration).
2. Incubate the reaction at 37°C for 2–4 h.
3. Add 0.6 mL of 0.5 M EDTA to stop the reaction.
4. Perform ethanol precipitation by adding 3 volumes of cold ethanol and 1/10 volume of 3 M sodium acetate (pH 5.2). Incubate for 30 min on ice. Centrifuge for 30 min at 15,000 × g.
5. Decant the supernatant and air-dry the pellet.
6. Resuspend the dried pellet in ~5 mL of Binding Buffer.

3.2. First Affinity Column

1. Prepare the affinity support by automated solid phase chemical DNA synthesis on 1 g of Oligo Affinity Support (Glen Research). The deprotected support is ready for use (see Note 1).
2. Pack the affinity support into the empty column.
3. Equilibrate with five column volumes (~10 mL) of Binding Buffer.

4. Load the RNA sample onto the affinity column (see Note 4).
5. Incubate at room temperature for 1 h.
6. Wash with five column volumes of Binding Buffer.
7. Elute the RNA sample with Elution Buffer and collect as a single fraction.
8. Measure the RNA concentration by the absorbance at 260 nm.
9. Re-equilibrate the column with Binding Buffer for the second affinity column in Subheading 3.4 (see Note 5).

3.3. DNAzyme Reaction

1. Combine the RNA with the DNAzyme in 0.1× DNAzyme reaction buffer. The ratio of DNAzyme to substrate RNA is 1:10 (see Note 6).
2. Incubate for 3 min in a 95°C water bath to denature the RNA and DNA.
3. Place on ice for 3 min.
4. Incubate for 10 min at 25°C.
5. Add an equal volume of 2× DNAzyme reaction buffer.
6. Add sufficient 1 M $MgCl_2$ to achieve a final concentration of 60 mM to start the DNAzyme reaction.
7. Incubate for 2 h at 37°C.
8. Add sufficient 0.5 M EDTA to achieve a concentration of ~100 mM EDTA to stop the DNAzyme reaction.

3.4. Second Affinity Column

1. Dialyze the RNA sample against binding buffer (see Note 7).
2. Load the RNA sample onto the affinity column that was regenerated at the end of Subheading 3.2 (see Notes 4 and 8).
3. Collect the flow-through containing the target RNA and DNAzyme.
4. Add RNase-free DNase I (~100 unit/100 μg DNA) to eliminate the DNAzyme DNA.
5. Incubate for 1 h at 37°C.
6. Add sufficient 0.5 M EDTA to achieve a final concentration of ~10 mM to stop the DNase I reaction (see Note 7).
7. Concentrate the sample using spin concentrator to a volume of less than 5 mL.
8. Apply to the Superdex-75 column on an FPLC system (see Note 9) and collect the target RNA fraction.
9. Analyze the purified RNA using 15% denaturing PAGE. Stain the gel in 0.1% toluidine blue for ~15 min and destain using water (see Note 10).

4. Notes

1. DNA-affinity chromatography has been used to purify DNA-binding proteins and the procedures for coupling oligonucleotides to silica or sepharose have been described (10). The Oligo Affinity Support used here functions as a normal solid-phase support during DNA synthesis except that the final oligo is not removed from the support when the bases are deprotected. The oligonucleotide synthesis can be ordered through a commercial synthesis service or can be made "in-house" on a standard automated DNA synthesizer using the standard cycles. The DNA oligonucleotide on the Oligo Affinity Support is deprotected as normal with ammonium hydroxide solution. This deprotected DNA-bound support is the affinity column to be used for RNA purification. The affinity column synthesized using 1 g of Oligo Affinity Support contains ~40 μmole equivalents of the oligo, which is sufficient for purifying 1 μmole of RNA transcripts.

2. The Binding Buffer should have a high ionic strength to hybridize the DNA-affinity column and the RNA-affinity tag. A low-ionic-strength Elution Buffer dissociates the RNA-affinity tag from the DNA-affinity column.

3. DNAzymes (or deoxyribozymes) are DNA molecules with a catalytic function. In vitro selection was used to develop the 10:23 and 8:17 DNAzymes (11). The RNA substrate is bound through Watson–Crick base-pairing and is cleaved next to an unpaired purine residue. Ca^{2+} ions produce higher reaction rates than Mg^{2+} ions in the case of 8:17 DNAzymes (12). The affinity tag added to the 3′-end of the target RNA is cleaved using the DNAzyme, which is more convenient and cost-effective than a ribozyme. The optimum arm lengths of the DNAzyme depend on the sequences and RNA secondary structures. The cleavage reaction is very efficient. However, there is one requirement for a specific sequence upstream of the reaction site; there must be a purine at the 3′-end (see Fig. 2).

4. Slowly load the RNA sample onto the column, or circulate it through the column to maximize the binding.

5. The affinity column is reusable. Wash the column with RNase-free water, and re-equilibrate it with Binding Buffer. For storage, wash the column with RNase-free water, and air-dry.

6. The ratio of the DNAzyme to the substrate RNA can be optimized depending on the activity and/or turnover rate of the DNAzyme.

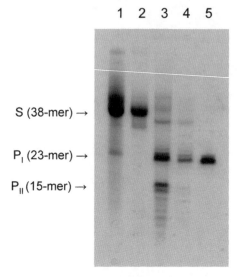

Fig. 3. Results of RNA purification with an affinity column and DNAzymes. A 15% polyacrylamide urea denaturing gel stained with toluidine blue is shown: *Lane 1*, crude RNA transcription mixture; *lane 2*, RNA purified using the affinity column; *lane 3*, the DNAzyme reaction products; *lane 4*, DNAzyme and the product purified using the affinity column; *lane 5*, RNA purified using size-exclusion chromatography.

7. Before the DNase I reaction, remove the remaining EDTA. After the DNase I reaction, add sufficient EDTA to achieve a concentration of ~10 mM to protect the RNA from degradation.
8. The cleaved affinity tag is removed using the second affinity column. The target RNA is released into the flow-through with the DNAzyme DNA, whereas the affinity tag binds to the column.
9. The DNAzyme is removed by DNase I followed by size exclusion chromatography. The gel filtration buffer should have at least 100 mM NaCl to reduce nonspecific interactions with the column. The target RNA elutes first as the main peak followed by the DNAzyme fragments.
10. The toluidine blue staining of RNA can detect about 50 ng of material. Toluidine blue is carcinogenic and great care must be taken in handling the solution. We have prepared 23-nt RNA using the protocol described here. After the final size-exclusion chromatography step, the product was very pure (>99%; Fig. 3).

References

1. Milligan JF, Groebe DR, Witherell GW, Uhlenbeck OC (1987) Oligoribonucleotide synthesis using T7 RNA polymerase and synthetic DNA templates. Nucleic Acids Res 15:8783–8798
2. Wyatt JR, Chastain M, Puglisi JD (1991) Synthesis and purification of large amounts of RNA oligonucleotides. Biotechniques 11:764–769
3. Lukavsky PJ, Puglisi JD (2004) Large-scale preparation and purification of polyacrylamide-free RNA oligonucleotides. RNA 10:889–893
4. Kao C, Zheng M, Rüdisser S (1999) A simple and efficient method to reduce nontemplated nucleotide addition at the 3 terminus of RNAs transcribed by T7 RNA polymerase. RNA 5:1268–1272
5. Shields TP, Mollova E, Ste Marie L, Hansen MR, Pardi A (1999) High-performance liquid chromatography purification of homogenous-length RNA produced by trans cleavage with a hammerhead ribozyme. RNA 5:1259–1267
6. Schürer H, Lang K, Schuster J, Mörl M (2002) A universal method to produce in vitro transcripts with homogeneous 3′ ends. Nucleic Acids Res 30:e56
7. Kim I, McKenna SA, Viani Puglisi E, Puglisi JD (2007) Rapid purification of RNAs using fast performance liquid chromatography (FPLC). RNA 13:289–294
8. Kieft JS, Batey RT (2004) A general method for rapid and nondenaturing purification of RNAs. RNA 10:988–995
9. Cheong HK, Hwang E, Lee C, Choi BS, Cheong C (2004) Rapid preparation of RNA samples for NMR spectroscopy and X-ray crystallography. Nucleic Acids Res 32:e84
10. Chockalingam PS, Jurado LA, Jarrett HW (2001) DNA affinity chromatography. Mol Biotechnol 19:189–199
11. Santoro SW, Joyce GF (1997) A general purpose RNA-cleaving DNA enzyme. Proc Natl Acad Sci U S A 94:4262–4266
12. Peracchi A (2000) Preferential activation of the 8–17 deoxyribozyme by Ca(2+) ions. J Biol Chem 275:11693–11697

Chapter 10

Preparation of λN-GST Fusion Protein for Affinity Immobilization of RNA

Geneviève Di Tomasso, Philipe Lampron, James G. Omichinski, and Pascale Legault

Abstract

Affinity purification of in vitro transcribed RNA is becoming an attractive alternative to purification using standard denaturing gel electrophoresis. Affinity purification is particularly advantageous because it can be performed in a few hours under non-denaturing conditions. However, the performance of affinity purification methods can vary tremendously depending on the RNA immobilization matrix. It was previously shown that RNA immobilization via an optimized λN-GST fusion protein bound to glutathione-Sepharose resin allows affinity purification of RNA with very high purity and yield. This Chapter outlines the experimental procedure employed to prepare the λN-GST fusion protein used for RNA immobilization in successful affinity purifications of RNA. It describes the details of protein expression and purification as well as routine quality control analyses.

Key words: RNA immobilization, Affinity purification of RNA, λN peptide, GSH-Sepharose, GST-fusion protein, λN-GST fusion protein

1. Introduction

Affinity chromatography has revolutionized the purification of recombinant proteins and still makes a vital contribution to proteomic research. For affinity purification of in vitro transcribed RNA to achieve a similar success, reliable RNA affinity matrices need to be identified. RNA immobilization can be achieved in several ways: (a) using an RNA-sequence tag captured by a complementary immobilized oligonucleotide (1–3); (b) using an RNA-aptamer tag captured by a ligand coupled to a solid support (4–8); and (c) using an RNA-motif tag captured via its immobilized RNA-binding protein (7, 9–16). In a previous study, we developed one such RNA-affinity matrix by exploiting the high-affinity interaction between the *boxB* RNA and the N peptide from bacteriophage λ (16).

For this affinity purification procedure, the RNA of interest is first transcribed in vitro with a 3′-ARiBo tag, which incorporates two functional elements: an activatable ribozyme, the *glmS* ribozyme, and the λ*boxB* RNA. The transcribed RNA is then bound to a λN-GST fusion protein and captured on glutathione-Sepharose (GSH-Sepharose) resin. Following several washes, the RNA is eluted by incubation with glucosamine-6-phosphate (GlcN6P), which activates self-cleavage of the *glmS* ribozyme. Several λN-GST fusion proteins were tested for affinity purification; however exceptionally high RNA purity (>99%) and yield were obtained using λN$^+$-L$^+$-GST, a fusion protein in which a G1N2K4 mutant of the λN$_{1-22}$ peptide (λN$^+$) that binds the λ*boxB* RNA with picomolar affinity (17) is attached to the N terminus of GST via a (GlyAla)$_{10}$ linker (L$^+$; Fig. 1a; (16)).

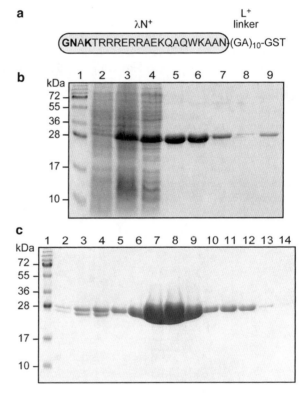

Fig. 1. Expression and purification of the λN$^+$-L$^+$-GST fusion protein. (a) Description of λN$^+$-L$^+$-GST, a fusion protein containing the G1N2K4 mutant of the bacteriophage λ N$_{1-22}$ peptide (λN$^+$) (17) and a (Gly-Ala)$_{10}$ linker (L$^+$) at the N terminus of GST (16). (b, c) Coomassie-stained SDS polyacrylamide gels of fractions collected at various stages of purification. In (b) lane 1: Molecular weight marker; lanes 2 and 3: preinduction (lane 2) and post-induction (lane 3) whole cell extract; lane 4: soluble *E. coli* lysate following ultracentrifugation; lanes 5–7: glutathione elutions 1–3 from the GSH-Sepharose; lanes 8 and 9: proteins still present in the supernatant (lane 8) and the resin (lane 9) following elution with glutathione. In (c) lane 1: Molecular weight marker; lanes 2–14: fractions 41–53 from the SP-Sepharose column. Fractions 44–51 (lanes 5–12), inclusively, were selected for dialysis and storage.

In this Chapter, we describe the detailed protocol for expression and purification of the λN⁺-L⁺-GST fusion protein. The λN⁺-L⁺-GST fusion protein is first overexpressed in *Escherichia coli* (*E. coli*) from a pET-42a vector. The bacteria are subsequently lysed, and the bacterial lysate cleared by ultracentrifugation. To achieve a high level of purity, a two-step purification procedure is performed that incorporates affinity batch purification on GSH-Sepharose resin and ion-exchange chromatography on an SP-Sepharose column. To remove nucleic acid contaminants that co-purify with the λN⁺-L⁺-GST fusion protein, a wash step with 2 M urea is included in the batch purification on GSH-Sepharose resin. Several quality controls are performed prior to using the protein for RNA affinity purification, including evaluations of protein purity and stability, a mass spectrometry analysis, and an RNase contamination assay. Using this protocol, approximately 200–300 mg of purified λN⁺-L⁺-GST can be obtained from 8 L of bacterial cell culture. Subsequently, this fusion protein can be used either for affinity purification of RNA or other applications that require RNA immobilization.

2. Materials

Prepare all solutions using ultrapure water, which is obtained by purifying deionized water to attain a sensitivity of at least 18 MΩ cm at 21°C. Sterilize all solutions either by autoclaving or filtering (0.22 μm filter). Store all reagents at room temperature, unless indicated otherwise, and follow proper disposal regulations when disposing waste materials.

2.1. Expression of the λN⁺-L⁺-GST Fusion Protein

1. BL21(DE3) *E. coli* cells transfected with the pET42a-λN⁺-L⁺-GST plasmid ((16); see Note 1). Store at −80°C.
2. LB Kan-50 medium: Luria–Bertani (LB) broth supplemented with 50 μg/mL kanamycin just before use.
3. Isopropyl β-D-1-thiogalactopyranoside (IPTG) solution. For 5-mL cultures, prepare fresh by dissolving 2 mg IPTG in 200 μL water (10 mg/mL). For the 8-L culture, prepare fresh by dissolving 2 g IPTG in 24 mL water.
4. Bacterial shaking incubator with a 15-mL tube rack and 4-L flask clamps.
5. Preparative centrifuge with rotor suitable for 500-mL bottles, e.g., Sorvall RC 6 Plus with Sorvall SLA-3000 rotor.
6. 500-mL Centrifuge bottles.

2.2. Protein Purification

All solutions for protein purification are stored at 4°C.

1. Homogenization buffer: 20 mM Tris-HCl pH 7.4, 0.2 mM EDTA pH 8.0, 1 M NaCl, and 1 mM DTT. Add 1 mM DTT just before use. For cell lysis, add 150 mg protease inhibitor cocktail (Sigma-Aldrich) to 80 mL of Homogenization buffer by first dissolving in 500 μL of DMSO.
2. Mechanical homogenizer, e.g., Ultra Turrax T25 Basic cell disrupter (IKA).
3. French Press with pressure cell.
4. Sonicator (e.g., Branson sonifier 450) with standard disruptor horn and cold metal beaker.
5. Ultracentrifuge with rotor for 30-mL ultracentrifuge tubes (e.g., Sorvall Discovery 100SE with T-1250 rotor).
6. 30-mL Ultracentrifuge tubes.
7. GSH-Sepharose 4B resin (GE Healthcare).
8. Tube rotator.
9. Centrifuge with swinging bucket rotor for 50-mL screw-cap conical tubes, e.g., IEC Centra CL2 with 215 economy swinging bucket rotor (Thermo Scientific).
10. Sintered glass Büchner funnel with 40–60 microns pore size.
11. Homogenization buffer with 2 M Urea: Add 12 g of urea directly to 100 mL of Homogenization buffer.
12. Phosphate-buffered saline (PBS): 10 mM Na_2HPO_4, 2 mM KH_2PO_4, 2.7 mM KCl, 140 mM NaCl and pH 7.4.
13. For PBS with 20 mM reduced L-glutathione: Just before use, add 0.61 g of reduced L-glutathione to 100 mL of PBS and adjust pH to 8.0 with NaOH (see Note 2).
14. A 0.22 μm filter unit, e.g., Steriflip (Millipore).
15. Dialysis tubing of 29 mm diameter and 12–14 kDa MWCO with closures.
16. Magnetic stir bar and plate.
17. FPLC-A buffer: 20 mM phosphate pH 7.4, 1 mM EDTA, and 1 mM fresh DTT.
18. FPLC-B buffer: FPLC-A buffer with 2 M NaCl.
19. SP-Sepharose column: Fill an empty column (~20 cm long and ~26 mm inner diameter) with 75 mL of SP-Sepharose High Performance resin (GE Healthcare). Store at 4°C.
20. FPLC system with a superloop, if available.
21. Storage buffer: 50 mM HEPES pH 8.0, 100 mM NaCl, 2 mM fresh DTT, and 20% glycerol.
22. UV/Vis spectrophotometer with a quartz cuvette.

2.3. Monitoring the Protein Induction and Purification by SDS Polyacrylamide Gels

1. Laemmli sample buffer (2×): Mix 1.2 mL 0.5 M Tris-HCl pH 6.8, 1.9 mL glycerol, 1 mL SDS 20%, 0.5 mL β-mercaptoethanol, and a pinch of bromophenol blue. Complete to 15 mL final volume with water. Store at −20°C.
2. Tabletop microcentrifuge with rotor.
3. Electrophoresis system for SDS-PAGE, e.g., Mini-PROTEAN 3 Cell (Bio-Rad).
4. 15% Sodium dodecyl sulfate (SDS) polyacrylamide gels for electrophoresis. The gels could be purchased (e.g., Bio-Rad Ready Gel Tris–HCl gels) or prepared according to Bio-Rad's protocol.
5. Tris–glycine running buffer: 0.024 M Tris-Base, 0.192 M glycine, and 0.1% SDS. Prepare first a 10× buffer solution without the SDS. Dilute 100 mL of 10× buffer into 890 mL of water and then add 10 mL of 10% SDS.
6. Molecular weight marker stored at −20°C.
7. Low voltage power supply, e.g., Thermo EC105.
8. Coomassie staining solution: 45% methanol, 10% acetic acid, and 0.25% Brilliant Blue G-250 in water.
9. Destaining solution: 10% methanol and 10% acetic acid in water.

2.4. Quality Control

1. Temperature-controlled water bath.
2. RNA sample (~150 pmol) stored at −20°C. Here, the terminal loop of the precursor let-7g miRNA (TL-let-7g RNA) was used ((18); see Note 3).
3. Equilibration buffer: 50 mM HEPES pH 7.5. Prepare as a 10× solution.
4. Proteinase K, 50 U/mL, stored at 4°C.
5. Gel loading buffer: Mix 0.02 g of bromophenol blue, 5 mL of 0.5 M EDTA pH 8.0, and 95 mL of formamide (see Note 4).
6. TBE buffer: 50 mM Tris-Base, 50 mM boric acid, and 1 mM EDTA. Prepare as a 10× solution.
7. 20% Gel solution: 20% acrylamide:bisacrylamide (19:1), 7 M urea, and TBE buffer. Store at 4°C. Unpolymerized acrylamide and bisacrylamide are strong neurotoxins. Protective equipment (gloves, mask, laboratory coat) should be worn and care should be taken when handling acrylamide powder and solutions.
8. 20% Analytical denaturing polyacrylamide gel: Mix 40 mL of gel solution with 200 μL ammonium persulfate 10% (w/v) and 40 μL TEMED. Immediately pour in a glass plate assembly using 20×20 cm glass plates and 0.7 mm thick comb and spacers.
9. High-voltage power supply, e.g., Thermo EC600-90.

10. SYBR Gold staining solution: Make a fresh 1:10,000 dilution of SYBR Gold nucleic acid gel stain in TBE buffer.
11. Molecular Imager and analysis software. Here, we use a Molecular Imager FX densitometer and ImageLab software version 3.0 (Bio-Rad).

3. Methods

All procedures are carried out at room temperature unless specified otherwise.

3.1. Expression of the λN⁺-L⁺-GST Fusion Protein

3.1.1. Small-Scale Induction Test (See Note 5)

1. At the end of the day, inoculate 5 mL of LB Kan-50 medium with 25 µL of a glycerol stock of the pET42a-λN⁺-L⁺-GST plasmid cloned into BL21 (DE3) ((16); see Note 1). Let it grow overnight at 37°C with shaking (see Note 6).
2. In the morning, dilute the culture by mixing 1 mL of culture with 3 mL LB Kan-50 medium.
3. Collect a 200-µL preinduction aliquot of the culture.
4. Induce protein expression by adding 100 µL of IPTG (10 mg/mL).
5. Incubate for 4 h at 30°C with shaking.
6. Collect a post-induction 200-µL aliquot of the culture.
7. Verify for efficient induction on a 15% SDS polyacrylamide gel (see Subheading 3.3 and Note 7).

3.1.2. Large-Scale Expression

1. In the morning, inoculate 5 mL of LB Kan-50 medium with 25 µL of a glycerol stock of the pET42a-λN⁺-L⁺-GST plasmid cloned into BL21 (DE3) ((16); see Note 1). Grow for 6–8 h at 37°C with shaking (see Note 6).
2. Use 1 mL of the small culture to inoculate 1 L of LB Kan-50 medium in a 4-L flask. Repeat to prepare a total of 2 L of culture. Grow overnight at 37°C with shaking (see Note 6).
3. Dilute the cultures in the morning by mixing each 1-L culture with 3 L of LB Kan-50 medium and distributing equally in three 4-L flasks (1,333 mL of culture per flask). Grow for 15 min at 30°C with shaking.
4. Collect a 500-µL preinduction aliquot of the culture.
5. Induce protein expression by adding to each flask 4 mL of IPTG (2 g/24 mL) and grow for 4 h at 30°C with shaking.
6. Collect a post-induction 500-µL aliquot of the culture.

7. Pellet the cells in six 500-mL bottles by centrifugation at 6,000 × g for 10 min and discard the supernatant. Store pellets at −80°C until purification.

8. Verify for efficient induction on a 15% SDS polyacrylamide gel (see Subheading 3.3, Fig. 1b, and Note 7).

3.2. Protein Purification

For protein purification, best results are generally obtained by keeping the overall purification time as short as possible. Even though the purification can be completed in 2.5 days, we suggest starting the purification at the beginning of the week in case additional time is needed. In the following steps, all solutions are stored at 4°C and protein-containing samples are kept on ice (see Note 8). If possible, the FPLC purification is conducted in the cold room. Starting at step 10, it is important to employ RNase-free methods.

1. Prepare 80 mL of Homogenization buffer with 150 mg of protease inhibitor cocktail.

2. Resuspend the bacterial culture pellets from an 8-L preparation (6 pellets) into the 80 mL of Homogenization buffer.

3. Process the resuspended cells with a mechanical homogenizer until all clumps are disrupted.

4. Lyse cells using a French press and a sonicator as follows. First wash the pressure cell by passing a solution of 50:50 water:ethanol through the French Press followed with two passes of water. After the washing steps, pass the cell slurry through the French Press at 800–1,000 psi and collect lysate on ice. Sonicate for 10 s. Pass the cell slurry through the French Press a second time. The cell lysate should become clear and take on a darker color.

5. Transfer the cell lysate to the ultracentrifuge tubes and centrifuge for 60 min at 138,000 × g and 4°C to pellet unbroken cells and insoluble material. When the spin is completed, take a 30-µL aliquot of the supernatant.

6. During the centrifugation, prepare the GSH-Sepharose resin as follows. Resuspend the GSH-Sepharose resin in the supplier bottle by vigorous mixing. Transfer 12.5 mL of GSH-Sepharose slurry to a 50-mL screw-cap conical tube and add 37.5 mL of water. Centrifuge for 3 min at 1,150 × g in a swinging bucket and decant supernatant (see Note 9). Then, wash the resin twice as follows: resuspend in Homogenization buffer, centrifuge for 3 min at 1,150 × g, and decant supernatant (see Note 10).

7. Add supernatant from the high-speed spin of cell lysate to the washed GSH-Sepharose resin, and transfer all supernatant and resin to a 250-mL plastic bottle. Rinse the 50-mL conical tube containing the resin with a small amount (~5 mL) of Homogenization buffer and transfer to 250-mL bottle to recover all the resin.

8. Incubate for 1 h on the rotator at 4°C.
9. After incubation, transfer the GSH-Sepharose resin with cell lysate back to a 50-mL screw-cap conical tube, 50 mL at a time. After each addition, centrifuge the resin for 3 min at $1,150 \times g$ and decant supernatant (see Note 9). Repeat until all the resin and lysate are removed from the 250-mL tube. Save all decanted supernatants (see Note 8).
10. Wash the resin twice with Homogenization buffer supplemented with 2 M Urea and twice with PBS by resuspension, centrifugation for 3 min at $1,150 \times g$, and decantation of the supernatant (see Notes 10 and 11).
11. Elute the λN^+-L^+-GST fusion protein as follows. Resuspend in PBS with 20 mM reduced glutathione pH 8.0 (see Note 2). Incubate on the rotator for 15 min at room temperature. Centrifuge the resin for 3 min at $1,150 \times g$ and decant supernatant. Take a 30-µL aliquot of the first elution supernatant. Repeat twice the elution by resuspension in PBS with 20 mM glutathione, centrifugation, and decantation (see Note 10). Take 30-µL aliquots of the second and third elution supernatants. Pool the elution supernatants (~100 mL) and filter through a 0.22-µm filter.
12. Resuspend the resin in PBS and take a 30-µL aliquot. Centrifuge for 3 min at $1,150 \times g$ and take a 30-µL aliquot of the supernatant.
13. Transfer the pooled elution supernatant to the dialysis tubing (MWCO of 12–14 kDa) and dialyze against 4 L of FPLC-A buffer overnight at 4°C with slow stirring.
14. Monitor the affinity batch purification on GSH-Sepharose resin using a 15% SDS polyacrylamide gel (see Subheading 3.3 and Fig. 1b).
15. The following day, carefully remove the sample from the dialysis tubing with a 10-mL serological pipette and transfer to a 250-mL flask.
16. Prepare the SP-Sepharose column by washing for 25 min with 100% FPLC-A buffer at 3 mL/min.
17. Load sample on the column through an FPLC pump or using a superloop at 3 mL/min.
18. Elute by first washing the column with 125 mL of FPLC-A buffer and then using a gradient of 0–100% FPLC-B buffer over 525 mL at 3 mL/min with UV detection at 280 nm. Collect 9-mL fractions (see Note 12).
19. Run a 15% SDS polyacrylamide gel to select the fractions containing the purified protein (see Subheading 3.3 and Fig. 1c).
20. Pool selected fractions (usually ~8 fractions), transfer to dialysis tubing (MWCO of 12–14 kDa), and dialyze against 2 L of Storage buffer overnight at 4°C with slow stirring.

21. The following day, carefully transfer the dialyzed sample with a 10-mL serological pipette to a 50-mL screw-cap conical tube. Determine the sample volume.
22. Determine the protein concentration by UV spectroscopy at 280 nm using an extinction coefficient of 48,610 cm^{-1} M^{-1} (19). Yields of 200–300 mg purified protein at a concentration of 5–7 mg/mL are typically obtained.
23. Distribute in 1–10 mL aliquots and store at −20°C.

3.3. Monitoring the Protein Induction and Purification by SDS Polyacrylamide Gels

1. Prepare samples to be loaded on the gel. For cell culture aliquots, pellet the aliquots by centrifugation at 16,000×g for 1 min, discard the supernatant, resuspend pellet with 50 μL of water, and then add 50 μL of 2× Laemmli sample buffer. For protein aliquots, add 30 μL of 2× Laemmli sample buffer directly to the 30 μL aliquots. Heat samples at 95°C for 3 min and spin down prior to loading (see Note 13).
2. Load samples to be analyzed on an analytical 15% SDS polyacrylamide gel. To verify the induction of the small-scale induction test, load 15-μL of the preinduction and post-induction samples (see Subheading 3.1.1). Load 7-μL samples to verify the induction of the large-scale culture (see Subheading 3.1.2), monitor the affinity batch purification on GSH-Sepharose (see Subheading 3.2), and examine fractions of the SP-Sepharose column purification (see Subheading 3.2). For all applications, load at least one lane with a molecular weight marker. Run the gel at 150 V for 1.25 h.
3. Stain the gel with Coomassie staining solution for 10 min. Destain the gel with Destaining solution for 30 min to overnight.

3.4. Quality Control

Four simple tests are performed to verify that the λN$^+$-L$^+$-GST fusion protein is of sufficient quality for affinity purification of RNA.

1. To evaluate the final protein purity, analyze 0.25, 0.5, 1.0, 2.0, 5.0, and 10 μg of purified protein on a 15% SDS polyacrylamide gel (see Subheading 3.3 and Fig. 2a). High purity (≥97.5%) is assessed by comparing the intensity of possible contaminants in the 10 μg lane with that of the 30-kDa band in the lanes containing small amounts of purified proteins.
2. To evaluate protein stability, incubate 5.0 μg of protein in Storage buffer at 37°C for 0, 1, 2, and 4 h, and assess the protein stability on the same 15% SDS polyacrylamide gel used to evaluate protein purity (see Fig. 2a). High stability (no visible degradation ≥5%) is determined by comparing the intensity of bands from degradation products, if detectable, with the intensity of the 30-kDa band in the lanes containing small amounts of purified proteins.

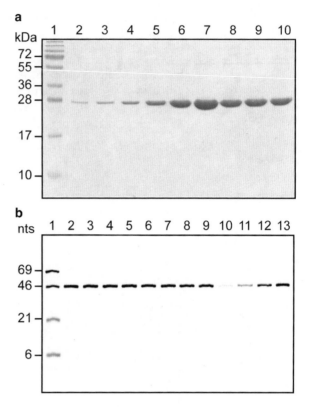

Fig. 2. Quality controls of the purified λN+-L+-GST fusion protein. (**a**) Purity and stability of the purified protein. Lane 1: Molecular weight marker; lanes 2–7: 0.25, 0.5, 1.0, 2.0, 5.0, and 10 μg of purified λN+-L+-GST; lanes 8–10: 5 μg of purified λN+-L+-GST following incubations for 1, 2, and 4 h at 37°C. (**b**) RNase contamination assay. Lane 1: Molecular weight marker with RNA size given in terms of the number of nucleotides (nts); lanes 2–5: 50 ng of TL-let-7g RNA following incubations for 0, 1, 2, and 4 h at 37°C; lanes 6–9: 50 ng of TL-let-7g RNA following incubations for 0, 1, 2, and 4 h at 37°C in the presence of purified λN+-L+-GST; lanes 10–13: 2.5, 10, 25, and 50 ng of gel-purified TL-let-7g RNA.

3. To ensure that the purified protein has the expected molecular weight (29,647 Da), send 200 μL of a 1 mg/mL sample (diluted in water) to a Mass Spectrometry facility for LC-MS analysis.

4. To ensure that the protein sample is RNase free:

    (a) Incubate 70 pmol of an RNA (here TL-let-7g (18); see Note 3) with 350 pmol of the purified protein (10.4 μg λN+-L+-GST) in 1× Equilibration buffer (8 μL final volume) for 0, 1, 2, and 4 h at 37°C. Perform the same incubations replacing the purified protein by an equivalent volume of Storage buffer.

    (b) Once the incubations are completed, add 0.05 U proteinase K to the protein-containing samples and leave at 37°C for an additional 15 min.

(c) Prepare samples to be analyzed by gel electrophoresis. First, dilute the RNase test samples 20-fold with water and mix the volumes of diluted samples corresponding to 50 ng RNA (7.55 μL for TL-let-7g RNA) with 10 μL of gel loading buffer. Also prepare control samples containing various amounts of purified RNA (2.5, 10, 25, and 50 ng RNA in sample volume ≤8 μL) and add 10 μL of gel loading buffer.

(d) Load samples to be analyzed on a 20% analytical denaturing polyacrylamide gel pre-run in TBE buffer at 600 V for 30 min. Run the gel in TBE buffer at 600 V for about 2 h, until the bromophenol blue is 2–4 cm from the bottom of the gel (see Note 4).

(e) Stain the gel with SYBR Gold staining solution for 10 min, scan on a Molecular Imager, and quantify band intensities. No visible RNA degradation (≤5%) is assessed by comparing the intensity of possible contaminants with the intensity of the RNA band of the control samples (see Fig. 2b).

4. Notes

1. The pET vectors use a T7 phage promoter for transcription of the cloned gene. For protein production, the recombinant plasmid must be used to transform a host *E. coli* strain that contains a chromosomal copy of the IPTG-inducible gene for T7 RNA polymerase, such as BL21(DE3) or BL21-Gold(DE3).

2. It is crucial to adjust the pH of the L-glutathione solution to 8.0 in order to maximize the elution efficiency. Otherwise, addition of L-glutathione at high concentration lowers the pH of the buffer.

3. For the RNase contamination assay, we used ~1 μg of TL-let-7g, a 46-nucleotide RNA derived from the terminal loop of the let-7g precursor miRNA (5′-GCA GAU UGA GGG UCU AUG AUA CCA CCC GGU ACA GGA GAU AUC UGC A-3′). It is important to select either the RNA to be purified by affinity and/or an RNA, like TL-let-7g, which contains single-stranded regions (internal loops and bulges) that are susceptible to RNase cleavage (18).

4. Here, the bromophenol blue dye is used to follow the RNA migration on the gel. RNA molecular weight markers can also be prepared using RNAs available in the laboratory (see Fig. 2b).

5. If the pET42a-λN⁺-L⁺-GST plasmid is a new clone in the laboratory, it is strongly recommended to send the plasmid for

sequencing and perform the small-scale induction test to insure that overexpression of the correct fusion protein is achieved with this clone. There is no need to perform this small-scale induction test on a routine basis.

6. Vigorous shaking is necessary for bacterial cell cultures; we routinely use 240 rpm for small cultures and 200–220 rpm for cultures in 4-L flasks. Slightly less vigorous shaking is used for 4-L flasks to prevent flasks from breaking.

7. Efficient induction of the λN$^+$-L$^+$-GST fusion protein is apparent from the increased intensity of the 30-kDa band in the post-induction aliquot lane (see Fig. 1b, lane 3).

8. It is a good idea to save all fractions considered to be "waste" (ultracentrifugation pellet, GSH-Sepharose resin, column flow throughs, etc.) at 4°C until the purification is successfully completed. This is just in case a purification step is not properly carried out (e.g., one forgets to adjust the pH of the glutathione solution). The protein could be recovered from the saved fraction and the purification continued from this step.

9. When washing large amounts of resin, the supernatant can be filtered using a sintered glass Büchner funnel to recover resin lost when decanting the supernatants.

10. All resin washes and elutions are done using a total volume of 50 mL (buffer and resin), except for the third elution where the total volume is 25 mL.

11. The urea is used to remove any bound nucleic acid. Do not use a concentration higher than 3.5 M as this is known to denature the GST protein (20).

12. After protein purification, wash the SP-Sepharose column for an additional 20 min with FPLC-B buffer. For long-term storage, wash the column for 20 min with a 20:80 ethanol:water solution.

13. Protein samples can be stored at –20°C in Laemmli sample buffer if needed. They should be heated just prior to loading on the gel.

Acknowledgments

We thank A. Desjardins and P. Dagenais for critical reading of the manuscript. This work was supported by the Canadian Institutes for Health Research (CIHR) to P. Legault (MOP-86502). P. Legault holds a Canada Research Chair in Structural Biology and Engineering of RNA.

References

1. Aviv H, Leder P. Purification of biologically active globin messenger RNA by chromatography on oligothymidylic acid-cellulose. Proc Natl Acad Sci USA. 1972;69:1408–12.
2. Cheong HK, Hwang E, Lee C, Choi BS, Cheong C. Rapid preparation of RNA samples for NMR spectroscopy and X-ray crystallography. Nucleic Acids Res. 2004;32:e84.
3. Pereira MJ, Behera V, Walter NG. Nondenaturing purification of co-transcriptionally folded RNA avoids common folding heterogeneity. PLoS One. 2010;5:e12953.
4. Bachler M, Schroeder R, von Ahsen U. StreptoTag: a novel method for the isolation of RNA-binding proteins. RNA. 1999;5:1509–16.
5. Srisawat C, Engelke DR. Streptavidin aptamers: affinity tags for the study of RNAs and ribonucleoproteins. RNA. 2001;7:632–41.
6. Hartmuth K, Urlaub H, Vornlocher HP, Will CL, Gentzel M, Wilm M, Luhrmann R. Protein composition of human prespliceosomes isolated by a tobramycin affinity-selection method. Proc Natl Acad Sci USA. 2002;99: 16719–24.
7. Hogg JR, Collins K. RNA-based affinity purification reveals 7SK RNPs with distinct composition and regulation. RNA. 2007;13:868–80.
8. Boese BJ, Corbino K, Breaker RR. In vitro selection and characterization of cellulose-binding RNA aptamers using isothermal amplification. Nucleosides Nucleotides Nucleic Acids. 2008;27:949–66.
9. Bardwell VJ, Wickens M. Purification of RNA and RNA-protein complexes by an R17 coat protein affinity method. Nucleic Acids Res. 1990;18:6587–94.
10. Srisawat C, Goldstein IJ, Engelke DR. Sephadex-binding RNA ligands: rapid affinity purification of RNA from complex RNA mixtures. Nucleic Acids Res. 2001;29:E4.
11. Kieft JS, Batey RT. A general method for rapid and nondenaturing purification of RNAs. RNA. 2004;10:988–95.
12. Czaplinski K, Kocher T, Schelder M, Segref A, Wilm M, Mattaj IW. Identification of 40LoVe, a Xenopus hnRNP D family protein involved in localizing a TGF-beta-related mRNA during oogenesis. Dev Cell. 2005;8:505–15.
13. Batey RT, Kieft JS. Improved native affinity purification of RNA. RNA. 2007;13:1384–9.
14. Bessonov S, Anokhina M, Will CL, Urlaub H, Luhrmann R. Isolation of an active step I spliceosome and composition of its RNP core. Nature. 2008;452:846–50.
15. Said N, Rieder R, Hurwitz R, Deckert J, Urlaub H, Vogel J. In vivo expression and purification of aptamer-tagged small RNA regulators. Nucleic Acids Res. 2009;37:e133.
16. Di Tomasso G, Lampron P, Dagenais P, Omichinski JG, Legault P. The ARiBo tag: a reliable tool for affinity purification of RNAs under native conditions. Nucleic Acids Res. 2011;39:e18.
17. Austin RJ, Xia T, Ren J, Takahashi TT, Roberts RW. Designed arginine-rich RNA-binding peptides with picomolar affinity. J Am Chem Soc. 2002;124:10966–7.
18. Piskounova E, Viswanathan SR, Janas M, LaPierre RJ, Daley GQ, Sliz P, Gregory RI. Determinants of microRNA processing inhibition by the developmentally regulated RNA-binding protein Lin28. J Biol Chem. 2008;283:21310–4.
19. Gill SC, von Hippel PH. Calculation of protein extinction coefficients from amino acid sequence data. Anal Biochem. 1989;182:319–26.
20. Kaplan W, Husler P, Klump H, Erhardt J, Sluis-Cremer N, Dirr H. Conformational stability of pGEX-expressed Schistosoma japonicum glutathione S-transferase: a detoxification enzyme and fusion-protein affinity tag. Protein Sci. 1997;6:399–406.

Chapter 11

Affinity Purification of RNA Using an ARiBo Tag

Geneviève Di Tomasso, Pierre Dagenais, Alexandre Desjardins, Alexis Rompré-Brodeur, Vanessa Delfosse, and Pascale Legault

Abstract

The increased awareness of the importance of RNA in biology, illustrated by the recent attention given to RNA interference research and applications, has spurred structural and functional investigations of RNA. For these studies, the traditional purification method for in vitro transcribed RNA is denaturing polyacrylamide gel electrophoresis. However, gel-based procedures denature the RNA and can be very tedious and time-consuming. Thus, several alternative schemes have been developed for fast non-denaturing purification of RNA transcribed in vitro. In a recent report, a quick affinity purification procedure was developed for RNAs transcribed with a 3′-ARiBo tag and shown to provide RNA with exceptionally high purity and yield. The ARiBo tag contains the λboxB RNA and the *glmS* ribozyme, allowing immobilization on GSH-Sepharose resin via a λN-GST fusion protein and elution by activation of the *glmS* ribozyme with glucosamine-6-phosphate. This Chapter outlines the experimental details for affinity batch purification of RNAs using ARiBo tags. Although the procedure was originally developed for purification of a stable purine riboswitch mutant, it is demonstrated here for purification of the terminal loop of the let-7g precursor miRNA, an important target of the pluripotency factor Lin28.

Key words: Affinity purification of RNA, ARiBo-fusion RNA, ARiBo tag, *glmS* ribozyme, *boxB* RNA/N peptide interaction, Let-7g microRNA

1. Introduction

The discovery of the enzymatic activity of RNA in the 1980s challenged the central dogma of molecular biology, provided new insights into the evolution of life, and stimulated several lines of RNA research. More recent discoveries implicating small regulatory RNAs, such as RNA interference involving miRNAs and siRNAs (1, 2) and metabolite-sensing gene regulation by riboswitches (3), have once again profoundly changed our views of gene regulation and have led to an explosion of research investigations on the roles and biomedical applications of small regulatory RNAs.

In vitro structural and functional investigations of RNAs are greatly benefiting from established procedures for in vitro synthesis and purification of RNA molecules (4–6). However, standard purification using gel electrophoresis denatures the RNA and can be very tedious and time-consuming, particularly when large amounts of RNA are needed (7–9). Over the past few years, several alternative schemes have been developed that allow non-denaturing and time-efficient purification of RNA transcribed in vitro, including size-exclusion and ion-exchange chromatography (9–14) as well as affinity purification methods (13, 15–21). Affinity purification represents a highly efficient strategy for protein purification and is likely to have a similar impact on RNA purification because it is very rapid and can be easily adapted to any molecular weight RNA as well as high-throughput applications.

In a recent report, we developed a quick and reliable procedure for affinity batch purification of in vitro transcribed RNA that provides highly pure RNA with yields that are comparable to denaturing gel electrophoresis (21). This procedure involves the synthesis of the RNA of interest with a novel RNA affinity tag, the ARiBo tag, at its 3′-end. The ARiBo tag contains an **A**ctivatable **Ri**bozyme, the *glmS* ribozyme, modified to incorporate the λBo*x*B RNA in its variable P1 stem. After in vitro transcription, the ARiBo-fusion RNA is immobilized on glutathione-Sepharose (GSH-Sepharose) resin via a λN$^+$-L$^+$-GST fusion protein, which incorporates a mutant of the λN$_{1-22}$ peptide (λN$^+$) that binds the λ*boxB* RNA with picomolar affinity (22) and is attached to the N terminus of GST via a (GlyAla)$_{10}$ linker (L$^+$) (21, 23). After several resin washes are performed to remove impurities from the transcription reaction, the RNA of interest is eluted by activation of the self-cleaving *glmS* ribozyme with glucosamine-6-phosphate (GlcN6P).

In this Chapter, we describe the experimental details for affinity purification of RNA using an ARiBo tag, including the cloning and preparation of the plasmid template, in vitro transcription, *glmS* ribozyme cleavage optimization, small-scale (3.5 nmol) and large-scale (0.25 μmol) affinity batch purifications, and quantitative analysis of the purification from denaturing gels stained with SYBR Gold. Although the procedure was originally developed for purification of a stable purine riboswitch aptamer mutant (21), it has since been exploited in our laboratory for purification of several other RNAs, including derivatives of the let-7g precursor miRNA (24). To further demonstrate the general applicability of the method, the procedure is applied here for the purification of the terminal loop of the let-7g precursor miRNA (TL-let-7g; see Fig. 1a), an important target of the pluripotency factor Lin28 (25).

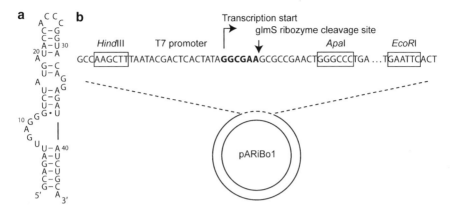

Fig. 1. Plasmid cloning for transcription of an ARiBo-fusion RNA. (a) The RNA of interest used here, the terminal loop of the let-7g precursor miRNA from *Mus musculus* (TL-let-7g). (b) The pARiBo1 plasmid used for cloning and transcription. The restriction sites (*Hind*III, *Apa*I, and *Eco*RI) are boxed and the T7 promoter is indicated.

2. Materials

Prepare all solutions using ultrapure water, which is obtained by purifying deionized water to attain a sensitivity of at least 18 MΩ cm at 21°C. Sterilize all solutions either by autoclaving or filtering (0.22 μm filter). Store all reagents at room temperature, unless indicated otherwise, and follow proper disposal regulations when disposing waste materials.

2.1. Preparation of Plasmid for Transcription of ARiBo-Fusion RNAs

1. The pARiBo1 plasmid (21) stored at 4°C.
2. Forward and reverse oligonucleotide primers for mutagenesis: 20 ng/μL stocks stored at 4°C. For purification of TL-let-7g, we used 5′-GCT TTA ATA CGA CTC ACT ATA GCA GAT TGA GGG TCT ATG ATA CCA CCC GGT ACA GGA GAT ATC TGC AGC GCC GAA CTG GGC C-3′ (TL-let-7g-fwd) and 5′-GGC CCA GTT CGG CGC TGC AGA TAT CTC CTG TAC CGG GTG GTA TCA TAG ACC CTC AAT CTG CTA TAG TGA GTC GTA TTA AAG C-3′ (TL-let-7g-rev).
3. Pfu high-fidelity DNA polymerase 2.5 U/μL supplied with 10× Pfu reaction buffer. Store at –20°C.
4. 10 mM dNTP mixture: Prepare by combining 1/10 dilution of 100 mM dATP, dTTP, dCTP, dGTP stocks in water. Store at –20°C.
5. Dimethyl sulfoxide (DMSO) for molecular biology ≥99.9%.
6. Thermal cycler.
7. *Dpn*I 20,000 U/mL restriction enzyme stored at –20°C.

8. Subcloning efficiency DH5α chemically competent *Escherichia coli* stored at −80°C.

9. LB-Amp plates and medium: Supplement Luria–Bertani (LB) plates and medium with 100 μg/mL ampicillin just prior to use.

10. Bacterial plate incubator.

11. Bacterial shaking incubator with a 15-mL tube rack, 500-mL flask clamps, and 4-L flask clamps.

12. 50% Glycerol.

13. DNA mini-prep kit.

14. Sequencing primer for pARiBo1: 5′-TCA CAC AGG AAA CAG CTA TGA CCA-3′. Prepare as a 5 pmol/μL stock and store at 4°C.

15. DNA plasmid purification kits, e.g., Qiafilter Plasmid Maxi Kit and/or Qiafilter Plasmid Giga Kit (Qiagen).

16. Preparative centrifuge with rotor suitable for 500-mL bottles, e.g., Sorvall RC 6 Plus with Sorvall SLA-3000 rotor.

17. 500-mL Centrifuge bottles.

18. *Eco*RI 100,000 U/mL restriction enzyme stored at −20°C.

19. *Eco*RI/HEPES buffer (10×): 0.5 M HEPES pH 7.5, 0.1 M $MgCl_2$, 1 M NaCl, 0.2% Triton X-100, and 1 mg/mL BSA (see Note 1). Store at −20°C.

2.2. In Vitro Transcription of ARiBo-Fusion RNAs and Cleavage Optimization

1. 400 mM HEPES pH 8.0.

2. 1 M DTT prepared fresh.

3. 1% Triton X-100.

4. 25 mM Spermidine stored at −20°C.

5. Nucleotide solutions: 100 mM ATP, 100 mM CTP, 100 mM GTP, 100 mM UTP, and 100 mM GMP. Prepare NTP solutions on ice and adjust to pH 8.0 using NaOH. Store at −20°C.

6. 0.5 M $MgCl_2$.

7. Ribonuclease inhibitor 40 U/μL, e.g., RNAsin Ribonuclease inhibitor (Promega). Prepare a 1:120 dilution (0.3 U/μL) in ribonuclease buffer (20 mM HEPES pH 7.6, 50 mM KCl, 8 mM DTT, and 50%v/v glycerol; see Note 1). Store at −20°C.

8. Linearized plasmid DNA template (~1.5 mg/mL) stored at 4°C.

9. In-house purified His-tagged T7 RNA polymerase (~6 mg/mL) stored at −20°C (see Note 1).

10. Optional: Yeast inorganic pyrophosphatase 2,000 U/mL (see Note 2) stored at −20°C.

11. Optional: Glucose-6-phosphate (see Note 3). Prepare on ice as a 40 mM stock and adjust to pH 8.0 using NaOH. Aliquot and store at −20°C.
12. 0.5 M EDTA pH 8.0.
13. 0.5 M Tris-HCl pH 7.6.
14. 40 mM GlcN6P: Prepare on ice and adjust to pH 7.6 using NaOH. Aliquot and store at −20°C.
15. Purified RNA control (100 ng; see Note 4) stored at −20°C.

2.3. Affinity Batch Purification

1. In-house purified λN$^+$-L$^+$-GST fusion protein [5–7 mg/mL; see refs. 21 and 23] stored at −20°C.
2. Equilibration buffer: 50 mM HEPES, pH 7.5. Adjust pH with NaOH.
3. Tube rotator.
4. Spin cups (Pierce).
5. GSH-Sepharose 4B resin (GE Healthcare) stored at 4°C.
6. Tabletop microcentrifuge with rotor.
7. Phosphate-buffered saline (PBS): 10 mM Na_2HPO_4, 2 mM KH_2PO_4, 2.7 mM KCl, 140 mM NaCl and pH 7.4.
8. Calf intestinal alkaline phosphatase (CIP), 1 U/μL, stored at 4°C.
9. CIP buffer: 50 mM HEPES pH 8.5 and 0.1 mM EDTA (see Note 1).
10. Elution buffer: 20 mM Tris-HCl pH 7.6, 10 mM $MgCl_2$, and 1 mM GlcN6P (or the concentration of GlcN6P determined by the cleavage assay). Prepare just before use from stock solutions (see Subheading 2.2).
11. 2.5 M NaCl.
12. PBS with 20 mM reduced L-glutathione: Just before use, add 0.61 g of reduced L-glutathione to 100 mL of PBS and adjust pH to 8.0 with NaOH (see Note 5).
13. Centrifugal filter device, e.g., Amicon Ultra-15 (Millipore).
14. Centrifuge with swinging-bucket rotor suitable for item 13.
15. UV/Vis spectrophotometer with a quartz cuvette.
16. 50-mL Sterile disposable vacuum filtration system, e.g., Steriflip filter unit (Millipore).

2.4. Quantitative Analysis of Affinity Batch Purification

All solutions used for denaturing gel electrophoresis are filtered through a 0.22 μm filter membrane to minimize detection of undesirable fluorescent speckles on the gel.

1. Gel loading buffer: 20 mg bromophenol blue, 5 mL EDTA 0.5 M pH 8.0, and 95 mL formamide.

2. TBE buffer: 50 mM Tris-Base, 50 mM boric acid, and 1 mM EDTA. Prepare as a 10× stock solution.
3. 10% Gel solution: 10% acrylamide:bisacrylamide (19:1) and 7 M urea in TBE buffer. Store at 4°C. Unpolymerized acrylamide and bisacrylamide are strong neurotoxins. Protective equipment (gloves, mask, laboratory coat) should be worn and care should be taken when handling acrylamide powder and solutions.
4. 10% Analytical denaturing polyacrylamide gel: Mix 40 mL of gel solution with 200 μL ammonium persulfate 10% (w/v) and 40 μL TEMED. Immediately pour in a glass plate assembly using 20×20 cm glass plates and 0.7 mm thick comb and spacers.
5. High-voltage power supply, e.g., Thermo EC600-90.
6. SYBR Gold staining solution: Make a fresh 1:10,000 dilution of SYBR Gold nucleic acid gel stain in TBE buffer.
7. Molecular Imager and analysis software. Here, we use a Molecular Imager FX densitometer and ImageLab software version 3.0 (Bio-Rad).

3. Methods

All procedures are carried out at room temperature unless specified otherwise.

3.1. Preparation of Plasmid for Transcription of ARiBo-Fusion RNAs

3.1.1. Cloning

For cloning the plasmid used for transcription of small RNAs (< 50 nucleotides), it is straightforward to use the modified QuikChange II site-directed mutagenesis procedure (Agilent Technologies), as described here for TL-let-7g (see Fig. 1a). For longer RNA sequences, other cloning procedures can be used. For example, a double-stranded DNA template insert (annealed synthetic oligonucleotides or PCR fragment) digested with *Hind*III and *Apa*I can be ligated within the pARiBo1 plasmid digested with the same two restriction enzymes and dephosphorylated (see Fig. 1b).

1. Design forward and reverse oligonucleotide primers for mutagenesis.
2. Prepare a PCR amplification reaction (50 μL) that includes 5 μL 10× Pfu reaction buffer, 100 ng of pARiBo1 supercoiled plasmid DNA, 125 ng of forward primer, 125 ng of reverse primer, 1 μL of 10 mM dNTP mixture, 3 μL DMSO, water to complete to 49 μL, and 1 μL of Pfu high-fidelity DNA polymerase.

3. Run the PCR reaction in the thermal cycler as follows: (1) 95°C for 2 min to start; (2) then 18 cycles of 95°C for 1 min, 60°C for 1 min, 68°C for 7 min; and (3) finish with 68°C for 7 min and 4°C for 5 min.

4. Add 30 U of *Dpn*1 to the PCR mixture and incubate at 37°C for 2 h in order to digest the parental DNA.

5. Transform 3 μL of the *Dpn*1-digested PCR mixture into 50 μL of DH5α competent cells, spread the transformation on the surface of an LB-Amp plate, and incubate overnight at 37°C. Store the plate at 4°C.

6. At the end of the next day, inoculate 5 mL of LB-Amp medium with an individual colony. Repeat for two other small cultures. Incubate overnight at 37°C with shaking (see Note 6).

7. The next day, prepare glycerol stocks for each culture by mixing 600 μL of the culture with 400 μL of 50% glycerol. Store at −80°C.

8. Purify plasmids using a mini-prep kit. Send for DNA sequencing using the pARiBo1 sequencing primer and select a clone with the right sequence.

3.1.2. Plasmid Preparation

Plasmid preparation can be performed at different scales depending on the anticipated needs for transcription. Small bacterial cultures (150 mL) are used for plasmid purification with a Maxi-prep kit to obtain 0.3–1 mg of plasmid, which is sufficient for several small-scale transcriptions. Large bacterial cultures (2.5 L) are used for plasmid purification with a Giga-prep kit to obtain 7.5–15 mg of plasmid, which is sufficient for large-scale transcriptions.

1. In the morning, inoculate 5 mL of LB-Amp medium with 25 μL of a glycerol stock of the new plasmid, here pTL-let-7g-ARiBo1, cloned into DH5α. Grow for 6–8 h at 37°C with shaking (see Note 6).

2. For Maxi preps, use 0.15 mL of the small culture to inoculate 150 mL LB-Amp in a 500-mL flask. For Giga preps, use 1.25 mL of the small culture to inoculate 1.25 L of LB-Amp medium in a 4-L flask and repeat to prepare a total of 2.5 L of culture. Grow overnight at 37°C with shaking (see Note 6).

3. Pellet the cells by centrifugation at $6,000 \times g$ for 10 min using 500-mL bottles. Discard the supernatant. The pellets can either be stored at −80°C until needed or processed immediately.

4. Extract the plasmid from the cell pellet using either a plasmid Maxi kit or a plasmid Giga kit, according to the supplier's protocol. Resuspend the purified plasmid in water. Determine the DNA concentration by UV spectroscopy ($\lambda = 260$ nm, 1 $OD_{260} = 50$ mg/mL double-stranded DNA).

5. Linearize the plasmid with the *Eco*RI restriction enzyme, keeping a small amount of undigested plasmid (~ 5 μg) for controls on agarose gels. For 300 μg of plasmid, use 300 U of *Eco*RI and 20 μL of 10× *Eco*RI/HEPES buffer (see Note 1) and complete the volume to 200 μL with water. Scale up this reaction as needed for larger quantities of plasmid. Incubate overnight at 37°C.

6. Verify that the plasmid is completely linearized on a 1% agarose gel (see Note 7).

7. Once the plasmid is completely cut, inactivate the restriction enzyme by heating at 65°C for 5 min and transferring on ice. Store the linearized DNA plasmid at 4°C.

3.2. In Vitro Transcription of ARiBo-Fusion RNAs and Cleavage Optimization

Several small-scale transcriptions (100 μL) are usually performed in order to optimize the yield for large-scale transcriptions (5–50 mL).

3.2.1. Small-Scale Transcription Optimization

1. Set up small-scale transcription reactions, typically six reactions of 100 μL. The standard reaction contains 40 mM HEPES pH 8.0 (see Note 1), 50 mM fresh DTT, 0.1% Triton X-100, 1 mM spermidine, 20 mM $MgCl_2$, 4 mM of each NTP (ATP, UTP, GTP, CTP), 8 μg of linearized plasmid DNA, 0.3 U ribonuclease inhibitor, and 1 μL of T7 RNA polymerase (6 mg/mL). The five other transcription reactions are as the standard reaction except that one factor is varied in each reaction: the concentration of $MgCl_2$ (15 mM and 25 mM instead of 20 mM), the template concentration (12 μg/100 μL instead of 8 μg/100 μL), the nucleotide concentration (4 mM GMP is added), or the enzyme concentration (2 μL instead of 1 μL T7 RNA polymerase 6 mg/mL). If needed, 0.01–0.05 U inorganic pyrophosphatase (see Note 2) and 5–10 mM glucose-6-phosphate (see Note 3) can be added.

2. Incubate for 3 h at 37°C.

3. Stop the transcription reaction by adding the necessary volume of 0.5 M EDTA pH 8.0 such that the EDTA concentration is equal to the $MgCl_2$ concentration. Store at −20°C.

4. Analyze samples (1.5 μL of a 1:200 dilution) on an analytical 10% denaturing polyacrylamide gel stained with SYBR Gold (see Subheading 3.4).

5. Scan the gel on a Molecular Imager and quantify the intensity of the high-molecular-weight band on the gel (see Subheading 3.4).

Select the transcription condition that produces the highest yield of ARiBo-fusion RNA according to the intensity of this band.

3.2.2. Optimization of Cleavage Conditions with GlcN6P

Once the small-scale transcription reactions are completed, the condition for *glmS* ribozyme cleavage is optimized. One can use either the transcription reaction that produces the highest yield or simply the standard transcription reaction (see Subheading 3.2.1).

1. Set up 100-µL cleavage reactions that contain 3 µL of the transcription reaction, 20 mM Tris-HCl pH 7.6, 10 mM $MgCl_2$, and varying concentrations (typically 1, 2, and 4 mM) of GlcN6P.

2. Incubate the cleavage reactions at 37°C. Remove 5-µL aliquots from the reaction mixture at specific times (0, 15, 30, and 60 min) and mix with 95 µL of gel loading buffer to stop the cleavage reaction.

3. Analyze cleavage samples (5–20 ng of cleaved RNA per well, here 10 µL of the stopped cleavage mix) together with control samples containing various amounts of purified RNA (2.5, 10, 25, and 50 ng RNA; see Note 4) on an analytical 10% denaturing polyacrylamide gel stained with SYBR Gold (see Subheading 3.4 and Fig. 2).

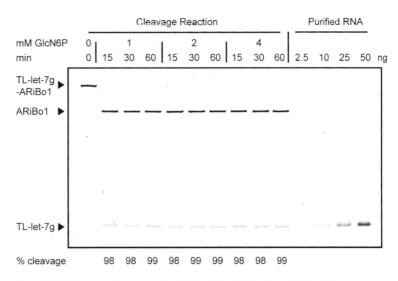

Fig. 2. *GlmS* ribozyme cleavage optimization of the ARiBo-fusion RNA. All cleavage reactions were performed at 37°C in 100-µL solution containing 3 µL of the standard transcription reaction, 10 mM $MgCl_2$, 20 mM Tris-HCl buffer pH 7.6, but with different concentrations of GlcN6P and for different amounts of time (in min), as indicated above each lane of the gel. The mobility of the RNA precursor and products is marked with arrows on the left side of the gel. The percentage of cleavage for each condition is given below the gel. Standard amounts of purified TL-let-7g were loaded for quantitative analysis of the transcription.

4. Scan the gel on a Molecular Imager and quantify the intensity of the gel bands corresponding to the ARiBo-fusion RNA and the ARiBo tag (see Subheading 3.4).

5. Determine the *% of cleavage* in solution:

$$\left[\left(BI_{ARiBo}/nt_{ARiBo}\right)/\left\{\left(BI_{ARiBo}/nt_{ARiBo}\right)+\left(BI_{Fusion}/nt_{Fusion}\right)\right\}\right] \times 100\% \quad (1)$$

where BI_{ARiBo} and BI_{Fusion} are the band intensities of the ARiBo tag and ARiBo-fusion RNA, respectively, whereas nt_{ARiBo} and nt_{Fusion} are the number of nucleotides of these RNAs.

6. Select the best cleavage condition (see Note 8).

7. Estimate the *expected yield* of RNA (in mg/mL transcription and nmol/μL transcription) for the selected cleavage condition. The data in the control lanes are used to derive a standard curve, from which is determined the quantity (in ng) of RNA (N_{RNA}) corresponding to the amount of transcription volume loaded on the gel (here, considering the several dilutions, this corresponds to 15 nL; see Fig. 2).

3.2.3. Large-Scale Transcription

The reaction conditions for the large-scale transcription (typically 5–50 mL) are determined from the small-scale transcription optimization and scaled up according to the RNA needs. The yield of the large-scale transcription (in mg RNA/mL transcription) should be the same as for the small-scale reaction if care is taken to use the same solutions for both reactions.

1. Perform the large-scale transcription reaction using the optimal conditions identified in Subheading 3.2.1.

2. Once the transcription is completed, compare the yield of the large-scale transcription to that of the small-scale transcription on a 10% denaturing polyacrylamide gel stained with SYBR Gold (see Subheading 3.4). Samples loaded on the gel are aliquots from the small-scale and large-scale transcription reactions (1.5 μL of a 1:200 dilution of the transcription reaction); small-scale and large-scale transcription reactions after cleavage of the ARiBo tag with GlcN6P under optimized conditions (see Subheading 3.2.1; 3 and 6 μL of a 1:10 dilution of the cleavage reaction); and control samples containing various amounts of purified RNA (2.5, 10, 25, and 50 ng RNA; see Note 4).

3. Scan the gel with a Molecular Imager and quantify band intensity (see Subheading 3.4).

4. Determine the *% of cleavage* in solution for the small-scale and large-scale transcription reactions using Eq. 1 (see Subheading 3.2.2). The *% of cleavage* should be similar for both transcriptions.

5. Estimate the *expected yield* of RNA (in mg/mL transcription and nmol/μL transcription) for the small-scale and large-scale transcription reactions, as described in Subheading 3.2.2. The *expected yield* should be similar for both reactions.

3.3. Affinity Batch Purification

In this section, the affinity batch purification procedure (Fig. 3a) is described in detail for small-scale (3.5 nmol) applications, and guidelines are provided for adapting the procedure to large-scale applications (0.25 μmol). Only one main modification has been made with respect to the original protocol (21). To circumvent the cumbersome process of decanting the supernatant after centrifugation of GSH-Sepharose resin, spin cups were introduced for small-scale purifications and disposable filter units for large-scale purifications. The use of these devices is not only straightforward, but it also improves time efficiency and prevents the loss of resin during the purification. For the procedure described below, all incubations are performed at room temperature with gentle rotation using a tube rotator, unless otherwise mentioned, and all centrifugation steps are performed for 1 min at $5,000 \times g$. For all incubations, the top of the spin cup may be covered with a parafilm to prevent RNase contamination.

3.3.1. Small-Scale Purification

1. Prepare the RNA–protein mix as follows: In a 1.5-mL Eppendorf tube, add 17.5 nmol of λN^+-L^+-GST fusion protein to a transcription volume that corresponds to 3.5 nmol of RNA to be purified (223 μg for the TL-let-7g RNA; see Note 9). Adjust to a total volume of 400 μL with Equilibration buffer. Incubate for 15 min.

2. In the meantime, prepare the GSH-Sepharose matrix in a spin cup (see Note 10). Add 125 μL of GSH-Sepharose resin (163 μL of the 77% slurry) to the spin cup. Wash twice by adding 400 μL of PBS and centrifuging immediately.

3. Add the RNA–protein mix to the washed resin directly in the spin cup. Incubate for 15 min and centrifuge. Keep the load eluate (LE) on ice for quantitative analysis on gel.

4. Wash the RNA-loaded resin three times as follows: Add 400 μL of Equilibration buffer, incubate for 5 min, and centrifuge. Keep the wash eluates (W1, W2, and W3) on ice for quantitative analysis (see Note 11).

5. Elute the RNA as follows: Add 400 μL of Elution buffer, incubate at 37°C for 15 min (or the optimal time determined from the cleavage assay; see Subheading 3.2.2) with periodic inversion of the tube, then at room temperature for 5 min, and centrifuge. Keep the RNA elution sample (E1) on ice for quantitative analysis and further processing. After elution with GlcN6P, wash the resin twice as follows: Add 400 μL of Equilibration buffer, incubate for 5 min, and centrifuge.

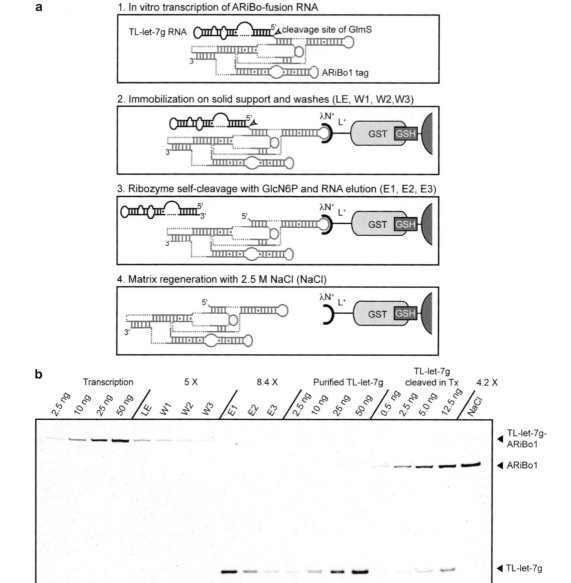

Fig. 3. Affinity batch purification of the TL-let-7g RNA. (a) General purification scheme. The TL-let-7g RNA is synthesized as an ARiBo1-fusion RNA (TL-let-7g-ARiBo1) and immobilized on GSH-Sepharose beads via a λN^+-L^+-GST fusion protein. RNA elution is triggered by addition of GlcN6P, which activates the *glmS* ribozyme of the ARiBo tag. The resin matrix is partly regenerated by incubation with 2.5 M NaCl. (b) Small-scale affinity purification of TL-let-7g RNA analyzed on a 10% denaturing polyacrylamide gel stained with SYBR Gold. Aliquots from each purification steps were loaded on the gel (LE: loading eluate; W1-3: washes; E1-3: RNA elutions; and NaCl: matrix regeneration with 2.5 M NaCl) in amounts shown, where 1× corresponds to 50 ng of TL-let-7g-ARiBo1 present in the transcription reaction or 11.9 ng of TL-let-7g to be purified. In addition, standard amounts of the TL-let-7g-ARiBo1 fusion RNA from the transcription reaction, purified TL-let-7g, and TL-let-7g after cleavage of the fusion RNA in the transcription reaction were loaded for quantitative analysis of the purification. Bands corresponding to the TL-let-7g-ARiBo1 fusion RNA, the ARiBo1 tag, and the desired RNA (TL-let-7g) are indicated on the right of the gel.

Keep the RNA elution samples (E2 and E3) on ice for quantitative analysis and further processing (see Note 12).

6. Wash the resin to remove residual RNA as follows: Add 400 μL of 2.5 M NaCl, incubate for 5 min, and then centrifuge. Keep the eluate (NaCl) on ice for quantitative analysis. Resuspend the resin in 125 μL PBS.

7. To completely regenerate the resin, first collect the used resin in a 50-mL screw-cap conical tube until a significant amount of resin is available (≥5 mL). Filter the resin in a Steriflip filter unit (see Note 13) and keep the same Steriflip for the subsequent wash steps. Wash the resin with 4× resin volume of solution: twice with PBS (incubate for 5 min and filter), three times with 20 mM L-glutathione in PBS (incubate for 15 min and filter; see Note 5), and once with 20% ethanol (incubate for 5 min and filter). Store the regenerated resin in 20% ethanol at 4°C.

8. Once the affinity purification is completed, evaluate the purification on a 10% denaturing polyacrylamide gel stained with SYBR Gold (see Subheading 3.4 and Fig. 3b). Samples loaded on the gel are (1) control samples containing various volumes of the transcription reaction corresponding to specific amounts of ARiBo-fusion RNA (2.5, 10, 25, and 50 ng RNA); (2) aliquots from load and wash eluates corresponding to 250 ng of ARiBo-fusion RNA assuming that 100% of the input RNA is present in each eluate (see Note 14); (3) aliquots from the RNA elution corresponding to 100 ng of the RNA assuming a 100% purification yield at each step (see Note 15); (4) control samples containing various amounts of purified RNA (2.5, 10, 25, and 50 ng RNA; see Note 4); (5) control samples containing various volumes of the transcription reaction cleaved with GlcN6P and corresponding to specific amounts of purified RNA (0.5, 2.5, 5.0, and 12.5 ng RNA); and (6) aliquot from the NaCl wash corresponding to 50 ng of the TL-let-7g RNA of interest assuming 100% RNA recovery at this step (see Note 15).

9. Combine the RNA elution samples (E1, E2, and E3), concentrate using an ultracentrifugation device, and exchange in appropriate storage buffer.

10. Determine the RNA concentration by UV spectroscopy at 260 nm using a conversion factor of 1 $OD_{260} = 40$ μg/mL or an extinction coefficient determined experimentally for the RNA of interest (8, 26).

3.3.2. Large-Scale Purification

Large-scale purifications are typically performed similarly as the small-scale purifications (Subheading 3.3.1), but in 50-mL screw-cap conical tubes, using a transcription volume corresponding to 0.25 μmol of ARiBo-fusion RNA, 1.25 μmol λN$^+$-L$^+$-GST fusion protein, 8.9 mL of GSH-Sepharose resin (11.6 mL of 77% resin slurry), and incubation volumes of 25 mL. A single Steriflip filter unit is used to recover the liquid phase of resin incubations at the various purification steps (see Note 13). In contrast to small-scale purifications, the large-scale purification needs to be evaluated by gel electrophoresis prior to discarding any wash or elution filtrate and performing any of the resin regeneration steps, including the wash with 2.5 M NaCl. This allows one to repeat the necessary steps in cases where the yield is not as high as expected.

3.4. Quantitative Analysis of Affinity Batch Purification

3.4.1. Denaturing Gel Electrophoresis

1. Prepare an analytical 10% denaturing polyacrylamide gel. Pre-run the gel in TBE buffer at 425 V for 20 min.
2. Prepare gel samples as needed in volumes ≤10 µL and add 10 µL of gel loading buffer.
3. Load samples and run the gel at 425 V for 1 h 45 min, until the bromophenol blue is 2 cm from the bottom of the gel.
4. Stain the gel for 10 min with 200 mL SYBR Gold staining solution.
5. Scan on a Molecular Imager and quantify band intensities.

3.4.2. Quantitative Analysis

The quantitative analysis described here is used for evaluating the affinity batch purifications using sample loading as described in Subheading 3.3.1. Six variables are defined for this analysis: the quantities (in ng) of purified RNA (N_{RNA}), ARiBo tag (N_{ARiBo}), and ARiBo-fusion RNA (N_{Fusion}) as well as the number of nucleotides in the purified RNA (nt_{RNA}), ARiBo tag (nt_{ARiBo}), and ARiBo-fusion RNA (nt_{Fusion}).

1. For each gel, four lanes were loaded with transcription reaction containing estimated quantities of intact ARiBo-fusion RNA (see Subheading 3.2.3). From these lanes, derive a standard curve relating band intensity to the quantity of ARiBo-fusion RNA (N_{Fusion}).
2. For each gel, four lanes were loaded with known quantities of the purified RNA of interest (TL-let-7g), derived from OD_{260} measurements. From these data, derive a standard curve relating band intensity with the quantity of purified RNA (N_{RNA}).
3. For each gel, four lanes were loaded with transcription reaction treated with GlcN6P and containing estimated quantities of TL-let-7g (see Subheading 3.2.3). Calculate the exact quantity of TL-let-7g (N_{RNA}) detected in these lanes using the standard curve for N_{RNA}. Subsequently, determine the exact quantity of ARiBo tag (N_{ARiBo}) detected in these same lanes from:

$$N_{ARiBo} = \left(N_{RNA} / nt_{RNA}\right) \times nt_{ARiBo}. \qquad (2)$$

Finally, use these lanes with the cleaved ARiBo-fusion RNA to derive a standard curve relating band intensity with the quantity of ARiBo tag (N_{ARiBo}).

4. Determine the *% of cleavage* in solution from a control lane in which the transcription reaction is treated with GlcN6P (see Fig. 3b, lane 19) using the equation

$$\{(N_{ARiBo}/\text{nt}_{ARiBo})/[(N_{ARiBo}/\text{nt}_{ARiBo})+(N_{Fusion}/\text{nt}_{Fusion})]\} \times 100\%. \quad (3)$$

5. Also using Eq. 3, determine the *% of cleavage* on the resin from the NaCl lane (see Fig. 3b, lane 20).

6. Determine the *% of unbound RNA* using:

$$\left[\left(\sum N_{Fusion}\right)/I_{Fusion}\right] \times 100\%, \quad (4)$$

where ΣN_{Fusion} represents the total amount of ARiBo-fusion RNA (ng) detected in lanes LE, W1, W2, and W3, and I_{Fusion} represents the input of the same RNA in equivalent volumes of affinity batch purification (250 ng; see Note 16).

7. Determine the *% of RNA eluted* using:

$$\left[\left(\sum N_{RNA}/I_{RNA}\right)\right] \times 100\%, \quad (5)$$

where ΣN_{RNA} represents the total amount of TL-let-7g (ng) detected in lanes E1, E2, and E3, and I_{RNA} represents the calculated amount of TL-let-7g expected from 100% cleavage in equivalent volumes of transcription (100 ng).

8. Determine the *% of RNA purity* from the E1 lane (see Fig. 3b, lane 9) using:

$$\left[N_{RNA}/(N_{RNA}+N_{ARiBo})\right] \times 100\%. \quad (6)$$

4. Notes

1. Although transcription reactions are generally performed in a Tris–HCl buffer, Tris is known to activate the *glmS* ribozyme (27, 28) and could lead to significant amount of *glmS* cleavage during the transcription reaction (17). Tris buffers should therefore be avoided in the transcription reaction and in buffers used for components of the reaction such as the DNA template, ribonuclease inhibitor dilution, and T7 RNA polymerase. Tris buffers should also be avoided in the first steps of affinity purification.

2. A white precipitate generally forms during the course of the transcription reaction, which results from the formation of an insoluble complex between Mg^{2+} and pyrophosphate. A large amount of precipitate is often associated with good transcription yields. Inorganic phosphatase can be added to the reaction to reduce the precipitate and can sometimes increase the yield of transcription (29).

3. *Glm*S ribozyme self-cleavage may be observed in transcription reaction if activators of the ribozyme are present in the reaction (27, 28, 30). Glucose-6-phosphate is an inhibitor of the *glmS* ribozyme (27, 30) that can be used to reduce ARiBo-tag cleavage without significantly affecting the transcription yield and subsequent GlcN6P-induced cleavage.

4. For the purified RNA control, it is preferable to use the same RNA as the one being purified. If this RNA is not available, a purified RNA of similar size can be used to estimate the expected yield of the RNA of interest.

5. It is crucial to adjust the pH of the L-glutathione solution to 8.0 in order to maximize the elution efficiency of the GST-fusion protein. Otherwise, addition of L-glutathione at high concentration lowers the pH of the buffer.

6. Vigorous shaking is necessary for bacterial cell cultures; we routinely use 240 rpm for small cultures (5 mL and 150 mL) and 200–220 rpm for cultures in 4-L flasks. Slightly less vigorous shaking is used for 4-L flasks to prevent flasks from breaking.

7. In order to maximize the yield of transcription, it is essential that the restriction enzyme digestion be performed to completion. Uncut plasmids allow efficient continuous transcription, giving rise to very long transcripts that use up the NTPs.

8. Although >95% cleavage is typically obtained with a 15-min incubation in 1 mM GlcN6P (see Fig. 2), efficient cleavage of some ARiBo-fusion RNA may require a higher concentration of GlcN6P and/or a longer incubation time. This is generally the case when the nucleotide at the 3′-end of the desired RNA is not an unpaired adenine (21). For RNAs with an unpaired adenine at their 3′-end, if little or no cleavage is observed after a 1-h incubation with 4 mM GlcN6P, this may indicate misfolding of the ARiBo-fusion RNA. In such case, one or more of the following conditions can be tested to help improve the cleavage yield: (1) use even longer incubation time and/or higher GlcN6P concentration; (2) increase or lower the concentration of $MgCl_2$; (3) refold the RNA by heating and subsequently cooling; (4) increase the cleavage temperature (e.g., 42°C); and (5) store the transcription reaction at 4°C (instead of −20°C) or perform purification immediately after

the transcription is completed. It is important to bear in mind that *glmS* ribozyme cleavage is typically performed at 37°C with 10 mM $MgCl_2$; incubations at higher temperatures and for longer periods of time may cause undesirable degradation of the RNA.

9. The protein:RNA ratio may need to be optimized to maximize RNA yield and purity. A 5:1 protein:RNA molar ratio is typically used to provide high RNA yield and purity. Ratios as low as 3:1 may be used without sacrificing sample purity but will likely result in lower yields, whereas higher ratios (e.g., 8:1) may provide slightly higher yields but require excessive amounts of purified fusion protein (21).

10. Spin cups are convenient tools for affinity batch purification with small volume of resin (20–400 µL), since they prevent the loss of resin and improve time efficiency.

11. If needed, an alkaline phosphatase step can be inserted between the first and second washes. For small-scale applications, standard reaction conditions can be used: Add 35 U of CIP (10 U/nmol RNA) in 400 µL CIP buffer, incubate at 37°C for 30 min with periodic inversion of the spin cup, then transfer to room temperature for 5 min, and centrifuge. For large-scale applications, reaction conditions can be modified to reduce enzyme cost by using 130 U/µmol RNA and incubating for 4 h at 37°C with periodic inversion of the 50-mL conical tube.

12. In some cases, although >95% *glmS* cleavage is obtained under optimized cleavage conditions, the RNA of interest may be difficult to elute because it remains bound to the resin. In these cases, RNA elution could be facilitated by adding NaCl to the RNA elution buffers, but care should be taken to minimize co-elution of the ARiBo tag. We suggest to modify the elution steps as follows: (1) after the E1 incubations, add 0.5 M NaCl and 50 mM EDTA, incubate for 5 min and centrifuge; (2) after the E2 and E3 incubations, add 0.1–0.25 M NaCl, incubate for 5 min, and centrifuge.

13. To use the Steriflip for washing resin and large-scale affinity batch purifications, proceed as follows. The Steriflip filter unit is first attached to the top of a 50-mL conical tube used for the incubation (tube 1) and flipped over, and a vacuum is applied. The bottom tube containing the eluate (tube 2) is capped, kept on ice, and replaced by a new 50-mL conical tube (tube 3). The Steriflip filter is then flipped over again, and the bottom tube (tube 1) is carefully detached from the filter unit, filled with the buffer used for the next incubation step, reattached to the Steriflip filter, and gently mixed several times to ensure that all the resin is recovered from the filter surface. During the following incubation period, the filter unit on tube 1 is replaced

by a screw cap and kept under RNase-free conditions for the next filtering step.

14. In the case of the ARiBo-fusion TL-let-7g (a 193-nucleotide RNA of 63.7 kDa), 3.5 nmol or 223 μg would be present in the 400 μL flow through, and thus 4.49 μL of the 1:10 dilution would represent 250 ng of this RNA.

15. In the case of the TL-let-7g RNA (a 46-nucleotide RNA of 15.2 kDa) 3.5 nmol or 53.15 μg of TL-let-7g would be present in the 400 μL RNA elution sample, and thus 7.52 μL of the 1:10 dilution would represent 100 ng of this RNA and 3.76 μL of the 1:10 dilution would represent 50 ng of this RNA.

16. Since the percentage of unbound RNA is based only on the quantity of fusion RNA, it represents a minimum value of the total unbound RNA. Although not observed for the TL-let-7g purification, slower migrating species in lanes LE, W1, W2, and W3 have been observed for purification of other RNAs.

Acknowledgments

We thank J. G. Omichinski for critical reading of the manuscript. This work was supported by grants from the Canadian Institutes for Health Research (CIHR HOP-83068 and MOP-86502) and the Natural Sciences and Engineering Council of Canada (NSERC) to P. Legault, a Ph.D. scholarship from CIHR to A.D., an M.Sc. scholarship from CIHR to P.D., and summer student scholarships from NSERC and The Mach-Gaensslen Foundation of Canada to A.R.-B. P. Legault holds a Canada Research Chair in Structural Biology and Engineering of RNA.

References

1. Fire A, Xu S, Montgomery MK, Kostas SA, Driver SE, Mello CC (1998) Potent and specific genetic interference by double-stranded RNA in Caenorhabditis elegans. Nature 391:806–811
2. Ambros V (2004) The functions of animal microRNAs. Nature 431:350–355
3. Winkler W, Nahvi A, Breaker RR (2002) Thiamine derivatives bind messenger RNAs directly to regulate bacterial gene expression. Nature 419:952–956
4. Milligan JF, Groebe DR, Witherell GW, Uhlenbeck OC (1987) Oligoribonucleotide synthesis using T7 RNA polymerase and synthetic DNA templates. Nucleic Acids Res 15:8783–8798
5. Wyatt JR, Chastain M, Puglisi JD (1991) Synthesis and purification of large amounts of RNA oligonucleotides. Biotechniques 11:764–769
6. Doudna JA (1997) Preparation of homogeneous ribozyme RNA for crystallization. Methods Mol Biol 74:365–370
7. Uhlenbeck OC (1995) Keeping RNA happy. RNA 1:4–6
8. Legault P (1995) Structural studies of ribozymes by heteronuclear NMR spectroscopy, University of Colorado at Boulder, Boulder
9. Lukavsky PJ, Puglisi JD (2004) Large-scale preparation and purification of polyacrylamide-free RNA oligonucleotides. RNA 10:889–893

10. Shields TP, Mollova E, Ste Marie L, Hansen MR, Pardi A (1999) High-performance liquid chromatography purification of homogenous-length RNA produced by trans cleavage with a hammerhead ribozyme. RNA 5:1259–1267
11. Kim I, McKenna SA, Puglisi EV, Puglisi JD (2007) Rapid purification of RNAs using fast performance liquid chromatography (FPLC). RNA 13:289–294
12. McKenna SA, Kim I, Puglisi EV, Lindhout DA, Aitken CE, Marshall RA, Puglisi JD (2007) Purification and characterization of transcribed RNAs using gel filtration chromatography. Nat Protoc 2:3270–3277
13. Keel AY, Easton LE, Lukavsky PJ, Kieft JS (2009) Large-scale native preparation of in vitro transcribed RNA. Methods Enzymol 469:3–25
14. Easton LE, Shibata Y, Lukavsky PJ (2010) Rapid, nondenaturing RNA purification using weak anion-exchange fast performance liquid chromatography. RNA 16:647–653
15. Cheong HK, Hwang E, Lee C, Choi BS, Cheong C (2004) Rapid preparation of RNA samples for NMR spectroscopy and X-ray crystallography. Nucleic Acids Res 32:e84
16. Kieft JS, Batey RT (2004) A general method for rapid and nondenaturing purification of RNAs. RNA 10:988–995
17. Batey RT, Kieft JS (2007) Improved native affinity purification of RNA. RNA 13:1384–1389
18. Boese BJ, Corbino K, Breaker RR (2008) In vitro selection and characterization of cellulose-binding RNA aptamers using isothermal amplification. Nucleosides Nucleotides Nucleic Acids 27:949–966
19. Vicens Q, Gooding AR, Duarte LF, Batey RT (2009) Preparation of group I introns for biochemical studies and crystallization assays by native affinity purification. Plos One 4(8):e6740
20. Pereira MJ, Behera V, Walter NG (2010) Nondenaturing purification of co-transcriptionally folded RNA avoids common folding heterogeneity. PLoS One 5:e12953
21. Di Tomasso G, Lampron P, Dagenais P, Omichinski JG, Legault P (2011) The ARiBo tag: a reliable tool for affinity purification of RNAs under native conditions. Nucleic Acids Res 39:e18
22. Austin RJ, Xia T, Ren J, Takahashi TT, Roberts RW (2002) Designed arginine-rich RNA-binding peptides with picomolar affinity. J Am Chem Soc 124:10966–10967
23. Di Tomasso G, Lampron P, Omichinski JG, Legault P (2012) Preparation of λN-GST fusion protein for affinity immobilization of RNA. Methods Mol Biol 941:123–135
24. Pasquinelli AE, Reinhart BJ, Slack F, Martindale MQ, Kuroda MI, Maller B, Hayward DC, Ball EE, Degnan B, Muller P, Spring J, Srinivasan A, Fishman M, Finnerty J, Corbo J, Levine M, Leahy P, Davidson E, Ruvkun G (2000) Conservation of the sequence and temporal expression of let-7 heterochronic regulatory RNA. Nature 408:86–89
25. Piskounova E, Viswanathan SR, Janas M, LaPierre RJ, Daley GQ, Sliz P, Gregory RI (2008) Determinants of microRNA processing inhibition by the developmentally regulated RNA-binding protein Lin28. J Biol Chem 283:21310–21314
26. Zaug AJ, Grosshans CA, Cech TR (1988) Sequence-specific endoribonuclease activity of the Tetrahymena ribozyme: enhanced cleavage of certain oligonucleotide substrates that form mismatched ribozyme-substrate complexes. Biochemistry 27:8924–8931
27. McCarthy TJ, Plog MA, Floy SA, Jansen JA, Soukup JK, Soukup GA (2005) Ligand requirements for glmS ribozyme self-cleavage. Chem Biol 12:1221–1226
28. Roth A, Nahvi A, Lee M, Jona I, Breaker RR (2006) Characteristics of the glmS ribozyme suggest only structural roles for divalent metal ions. RNA 12:607–619
29. Cunningham PR, Ofengand J (1990) Use of inorganic pyrophosphatase to improve the yield of in vitro transcription reactions catalyzed by T7 RNA polymerase. Biotechniques 9:713–714
30. Watson PY, Fedor MJ (2011) The glmS riboswitch integrates signals from activating and inhibitory metabolites in vivo. Nat Struct Mol Biol 18:359–363

Chapter 12

Plasmid Template Design and In Vitro Transcription of Short RNAs Within a "Structure Cassette" for Structure Probing Experiments

Virginia K. Vachon and Graeme L. Conn

Abstract

Chemical and enzymatic RNA structure probing methods are important tools for examining RNA secondary and tertiary structures and their interactions with proteins, small molecules, and ions. The recently developed "Selective 2'-Hydroxyl Acylation Analyzed by Primer Extension" (SHAPE) approach has proven especially useful for uncovering details of secondary structures, complex tertiary interactions, and RNA dynamics. Analysis of short RNAs using SHAPE or other probing methods that require reverse transcription to detect RNA modifications presents a technical hurdle in that intense bands corresponding to abortive transcription during primer extension and the full-length RT product may obscure information corresponding to the 3' and 5' ends of the molecule, respectively. This chapter describes the design and use of an RNA "structure cassette" that addresses these issues. First, we describe methods by which any RNA of interest may be cloned into a new plasmid preloaded with sequences that encode a structure cassette surrounding the short internal target RNA. Next, we outline key considerations and analyses of the RNAs produced that should be performed prior to SHAPE or other structure probing experiments.

Key words: Structure cassette, In vitro transcription, RNA structure probing, SHAPE, Reverse transcriptase

1. Introduction

The ability to thoroughly dissect RNA structures and how they govern interactions with other regulatory molecules is critical for understanding their varied biological roles and functions. Well-established approaches to RNA structure probing in solution include enzymatic, e.g., RNase V1, T1, and A, and chemical probing with reagents such as dimethyl sulfate (DMS), kethoxal, 1-cyclohexyl-3-(2-morpholinoethyl)-carbodiimide metho-p-toluene sulfonate (CMCT), Pb^{2+}, or hydroxyl radical. More recently, a new approach termed "Selective 2'-Hydroxyl Acylation Analyzed by Primer Extension"

(SHAPE), pioneered by Kevin Weeks' laboratory (1), has added a new and powerful dimension to such analyses. Together these methods can interrogate RNA secondary and tertiary structures, solvent accessibility, and, in the case of SHAPE, flexibility of each individual nucleotide in an RNA molecule. The quantitative analysis of each nucleotide that is possible with SHAPE is especially useful for identifying the overall architecture of an RNA molecule, tertiary interactions, and changes in nucleotide flexibility upon protein or aptamer binding and is a valuable tool for exploring the nature of RNA folding (2–4). The purpose of this chapter is to provide a method by which short RNAs can be efficiently produced for SHAPE or any other structure probing method that exploits reverse transcriptase (RT) primer extension for analysis.

RNA for structure probing can be obtained in various ways. For SHAPE analysis of the entire HIV-1 genome, the RNA was obtained by direct purification from virions (5). In many cases, however, the RNA must be produced in vitro. For structure probing of longer RNAs, primers may be designed to anneal to different regions along the RNA so that primer extension products for the entire RNA can be visualized on a denaturing polyacrylamide sequencing gel or using capillary electrophoresis (6, 7). In either case, a limitation for shorter RNAs arises because aborted RT DNA transcripts and full-length products obscure the results of primer extension at the 3′ and 5′ ends of the molecule, respectively. In order to obtain structural information for the entirety of a short RNA, a "structure cassette" has been adopted (1, 3, 6, 8) which introduces linker regions encoding short stable RNA hairpins to both the 5′ and 3′-end of the RNA of interest. The 3′-end extension additionally provides an invariant RT primer binding site (Fig. 1), so only a single DNA RT primer needs to be synthesized and labeled for all samples. Finally, this approach also alleviates problems of 5′- and 3′-end heterogeneity. Although potentially still present, heterogeneity at the 3′ end of the RNA is of no consequence to the data obtained via primer extension since the heterogeneity exists beyond the primer-annealing site. Similarly, heterogeneity at the RNA 5′ end lies beyond the area of interest in the reverse transcription reaction analysis. The structure cassette's linker regions were designed with stable tetraloops intended to avoid interference with the folding and structure of the internal RNA of interest (8). Although initially intended for use in SHAPE probing experiments, its usefulness extends to any RNA probing experiment in which short RNAs are analyzed by RT primer extension.

Typically the structure cassette is incorporated into the DNA in vitro transcription template via the forward and reverse primers of a polymerase chain reaction (PCR). Although widely applicable, this approach has some drawbacks. For example, long primers need to be synthesized for each new RNA to be studied and we have

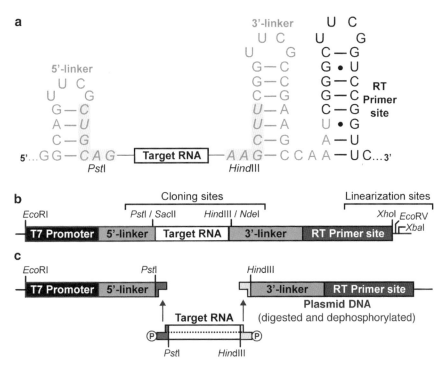

Fig. 1. A plasmid system for in vitro transcription of RNAs within a "structure cassette." (**a**) Sequence and structure of the 5′ and 3′ hairpin linkers (*grey*) and 3′-end RT site (*black*). The structure cassette is shown with *Pst*I and *Hin*dIII sequences (shaded regions); for the alternative cloning sites (*Sac*II and *Nde*I) both strands of the hairpin stem are altered to maintain Watson–Crick base-pairing. (**b**) Organization of the structure cassette plasmid with all unique restriction enzyme sites for cloning and linearization for run-off transcription labeled. (**c**) Generation of new transcription templates by ligation of paired 5′ end phosphorylated DNA oligonucleotides synthesized with matching "sticky ends" (shown here for *Pst*I and *Hin*dIII double-digested plasmid).

found that for some RNAs, these PCR reactions require significant troubleshooting and optimization. Generating templates for short or G-C-rich RNAs may be particularly challenging via PCR. PCR is also a potentially error-prone process which may lead to the production of fully altered or heterogeneous template DNA, and thus equivalent issues in the final transcribed RNA present in the structure probing reaction. Thus, an appealing alternative is a plasmid-based template system which can circumvent these issues. In such a system, the structure cassette elements may be pre-loaded onto the plasmid with suitable restriction enzyme sites built into the linker regions to allow simple cloning of only the RNA-encoding sequence. New constructs can be sequenced prior to use and protocols are well established that produce plasmid template of consistent yield and quality suitable for all structure probing applications.

We have created a structure cassette plasmid by modifying a general in vitro transcription system based on pUC19 that our laboratory previously developed (9). So that they may be utilized as internal restriction sites for the SHAPE plasmid, existing *Pst*I and *Hin*dIII restriction sites were removed by digesting the vector backbone with these enzymes, removal of the resulting 5′ overhangs with T4 exonuclease and subsequent re-ligation of the plasmid. Following these modifications, the first RNA of interest, the ~155 nt adenovirus VA RNA$_I$, was amplified by PCR using primers encoding the structure cassette linkers and cloned into the plasmid at its *Eco*RI and *Xho*I restriction sites. This process was performed using each combination of forward and reverse primers containing one of the two unique internal restriction sites within the 5′ and 3′ linkers (*Pst*I or *Sac*II and *Hin*dIII or *Nco*I, respectively) to create a total of four structure cassette plasmids (Fig. 1). These multiple options for cloning, in addition to three unique 3′-end run-off transcription linearization sites (*Xho*I, *Eco*RV, and *Xba*I) derived from the original transcription plasmid (9), significantly reduce the likelihood that sequences within any new target RNA will make it incompatible with this plasmid-based structure cassette system. We have subsequently cloned and tested multiple VA RNA$_I$ sequence variants and a second noncoding viral RNA, Epstein–Barr EBER1, into this system using the protocols described here.

First, this chapter describes approaches to cloning new RNA-encoding sequences into this structure cassette plasmid system using either PCR (Cloning Method 1) or direct ligation of pairs of complementary chemically synthesized DNA oligonucleotides (Cloning Method 2). Once sequence-verified clones are obtained, plasmid DNA can be purified and used in RNA in vitro transcription reactions using other established protocols (e.g., see Chapter 4). Both the chemical purity and conformational homogeneity of the RNA-structure cassette transcripts should be assessed before use in probing experiments, using denaturing and native polyacrylamide gel electrophoresis, respectively. The key steps involved are described in the final protocols of this chapter using both VA RNA$_I$ and EBER1 RNA as examples.

2. Materials

2.1. Generating a Structure Cassette Plasmid Containing a Target RNA Sequence

1. Plasmid containing the structure cassette with the appropriate internal restriction sites (see Fig. 1 and Note 1).
2. Competent cells of an *Escherichia coli* strain suitable for plasmid propagation, such as DH5α.
3. 50 mg/ml Ampicillin solution in water. This is a 1,000× stock for 50 μg/ml final concentration.
4. LB-agar plates: 10 g peptone from casein, 5 g yeast extract, 10 g sodium chloride, and 12 g agar dissolved in water to a total volume of 1 L. Divide into media bottles and autoclave. LB-agar can be stored after autoclaving; melt solid LB-agar in a microwave on low power. After autoclaving or microwaving, allow to

cool to <60°C, add 50 mg/ml ampicillin to a suitable final concentration (e.g., 50 or 100 μg/ml), and pour into plates.

5. LB broth: 2.5 g peptone from casein, 1.25 g yeast extract, and 2.5 g sodium chloride dissolved in water to a total volume of 250 mL. Autoclave immediately after preparation.

6. Restriction enzymes and corresponding 10× buffer provided by the supplier. An appropriate combination of *Pst*I or *Hind*III and *Sac*II or *Nco*I is needed depending on the plasmid being used. For the example protocol here, we use *Pst*I and *Hind*III.

7. Calf intestinal alkaline phosphatase (CIAP).

8. Agarose gel DNA extraction kit.

9. DNA ligase with corresponding ligase buffer.

2.1.1. Cloning Method 1: PCR

1. Forward and reverse DNA oligonucleotide PCR primers that contain (a) regions complementary to the target RNA-encoding sequence to be amplified and (b) the desired restriction enzyme sites to be used for cloning into the structure cassette plasmid (see Note 2).

2. *Taq* and Vent DNA polymerases: Mix at 60:1 unit ratio (see Note 3).

3. 10 μM dNTPs (i.e., a mixture of 10 μM dATP, 10 μM dCTP, 10 μM dGTP, and 10 μM dTTP).

4. *Optional*: PCR cloning kit for use with *Taq* polymerase (see Note 4).

5. *Optional*: 20 mg/ml X-Gal for blue-white screening if using the cloning kit.

2.1.2. Cloning Method 2: Direct Ligation of Chemically Synthesized DNA Oligonucleotides

1. Two chemically synthesized DNA oligos of sequence corresponding to the coding and complementary strands of the target RNA. The 5′ and 3′ ends of each DNA strand are designed to match the sticky ends produced by restriction enzyme digest of the desired target plasmid (see Fig. 1 and Note 5).

2. T4 polynucleotide kinase (T4 PNK).

3. DNA ligase buffer (see Note 6).

2.2. Analysis of Transcribed RNA

1. Purified product of in vitro transcription resuspended in TE buffer. For descriptions of RNA in vitro transcription and purification see Chapters 4–6. Generally, one 50–100 μl transcription reaction will yield sufficient RNA for approximately 50 structure probing reactions.

2. Tris–Boric acid–EDTA Buffer (TBE, 10×): 1 M Tris, 1 M boric acid, and 10 mM EDTA.

3. Denaturing polyacrylamide gel solution: Acrylamide/N,N'-methylene-bis-acrylamide (19:1 ratio) and 50% (w/v) urea dissolved in 1× TBE (see Note 7).

4. Native polyacrylamide gel solution: Acrylamide/ N,N'-methylene-bis-acrylamide (19:1 ratio) in 1× TBE.

5. 10% (w/v) Ammonium persulfate solution.

6. Tetramethylethylenediamine (TEMED).

7. Denaturing Gel Loading Dye (2×): 50% (w/v) urea, 0.25% (w/v) bromophenol blue, and 0.25% (w/v) xylene cyanol dissolved in 1× TE Buffer (10 mM Tris pH 7.5 and 1 mM EDTA pH 8).

8. Native Gel Loading Dye: 40% (w/v) sucrose, 0.17% (w/v) xylene cyanol, and 0.17% (w/v) bromophenol blue.

3. Methods

3.1. Generating Structure Cassette Plasmids with New Target RNAs

We have used two approaches to cloning target RNAs into the structure cassette plasmid: DNA amplification via a standard PCR and chemical synthesis of paired DNA oligonucleotides encoding the desired RNA target. PCR requires a DNA template corresponding to the target RNA and primers containing appropriate flanking restriction sites (e.g., PstI and HindIII; see Fig. 1). The resulting PCR product may either be digested and ligated directly into the structure cassette vector or cloned via an intermediate vector using a PCR cloning kit. The second method uses chemically synthesized DNA oligonucleotides that are 5′-phosphorylated with T4 PNK, annealed, and ligated directly into the structure cassette plasmid. This approach has proven to be especially useful for the introduction of mutations that were difficult to obtain using site-directed mutagenesis and for creating templates for many RNA variants in parallel.

1. In a total volume of 20 µl, digest 1 µg of the structure cassette plasmid with PstI and HindIII restriction enzymes (see Note 8).

2. Add 1 unit of CIAP and incubate for an additional hour at 37°C.

3. Dilute to 100 µl final volume with water and then purify the digested plasmid DNA using an agarose gel DNA extraction kit following the manufacturer's instructions (see Note 9).

4. Measure the concentration of the plasmid at 260 nm using a Nanodrop or other spectrophotometer (if necessary, use the conversion 1 OD_{260} = 50 µg/ml plasmid DNA). Ideally, the concentration should be > 25 ng/µl.

5. Prepare the insert DNA as described in Subheading 3.1.1 or 3.1.2, below.

6. Calculate the amount of insert DNA required for ligation reactions containing 50 ng of vector DNA and with a molar ratio

of vector to insert of 1:1 and 1:3. For example, for a 3,000 base pair plasmid and 150 base pair insert, 2.5 and 7.5 ng of insert is required, respectively.

7. Perform ligation reactions with vector:insert molar ratios of 1:0 (background control), 1:1, and 1:3, using a standard ligation with T4 ligase enzyme or a rapid ligation kit, according to the manufacturer's instructions.

8. Use 1–3 μl of ligation reaction to transform 30–50 μl aliquots of competent *E. coli* DH5α cells (see Note 10). Following incubation on ice for 30 min, heat shock at 42°C for 90 s and then return to ice for 5–10 min. Add 500 μl of LB broth to each and incubate at 37°C with gentle agitation for 45–60 min. Plate 100 μl of each transformation onto an LB-agar plate containing 100 μg/ml ampicillin.

9. Assess the efficiency of ligation by comparing the number of colonies on each plate. For a successful reaction expect to see at least twice as many colonies on one or both of the plates containing insert DNA compared to the background control.

10. Miniprep plasmid DNA from two to three colonies grown overnight in LB medium with 100 μg/ml ampicillin and confirm the presence of the correct insert using an automated DNA sequencing service.

3.1.1. Cloning Method 1: PCR

1. Perform a standard PCR reaction using the RNA-encoding template and primers incorporating the *Pst*I and *Hin*dIII restriction sites (see Notes 8 and 11).

2. Run the PCR reaction on a 1% agarose gel, cut out the band (DNA insert) using a clean blade, and recover the DNA using the agarose gel extraction kit.

3. Directly following purification of the DNA insert, double digest with *Pst*I and *Hin*dIII restriction enzymes (see Note 8).

4. Clean up the digested DNA using the agarose gel extraction kit (omitting the initial steps required to melt the gel slice) or a PCR reaction purification kit. Alternatively, heat deactivate the restriction enzymes following the enzyme supplier's instructions and use the digested DNA directly.

5. Determine the concentration of the insert using a Nanodrop spectrophotometer or by comparison of the purified insert to standards of known mass on an agarose gel.

3.1.2. Cloning Method 2: Direct Ligation of Chemically Synthesized DNA Oligonucleotides

1. Using the estimate of DNA yield provided by the supplier, dissolve each DNA oligonucleotide in sterile water to a final concentration of 1 μg/μl (see Note 12).

2. Individually phosphorylate 1 μg of each DNA using T4 PNK in a 20 μl reaction (see Note 6).

3. Mix the phosphorylated DNA oligonucleotides, anneal by heating at 95°C for 5 min, then turn off the heat block, and allow to cool to 30°C.

4. Dilute the phosphorylated DNA oligos with 960 μl of water to make the final DNA duplex concentration 1 ng/μl (see Note 13).

3.2. Analysis and Preparation of Transcribed RNA for Probing Experiments

After RNA has been transcribed and purified, it is important to verify that it is both chemically pure and that it exists in a single conformation prior to carrying out structure probing experiments. The purity and integrity of the RNA can be verified using denaturing gel electrophoresis, and its conformational homogeneity prior to and after annealing can be examined using native polyacrylamide gel electrophoresis.

1. Prepare a stock of the purified RNA at a concentration of 50 ng/μl.

2. Evaluate the purity of the isolated RNA by running 200 ng of each RNA on a 50% urea denaturing polyacrylamide gel of appropriate percentage for the RNA size. Stain the gel by adding 10 μl of 2 μg/ml of ethidium bromide to 20 ml of 1× TBE and soaking for 10 min. Visualize the bands using a UV gel imaging system; a single band corresponding to the full-length RNA within the structure cassette is expected (see Note 14 and Fig. 2).

3. Determine the optimal annealing temperature and conditions to ensure that the RNA is folded and conformationally homogeneous. These must be experimentally determined; a good starting point is to incubate 100 ng of RNA for 10 min at 25, 37, and 65°C and allow the sample to cool slowly to room

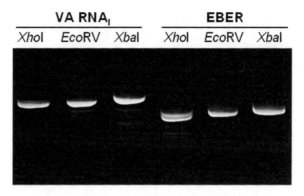

Fig. 2. Denaturing polyacrylamide gel analysis of target RNAs within the structure cassette. Purified samples of VA RNA$_I$ and EBER1 within the structure cassette prepared by run-off transcription from plasmid templates linearized with each of the three available restriction sites (XhoI, EcoRV, and XbaI). Note that transcription of EBER1 RNA from plasmid linearized with XhoI produces two closely spaced bands indicating the presence of $n+1$ transcript; this is absent in the equivalent VA RNA$_I$ sample and with the other linearization sites for EBER1 RNA.

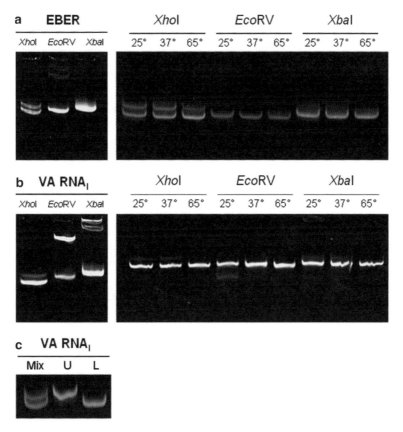

Fig. 3. Native polyacrylamide gel analysis of RNAs within the structure cassette. (a) EBER1 RNA within the structure cassette produced using each possible run-off site, immediately after denaturing purification (*left panel*) and following annealing at the indicated temperatures (*right panel*). (b) As panel (a) but for VA RNA$_I$. (c) Separation of the two differently migrating conformations of VA RNA$_I$ within the structure cassette produced by run-off transcription at the *XhoI* site.

temperature on the bench top for 10 min before placing on ice (see Note 15). Compare each sample of RNA on a native polyacrylamide gel at 4°C (see Note 16) and visualize by staining with ethidium bromide as described in step 2.

Many RNAs exist in multiple conformations, particularly after denaturing purification, and will appear as multiple bands on a native polyacrylamide gel (Fig. 3a, b, left panels). However, typically some combination of annealing at an empirically determined temperature in step 3 in the above protocol and solution conditions, e.g., varying monovalent salt or Mg^{2+} concentrations, will result in a homogeneous sample demonstrated by a single band on a native gel (see Fig. 3a, b, right panels). Alternatively, if the different RNA conformers are sufficiently well resolved on the native gel, they may be separately excised and recovered (they should then be rerun on a native gel to ensure that they are conformationally unique and not two structures in equilibrium). In the example shown in Fig. 3c for VA RNA$_I$, only the faster running form gave significant RT products after probing experiments, suggesting a misfolding that occluded the RT primer binding site. Once a homogeneous sample is obtained, it can be used for SHAPE or other RNA structure probing using detailed protocols provided elsewhere (6, 9).

4. Notes

1. Each SHAPE structure cassette plasmid contains a single internal restriction site on each side of the target RNA for cloning. Each possible combination of two different 5′ and 3′ sites has been generated, *Pst*I or *Sac*II and *Hind*III or *Nco*I, respectively, to produce a collection of four plasmids designed to accommodate a wide range of target RNAs (see Fig. 1). Plasmids are available from the authors upon request.

2. In the primer design, additional 5′-end nucleotides may be required for efficient direct restriction enzyme digestion of the PCR product (check the supplier's recommendation for each enzyme).

3. A 60:1 mixture of *Taq* and a proofreading polymerase, such as Vent, ensures high fidelity but still allows sufficient addition of 3′-end nontemplated adenine onto the PCR product by *Taq* for initial cloning into a commercial "TA Cloning" vector.

4. Although it adds an additional cloning step, using an intermediate commercial cloning kit can greatly simplify the process of sequence verification and propagation for purification of insert to transfer to the structure cassette plasmid.

5. It is also possible to exploit a unique internal restriction site within the RNA-encoding sequence if one is present. This can be useful, for example, to clone RNAs beyond the limit of economical DNA synthesis (>100 nts). In this case a set of four DNA oligonucleotides corresponding to the coding and complementary strands of the 5′ and 3′ halves of the RNA should be individually phosphorylated, annealed in pairs, and mixed together with vector in ligation reactions. Once the initial construct is prepared the internal site can also be used to generate RNA sequence variants.

6. When using PNK to phosphorylate the oligonucleotides, it is important to use a buffer containing 10 mM ATP. Supplied T4 PNK buffer typically does not contain ATP whereas the similar T4 DNA ligase buffer does, making it a convenient substitute.

7. Acrylamides can be purchased as powders or in a premixed solution. Acrylamide is a neurotoxin that is easily absorbed

through the skin and is more dangerous when handled in powder form. For this reason, we use premixed solutions (30 or 40%). Here, we used denaturing (50% urea) gels with 8% acrylamide in 1× TBE buffer; the appropriate percent depends on the size of the RNA of interest.

8. *Pst*I and *Hind*III are used in this example protocol; when using structure cassette plasmids with the alternate restriction sites, simply substitute the appropriate restriction enzymes. Use an appropriate 10× buffer provided with the enzymes (at 1× final concentration) and incubate at 37°C for one hour, unless otherwise directed by the enzyme supplier. During this incubation, preparation of the insert can be started in parallel (see Subheading 3.1.1 or 3.1.2).

9. Running the plasmid over the column of a gel extraction kit will remove any CIAP and restriction enzymes present in the digest. Because the digested plasmid has not actually been cut from a gel, there is no need to heat the sample as one would for an actual gel extraction. Simply add the required volume of buffer for a 100 mg gel slice and then follow the manufacturer's instructions.

10. As the resulting number of colonies on each plate will later be compared to gauge the success of the ligation reaction, it is critical that all three transformations are prepared and treated identically. Ideally, a single stock of competent cells is thawed on ice, gently resuspended, and divided into equal volumes in three separate prechilled tubes. Volumes of ligation reaction and cells used can be increased to obtain more colonies but do not add ligation reaction volume corresponding to more than 10% of the volume of competent cells used. If a low ligation efficiency is expected, each transformation, after plating 100 μl of each transformation, microcentrifuge each aliquot of transformed cells, leaving <200 μl of supernatant in which cells are gently resuspended for plating on a second set of LB-agar plates.

11. A suitable starting point for the PCR is 25 cycles of denaturing (95°C, 45 s), annealing (57°C, 30 s), and extension (72°C, 90 s). The annealing temperature and magnesium concentration can be optimized to get a single intense band as the product of the reaction.

12. It is advisable to confirm the DNA oligonucleotide concentration using a spectrophotometer after redissolving in water.

13. Heat inactivation of the phosphorylation reaction is not necessary as the subsequent large dilution of the annealed oligos eliminates any effect the enzyme might have on the ligation reaction.

14. Denaturing gels should be used to assess the products of initial transcription experiments used to determine the optimal restriction site for run-off transcription, each new RNA in vitro transcription reaction, and purified RNA after extended storage. This analysis should be done prior to use in probing experiments to ensure that degradation of the RNA sample has not occurred. Although of little consequence to probing experiments, this type of gel can also show if there is any tendency for T7 RNA polymerase to add nontemplated nucleotides to the end of the RNA (e.g., see Fig. 2, lane corresponding to EBER RNA prepared from *Xho*I linearized template).

15. The annealing conditions suggested in the protocol are a convenient starting point; however the annealing temperature, time of incubation, and method/speed of cooling can all be varied in addition to the buffer conditions to identify the optimal annealing protocol for a new RNA. Higher temperatures are possible but we have found that VA RNA_I begins to degrade extensively at temperatures above 85°C. Problems of degradation at higher temperatures or extended incubation times will be exacerbated if divalent ions such as Mg^{2+} are required in the buffer. We have also found that the protocol producing a single RNA species may depend on the restriction enzyme that was used to linearize the plasmid for in vitro transcription (and thus the sequence of the RNA at its 3′-end beyond the RT primer binding site). Because of this variability, we recommend that for each new RNA, test transcriptions using each of the three possible linearization enzymes are performed and the resulting RNA tested (as shown for VA RNA_I and EBER1 in Fig. 3). It is worth noting that it is not always the run-off site producing the greatest RNA yield in the transcription reaction that produces the best RNA for structure probing.

16. For the best results, native gels should be run at 4°C. Prechill the buffer, assembled electrophoresis apparatus, and gel prior to running.

Acknowledgements

This work was supported by laboratory start-up funds from the Department of Biochemistry, the University Research Council of Emory University (grant 2010050), and the Microbiology and Molecular Genetics (MMG) NIH Training Grant (T32-AI007470). We thank Dr. Christine Dunham for critical comments on the manuscript during its preparation.

References

1. Merino EJ, Wilkinson KA, Coughlan JL, Weeks KM (2005) RNA structure analysis at single nucleotide resolution by selective 2′-hydroxyl acylation and primer extension (SHAPE). J Am Chem Soc 127:4223–4231
2. Reymond C, Levesque D, Bisaillon M, Perreault JP (2010) Developing three-dimensional models of putative-folding intermediates of the HDV ribozyme. Structure 18:1608–1616
3. Wilkinson KA, Merino EJ, Weeks KM (2005) RNA SHAPE chemistry reveals nonhierarchical interactions dominate equilibrium structural transitions in tRNA(Asp) transcripts. J Am Chem Soc 127:4659–4667
4. Mortimer SA, Weeks KM (2009) Time-resolved RNA SHAPE chemistry: quantitative RNA structure analysis in one-second snapshots and at single-nucleotide resolution. Nat Protoc 4:1413–1421
5. Watts JM, Dang KK, Gorelick RJ, Leonard CW, Bess JW Jr, Swanstrom R, Burch CL, Weeks KM (2009) Architecture and secondary structure of an entire HIV-1 RNA genome. Nature 460:711–716
6. Wilkinson KA, Merino EJ, Weeks KM (2006) Selective 2′-hydroxyl acylation analyzed by primer extension (SHAPE): quantitative RNA structure analysis at single nucleotide resolution. Nat Protoc 1:1610–1616
7. Vasa SM, Guex N, Wilkinson KA, Weeks KM, Giddings MC (2008) ShapeFinder: a software system for high-throughput quantitative analysis of nucleic acid reactivity information resolved by capillary electrophoresis. RNA 14:1979–1990
8. Badorrek CS, Weeks KM (2005) RNA flexibility in the dimerization domain of a gamma retrovirus. Nat Chem Biol 1:104–111
9. Walker SC, Avis JM, Conn GL (2003) General plasmids for producing RNA *in vitro* transcripts with homogeneous ends. Nucleic Acids Res 31:e82

Chapter 13

In Vitro Transcription of Modified RNAs

Stephanie L. Moon and Jeffrey Wilusz

Abstract

RNAs containing a variety of terminal and internal modifications can be produced using bacteriophage polymerases often with a few simple adjustments to standard transcription protocols. RNAs containing a single phosphate or a cap structure at their 5′ ends can readily be generated either co-transcriptionally or through enzymatic treatments of transcription products. Likewise, a variety of modified bases, including fluorescent or biotinylated species, can be effectively incorporated co-transcriptionally. The key to effective co-transcriptional incorporation lies in determining the efficiency of incorporation of modified base relative to its standard counterpart. Finally, an approach to place a poly(A) tail at the exact 3′ end of a desired transcription product is presented. Collectively, these protocols allow one to synthesize RNAs with a variety of modifications to serve as versatile molecules to analyze biological questions.

Key words: Transcription, Capping, 5′ Monophosphate, Fluorescent nucleotides, Poly(A) tail, Modified bases

1. Introduction

The efficient production of RNA by bacteriophage polymerases (e.g., T7, SP6, T3) using commercially available vectors or oligonucleotide-derived templates has provided an enormous boost to posttranscriptional research and molecular biology in general over the last 25 years (1, 2). A key aspect of this technology is the ability to produce RNAs containing directed physiological or synthetic modifications for specific applications. The goal of this chapter is to provide a discussion of key methodologies to produce transcripts with 5′, 3′, or internal modifications.

RNA substrates containing a *bona fide* 5′ cap structure and/or a 3′ poly(A) tail, for example, are invaluable for translation, RNA stability, and other mRNA functional analyses. RNAs with a 5′ monophosphate at their 5′ ends are extremely useful as efficient ligation substrates and for exonuclease assays. Transcripts with internally modified nucleotides have a plethora of applications. Internal biotin modifications, for example, can be used for affinity purification of RNA-binding proteins. The incorporation of radioactive rNTPs is used routinely for detection probes, protein–RNA interaction analyses, and substrates for a variety of cell-free RNA processing assays. The substitution with fluorescent bases creates opportunities for non-isotopic detection for a variety of assays, including protein–RNA interaction, RNA structural perturbations, and drug screening. Finally, the inclusion of a poly(A) tail at the precise 3′ end of an RNA creates a physiologically relevant substrate molecule for translation, deadenylation, and mRNA structure/function assays. Therefore, collectively the protocols described below should provide the RNA researcher with the ability to produce a variety of RNA modification to tailor the transcript to the desired application.

2. Materials

2.1. Production of RNAs with a Modified 5′ End

1. rNTP solution: 0.5 mM rGTP and 5 mM each of rCTP, rATP, rUTP (see Note 1). Store at −20°C or colder.
2. Guanosine-5′-monophosphate (5′-GMP) solution: 5 mM 5′-GMP dissolved in dd H_2O. Store at −20°C or colder.
3. Double-distilled H_2O (dd H_2O).
4. 5× Transcription Buffer: 200 mM Tris–HCl (pH 7.9), 30 mM $MgCl_2$, 10 mM spermidine, and 50 mM dithiothreitol.
5. Commercial RNase inhibitor, e.g., Ribolock RNAse Inhibitor, 40 u/μL (Fermentas).
6. SP6 or T7 RNA Polymerase, 50 u/μL.
7. Phenol–chloroform–isoamyl alcohol. Mix components in a 25:24:1 ratio.
8. 20 mg/mL glycogen in ddH_2O.
9. 10 M ammonium acetate.
10. Ethanol. Stock solutions of 100% (200 proof) and 80% (prepared with water) are required.
11. RNA Loading Dye: Mix 12 g urea, 0.185 g EDTA, 125 μL 1 M Tris–HCl (pH 7.5 at 25°C), 0.125 g bromophenol blue, and 0.125 g xylene cyanol. Dissolve all to a final volume of 25 mL with dd H_2O.
12. 40% acrylamide/bisacrylamide mix: Bisacylamide represents 5% of the total acrylamide in this solution prepared in water and filtered to remove any particulates (see Note 2).
13. TBE Gel Running Buffer: 450 mM Tris base, 445 mM boric acid, and 10 mM EDTA.

14. Urea/TBE Gel Mix: Mix 240 g urea (final concentration 7 M), 50 mL 10× TBE running buffer, and 200 mL distilled water.
15. 10% ammonium persulfate solution. Prepare in water and store at 4°C (see Note 3).
16. N,N,N,N′-tetramethyl-ethylenediamine (TEMED). Store at 4°C.
17. HSCB Buffer: 25 mM Tris–HCl (pH. 7.6 at 25°C), 400 mM NaCl, and 0.1% SDS.
18. 1 mg/mL proteinase K solution in water. Store at −80°C.

2.2. Production of RNAs with Internal Modifications

1. rNTP-flATP Labeling Solution: 0.5 mM rATP and 5 mM each of rCTP, rGTP, rUTP (see Note 4). Store at −20°C or colder.
2. Fluorescein-ATP Solution: 5 mM Fluorescein-12-ATP dissolved in ddH$_2$O. Store at −20°C or colder.
3. Other transcription-related reagents (items 3–18) described in Subheading 2.1.

2.3. Production of RNAs with a poly(A) Tail at Precisely the 3′ End

1. DNA oligonucleotides.
2. T4 polynucleotide kinase (10 U/μL).
3. 10× T4 kinase reaction buffer: 700 mM Tris–HCl (pH 7.6 at 25°C), 100 mM MgCl$_2$, and 50 mM dithiothreitol.
4. Oligonucleotide hybridization buffer: 10 mM Tris–HCl (pH 8.0 at 25°C), 50 mM NaCl, and 1 mM EDTA.
5. Ligation buffer: 20 mM Tris–Cl (pH 7.6 at 25°C), 10 mM MgCl$_2$, 10 mM dithiotreitol, and 0.6 mM ATP.
6. T4 DNA Ligase (400 U/μL).
7. 10 mM dNTPs dissolved in water. Store at −20°C.
8. 10× PCR reaction buffer: 100 mM Tris–HCl (pH 8.3 at 25°C), 15 mM MgCl$_2$, and 500 mM KCl.
9. Taq DNA polymerase.
10. *Nsi*I restriction enzyme.
11. Other transcription-related reagents (items 3–18) described in Subheading 2.1.

3. Methods

3.1. Production of RNAs Containing a Modified 5′ End

While standard transcription reactions using phage polymerases yield RNAs with a 5′ triphosphate, it is often desirable to generate RNAs with alternative 5′ ends. The production of an RNA with a 5′ m^{7}GTP cap, for example, is necessary for efficient in vitro translation (3), polyadenylation (4), RNA decay assays (5), and for many RNA transfection studies (6). The capping of the 5′ end of a transcript can readily be performed co-transcriptionally. Alternatively, an RNA containing a 5′ triphosphate can be capped using GTP and recombinant vaccinia capping enzyme (7), albeit at a much lower efficiency than what can be obtained by adding cap analogs directly to transcription reactions.

One common 5′ end modification that we have used for a variety of applications is the production of RNAs containing a 5′ monophosphate. These transcripts can be used directly in ligation reactions (8) and exonuclease assays (9). This protocol is presented below to serve as a model for the co-transcriptional modification of RNA 5′ ends.

1. In a 1.5 mL microfuge tube, mix together 3.5 µL of ddH$_2$O, 2 µL of 5× transcription buffer, 1 µL of rNTP solution, 1 µL of DNA template (1 µg/µL of plasmid or ~0.5 pmol of oligonucleotide template), 1 µL 5′ GMP solution, 0.5 µL (~20 units) of RNase inhibitor, and 1 µL of SP6 or T7 polymerase. Give the mixture a brief spin in a tabletop microfuge (e.g. ~500 × g for 3 s) to ensure that all of the reaction contents are at the bottom of the tube (see Notes 5 and 6).

2. Incubate reaction at 37°C for 1–3 h.

3. Add 150 µL of ddH$_2$O and 150 µL of phenol–chloroform–isoamyl alcohol (25:24:1). Vortex until the mixture goes from clear to white. Centrifuge in a table top microcentrifuge at 16,000 × g room temperature for 1 min, and pipet the aqueous top layer into a fresh 1.5 mL tube.

4. Add 1 µL glycogen (20 mg/mL) and 40 µL 10 M ammonium acetate (see Note 7). Add 500 µL ice cold 100% ethanol and vortex. Incubate at least 10 min at –80°C.

5. Spin in a microcentrifuge at full speed for 10 min at room temperature to pellet the RNA. Carefully remove supernatant without disturbing the white pellet.

6. Wash the pellet with 150 µL ice cold 80% ethanol. Remove as much of the ethanol as possible without disturbing the pellet and dry the pellet either under vacuum in a Speed Vac system or for 5–10 min on the bench top.

7. Resuspend the RNA either in 5 µL of RNA loading dye and proceed to purification (see step 8) or in 20 µL of ddH$_2$O for storage at –80°C if desired (see Note 8).

8. To gel purify the RNA, electrophorese the pellet resuspended in RNA loading dye on a vertical 5% denaturing acrylamide gel containing 7 M urea. Set up the glass plates and spacers to form the gel mold. In a 50 mL beaker, add 3.75 mL 40% acrylamide/bisacrylamide mix, 21.25 mL urea/TBE gel mix, 300 µL 10% ammonium persulfate, and 30 µL TEMED. Quickly pour the solution between the glass plates and insert the desired gel comb.

9. Pre-run the gel in 1× TBE buffer for 20–30 min before loading (see Note 9).

10. Heat the RNA sample to 95°C for 30 s, quick chill on ice and load onto the gel using a standard micropipette tip. Run the gel approximately 1 h using the migration of the marker dyes to determine the approximate position of the RNA transcript (see Note 10).

11. Visualize the position of the RNA by either UV shadowing the gel (see Note 11) or using X-ray film or a phosphorimager if the RNA product is labeled with radioactivity or a fluorescent dye.

12. Cut out desired products, and let the gel slice incubate at room temperature in 400 µL HSCB buffer overnight to allow for passive diffusion of the RNA from the gel fragment.

13. Pipet the supernatant into a fresh tube. Add 400 µL of phenol–chloroform–isoamyl alcohol (25:24:1). Vortex until the mixture goes from clear to white. Centrifuge in a table top microcentrifuge at 16,000×g room temperature for 1 min, and pipet the aqueous top layer into a fresh 1.5 mL tube.

14. Add 1 µL glycogen (20 mg/mL) and 1 mL of ice cold 100% ethanol and vortex. Precipitate and wash the RNA pellet as described in steps 5–7 above, and resuspend the pellet in 20 µL of ddH$_2$O.

3.2. Production of RNAs with Internal Modifications

The incorporation of modified ribonucleotides into transcripts generated by conventional run-off transcriptions is an effective approach to produce large amounts of RNA for a variety of applications. A co-transcriptional incorporation procedure is described below. Note that a variety of modifications can also be added by splinted ligation approaches (8) that are described elsewhere in this book. The incorporation of fluorescently labeled ribonucleic acids into reporter transcripts using in vitro transcriptions is particularly useful in determining changes in RNA structure and binding affinity to particular ligands, including therapeutic compounds, using fluorescence spectroscopy (10). Although the attachment of fluorescent analogs to pyrimidines has traditionally not been pursued in favor of the use of purine analogues (particularly 2-aminopurine), the efficient incorporation of furan-containing ribonucleic acids via T7 run-off transcription has been described (10). Similarly, modified UTP containing positively charged, hydrophobic groups at the 5-position have also been shown to be permissive to T7-mediated incorporation into run-off transcription products (11). Interestingly, efforts are being made to expand the capacity of the T7 polymerase to incorporate modified nucleotides into nascent RNA transcripts by manipulating the enzyme itself (12). Chelliserrykattil and Ellington reported the generation of a variant T7 RNA polymerase with improved ability to incorporate 2′-O-methyl ribose nucleotides with the goal of enhancing RNA stability with removal of the 2′ hydroxyl group (12, 13).

Table 1
A survey of commercially available modified nucleotides that can be incorporated into RNA co-transcriptionally

Company	Hapten nucleotide analogs	Fluorescent analogs
PerkinElmer	Haptens: Biotin-ATP, -CTP, -GTP, -UTP Dinitrophenol-UTP	Fluorescent-labeled: Fluorescein-ATP, -CTP, -GTP,-UTP Cyanine-3 (UTP, GTP, ATP, CTP) Cyanine-5 (UTP, GTP, ATP, CTP)
Invitrogen (Life Technologies)		ChromaTide™ UTPs: Alexa Fluor 488, AlexaFluor 546, Fluorescein, Rhodamine Green
Applied Biosystems (Life Technologies)		Aminoallyl-UTP (transcript can be labeled subsequently with amine-reactive fluor or hapten of choice)
Fermentas (Thermo Fisher Scientific)		Aminoallyl-UTP (transcript can be labeled subsequently with amine-reactive fluor or hapten of choice)
Roche Applied Science	Haptens: Biotin-UTP Dinitrophenol-UTP	

Although the following protocol is described using fluorescein-ATP, it can be readily adapted for the incorporation of many other modified NTPs. Table 1 outlines some of the modified rNTPs that can be added by simply substituting the desired modified base for fluorescein-ATP. Note that if one chooses to incorporate aminoallyl-UTP using T7, T3, or SP6 polymerase, the RNA can subsequently be labeled with any amine-reactive fluor or hapten.

1. In a 1.5 mL microfuge tube, mix together 3.5 µL of ddH$_2$O, 2 µL of 5× transcription buffer, 1 µL of rNTP-flATP labeling solution, 1 µL of DNA template (1 µg/µL of plasmid or ~0.5 pmol of oligonucleotide template), 1 µL Fluorescein-ATP solution, 0.5 µL (~20 units) of RNase inhibitor and 1 µL of SP6 or T7 polymerase. Give the mixture a brief spin in a tabletop microfuge (e.g. ~500 ×g for 3 s) to ensure that all of the reaction contents are at the bottom of the tube.

2. Proceed as described in the protocol of Subheading 3.1, steps 2–13.

3.3. Production of RNAs with a poly(A) Tail at Precisely the 3' End

Commercial vectors for in vitro transcription reactions do not provide a means to generate an RNA with a poly(A) tail at precisely the 3' end of the transcript. The production of such a transcript could be highly desirable since it makes the in vitro synthesized RNA as biologically relevant as possible. Plasmid vectors have been described that encode a 60 base poly(A) tail followed immediately by an *Nsi*I site (14). Cleavage using this restriction enzyme and subsequent run off transcription allows the poly(A) stretch to be located at precisely the 3′ end of the RNA. Alternatively, one can add poly(A) stretches posttranscriptionally using yeast or bacterial poly(A) polymerases (see Note 12). However if one desires to avoid extra cloning and RNA modification steps, below is a straightforward PCR-based approach that will allow a fragment encoding a poly(A) tail to be attached onto any DNA fragment such that the adenosine stretch will appear at the precise 3′ end of the subsequent run-off transcription product.

1. Synthesize a complementary pair of oligonucleotides containing the following structure:

   XXXXAAAAA(n)AAAAATGCATTACCTCGAGCACTC
       TTTTT(n)TTTTTACGTAATGGAGCTCGTGAG

   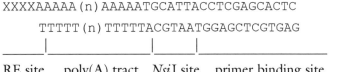

   RE site   poly(A) tract   *Nsi*I site   primer binding site

   See Note 13 for a complete description of the roles of the four regions of this oligonucleotide.

2. Change the 5′ end of the oligonucleotides from a 5′ hydroxyl to a 5′ phosphate using 1 μL of T4 polynucleotide kinase and 1 μL 10× kinase reaction buffer in a 10 μL reaction for 1 h at 37°C.

3. Hybridize the synthetic oligonucleotides by adding 100 pmol of each strand in 100 μL of oligo hybridization buffer. Place the tube in a heating block at 100°C, turn off the block and allow it to slowly cool to room temperature to ensure that the most stable hybrid is formed.

4. Ligate the hybridized oligonucleotides to the target DNA fragment. Mix 1 pmol of restriction enzyme-cut target DNA (or 1 pmol of oligonucleotide transcription template containing a four base single-stranded overhang) with 1 pmol of hybridized oligos in a 10 μL reaction containing 1 μL of ligation buffer and 10 units of T4 DNA ligase. Incubate at room temperature for at least 1 h or overnight at 15°C.

5. To amplify the ligated products by PCR, mix 5 μL of the ligation reaction, 50 pmol of an SP6 or T7 promoter primer (e.g. SP6 = 5′-CATACGATTTAGGTGACACTATAG), 50 pmol of a downstream primer (5′-GAGTGCTCGAGGTA); note—this is specific for the primer binding site region of the ligated oligonucleotide), 10 mM dNTPs, 10 mM Tris–Cl (pH 8.3), 1.5 mM $MgCl_2$, 50 mM KCl, and 20–25 units of Taq polymerase in a 500 μL reaction. Perform at least 30 cycles of amplification in a thermocycler: denaturation at 94°C for 1 min; annealing at 43°C for 1 min; and extension at 72°C for 1 min, for the example presented here.

6. Extract the PCR reaction mixture with phenol–chloroform–isoamyl alcohol (25:24:1) and concentrate the DNA by ethanol

precipitation as described in Subheading 3.1, steps 3–7. Alternatively, amplified products can also be purified from agarose gels or using spin columns if desired.

7. Resuspend the DNA in 100 µL of TE buffer. Treat the DNA with *Nsi*I according to the manufacturer's recommendations in order to place the A/T tract at the precise 3′ end of the transcription template.

8. Following digestion, add 400 µL of HSCB buffer along with 20–30 µg of proteinase K. Incubate at 37°C for 15 min (see Note 14).

9. Phenol–choroform–isoamyl alcohol extract and ethanol precipitate the DNA as described in Subheading 3.1, steps 3–7. Resuspend the DNA in 100 µL of TE buffer.

10. Transcribe the DNA template as described in Subheading 3.1 or 3.2 depending on the application of the RNA that will be generated.

4. Notes

1. The amount of rGTP is reduced tenfold relative to other rNTPs to allow for efficient incorporation of the 5′GMP at the initiation step of transcription. Since phage polymerases strongly prefer to begin transcription with a G residue, this nucleotide mixture is generally applicable for all 5′ modifications. Note that for internal modifications, the relative concentrations of rNTPs are adjusted to accommodate the efficient incorporation of modified bases.

2. Unpolymerized acrylamide is a neurotoxin and should be handled carefully.

3. Solution will lose potency over time. Best results are obtained with solutions less than a week old.

4. The concentration of rGTP in the solution should be lowered to 0.5 mM if the transcript is to be capped co-transcriptionally.

5. The two largest sources of problems that affect the yield of transcription reactions in our hands has been the quality of the reagents used and the quality of the DNA template. These can be minimized by purchasing high-quality chemicals from a reputable supplier, using double-distilled water and ensuring the purity and concentration of the DNA template.

6. Ten times more 5′ GMP (or m7GpppG cap analog) than 5′ GTP is added to the reaction since it is utilized less efficiently than the nucleotide triphosphate by the phage polymerase.

This is common with modified bases and we use the 10× concentration as an empirical starting point when coaxing the polymerase to add modified bases.

7. The use of ammonium acetate is preferred over sodium salts in this step since unincorporated rNTPs will not be effectively precipitated in the presence of ammonium salts. This aids in the purification of the RNA product away from the reaction components.

8. Note that the reaction can be stored at −80°C for extended periods of time in ethanol without loss of RNA quality.

9. The acrylamide gel is pre-run to allow the ion front that develops during the preparation of the gel to move down the gel. If this is not done, it could influence the migration of RNAs of interest.

10. On a 5% denaturing gel, the bromophenol blue dye runs approximately at the position of a 27–30 base RNA. The xylene cyanol runs at approximately the site of a 120 base RNA.

11. To UV shadow RNA on a gel, carefully place the gel on a piece of Saran Wrap and overlay this onto a TLC plate that contains a fluor which will absorb at 260 nm light. When the gel is irradiated with short wave UV light, the RNA will appear as a black shadow on the gel as it absorbs the light and prevents it from hitting the fluor below it.

12. In our hands, it has been very difficult to control the size of the poly(A) tail added to the ends of RNA using yeast poly(A) polymerase. This product heterogeneity requires an extra gel purification step which often results in low yields of RNAs containing defined lengths of poly(A).

13. The sequence of the restriction enzyme overhang in the oligo is used to hybridize with a convenient restriction enzyme site at the downstream end of the target DNA fragment for ligation purposes. If oligonucleotides instead of plasmid DNA are being used as the parent template, then any 4 base sequence can be used here as long as it hybridizes to the template. The A/T tract will serve as template for the poly(A) tail upon transcription. The length of the tract used can be determined by the researcher. We have successfully used A/T tracts up to 120 nucleotides long in this procedure. *Nsi*I is used to cleave the template so that the run off transcription product ends precisely with the poly(A) tail. The primer binding site is used for amplification of ligation products via PCR. The sequence of this primer binding site can be varied if necessary.

14. This step will degrade any proteins (including ribonucleases) in your reaction mixture and allow for transcription templates that will give consistently good results.

Acknowledgments

We wish to thank members of the Wilusz Laboratories for their input and helpful comments. RNA research in the laboratory is supported by grants from the NIH (R01-GM072481 and U54-AI-065357) to J.W. S.L.M. is supported by a training grant from the USDA (2010-38420-20367).

References

1. Melton DA, Krieg PA, Rebagliati MR, Maniatis T, Zinn K, Green MR (1984) Efficient in vitro synthesis of biologically active RNA and RNA hybridization probes from plasmids containing a bacteriophage SP6 promoter. Nucleic Acids Res 12:7035–7056
2. Milligan JF, Groebe DR, Witherell GW, Uhlenbeck OC (1987) Oligoribonucleotide synthesis using T7 RNA polymerase and synthetic DNA templates. Nucleic Acids Res 15:8783–8798
3. Olliver L, Boyd CD (1998) In vitro translation of messenger RNA in a rabbit reticulocyte lysate cell-free system. Methods Mol Biol 86:221–227
4. Flaherty SM, Fortes P, Izaurralde E, Mattaj IW, Gilmartin GM (1997) Participation of the nuclear cap binding complex in pre-mRNA 3′ processing. Proc Natl Acad Sci USA 94:11893–11898
5. Sokoloski KJ, Wilusz J, Wilusz CJ (2008) The preparation and applications of cytoplasmic extracts from mammalian cells for studying aspects of mRNA decay. Methods Enzymol 448:139–163
6. Yunus MA, Chung LM, Chaudhry Y, Bailey D, Goodfellow I (2010) Development of an optimized RNA-based murine norovirus reverse genetics system. J Virol Methods 169:112–118
7. Shuman S, Moss B (1990) Purification and use of vaccinia virus messenger RNA capping enzyme. Methods Enzymol 181:170–180
8. Solomatin S, Herschlag D (2009) Methods of site-specific labeling of RNA with fluorescent dyes. Methods Enzymol 469:47–68
9. Mukherjee D, Fritz DT, Kilpatrick WJ, Gao M, Wilusz J (2004) Analysis of RNA exonucleolytic activities in cellular extracts. Methods Mol Biol 257:193–212
10. Srivatsan SG, Tor Y (2007) Fluorescent pyrimidine ribonucleotide: synthesis, enzymatic incorporation, and utilization. J Am Chem Soc 129:2044–2053
11. Vaught JD, Dewey T, Eaton BE (2004) T7 RNA polymerase transcription with 5-position modified UTP derivates. J Am Chem Soc 126:11231–11237
12. Chelliserrykattil J, Ellington AD (2004) Evolution of a T7 polymerase variant that transcribes 2′ O methyl RNA. Nat Biotechnol 22:1155–1160
13. Chelliserrykattil J, Cai G, Ellington AD (2001) A combined in vitro/in vivo selection for polymerases with novel promoter specificities. BMC Biotechnol 22:1155–1160
14. Garneau NL, Sokoloski KJ, Opyrchal M, Neff CP, Wilusz CJ, Wilusz J (2008) The 3′ untranslated region of sindbis virus represses deadenylation of viral transcripts in mosquito and mammalian cells. J Virol 82:880–892

Chapter 14

End-Labeling Oligonucleotides with Chemical Tags After Synthesis

N. Ruth Zearfoss and Sean P. Ryder

Abstract

Many experimental strategies for determining nucleic acid function require labeling the nucleic acid with radioisotopes or a chemical tag. Labels enable nucleic acid detection, yield information about its state, and can serve as a handle by which the nucleic acid and associated factors can be purified from a mixture. Radioactive phosphate is commonly added to the 5′ or 3′ end of an oligonucleotide post synthesis using enzyme-catalyzed reactions. In contrast, chemical tags are usually added during synthesis or using reactive groups that are incorporated during synthesis. Here, we present protocols for post-synthetic conjugation of chemical tags to unmodified RNA or DNA oligonucleotides. The approach can be used to attach fluorescent dyes and biotin groups to oligonucleotides and to immobilize oligonucleotides to a solid support. Oligonucleotides tagged with fluorescent dyes are readily detected in both gel- and plate reader-based assays, while biotin- or resin-conjugated oligonucleotides are useful tools for affinity purification. Fluorescent end-labeling provides several advantages over radioactive labeling, reducing radioactivity-associated hazards and yielding a labeled molecule that does not decay while providing the sensitivity required for many procedures.

Key words: Nucleic acids, RNA, Oligonucleotides, End-labeling, Fluorescent dyes, Biotin

1. Introduction

Nucleic acids are routinely labeled with isotopes or chemical tags to facilitate a wide variety of experiments. Radioactive labels have the advantage of providing a high level of detection sensitivity and can be added to any oligonucleotide post synthesis (1), but their use is complicated by the hazardous nature of radiochemicals, the regulations surrounding them, and their limited lifetimes. Chemical tags offer an alternative to radioactive labeling and provide sufficient sensitivity for many experiments. For example, fluorescent ribonucleic acids have been used to quantitatively assess binding affinity in electromobility shift and fluorescence polarization (FP) assays

(2–5) and fluorescent DNA primers to monitor product formation in semiquantitative PCR (6). Modification of nucleic acids with chemical tags also expands the range of experiments that can be performed. For example, both FP and fluorescence resonance energy transfer assays rely on the chemical properties of fluorescent dyes and cannot be performed using radioisotope labels. RNA oligonucleotides can be labeled with biotin, allowing them to interact with streptavidin-conjugated resins, facilitating purification of associated factors (7). Oligonucleotides can also be directly coupled to solid supports for a similar purpose (8).

Chemical tags and chemically reactive groups are often added to oligonucleotides during synthesis. Although convenient, this strategy adds cost, especially if the experiment requires both labeled and unlabeled variants of the same sequence. End-labeling oligonucleotides after synthesis offers a simple and easily adapted alternative. We describe protocols for the labeling reactions below. The protocols are applicable to several types of chemical tags, and options are available for modifying both DNA and RNA.

For labeling the 5′ end of an oligonucleotide, we employ a two-step strategy, following a method described by Czworkowski et al. (9). The strategy makes use of the ability of bacteriophage T4 polynucleotide kinase (T4 PNK) to transfer a phosphate to the 5′ end of RNA or DNA oligonucleotides. In the reaction, ATP is substituted with adenosine 5′-(γ-thio)triphosphate (ATPγS), an ATP analog where the gamma phosphate is replaced with a phosphorothioate. The product is a phosphorylated oligonucleotide with a unique reactive sulfur at the 5′ end. The oligonucleotide can then be incubated with a haloacetamide derivative of a chemical tag, which reacts with the phosphorothioate to produce a labeled oligonucleotide (Fig. 1). We routinely use 5-(iodoacetamido)fluorescein (5-IAF) to conjugate a fluorophore to the 5′-end of DNA and RNA oligonucleotides; however, other reagents can be employed should different chemical properties be required. Several commercially available fluorescent haloacetamides are listed in Table 1, along with their absorbance and emission maxima. Note that these reagents have not all been tested in our protocol; therefore, optimization may be necessary.

The 3′ end-labeling strategy also makes use of two steps, as described by Reines and Cantor (10). First, sodium periodate is used to oxidize the 3′ terminal ribose sugar, forming reactive aldehydes. Second, the oxidized sugar is conjugated to an aldehyde-reactive chemical tag, such as fluorescein 5-thiosemicarbazide (FTSC; Fig. 2). Because periodate oxidation requires vicinal hydroxyls, the reaction is specific for RNA and only modifies the 3′ terminal ribose. The abundance of aldehyde-reactive chemical tags enables conjugation of a wide variety of fluorophores (Table 2). Additionally, oligonucleotides can be conjugated to biotin, using (+)-biotinamidohexanoic acid hydrazide (BACH), or to a solid

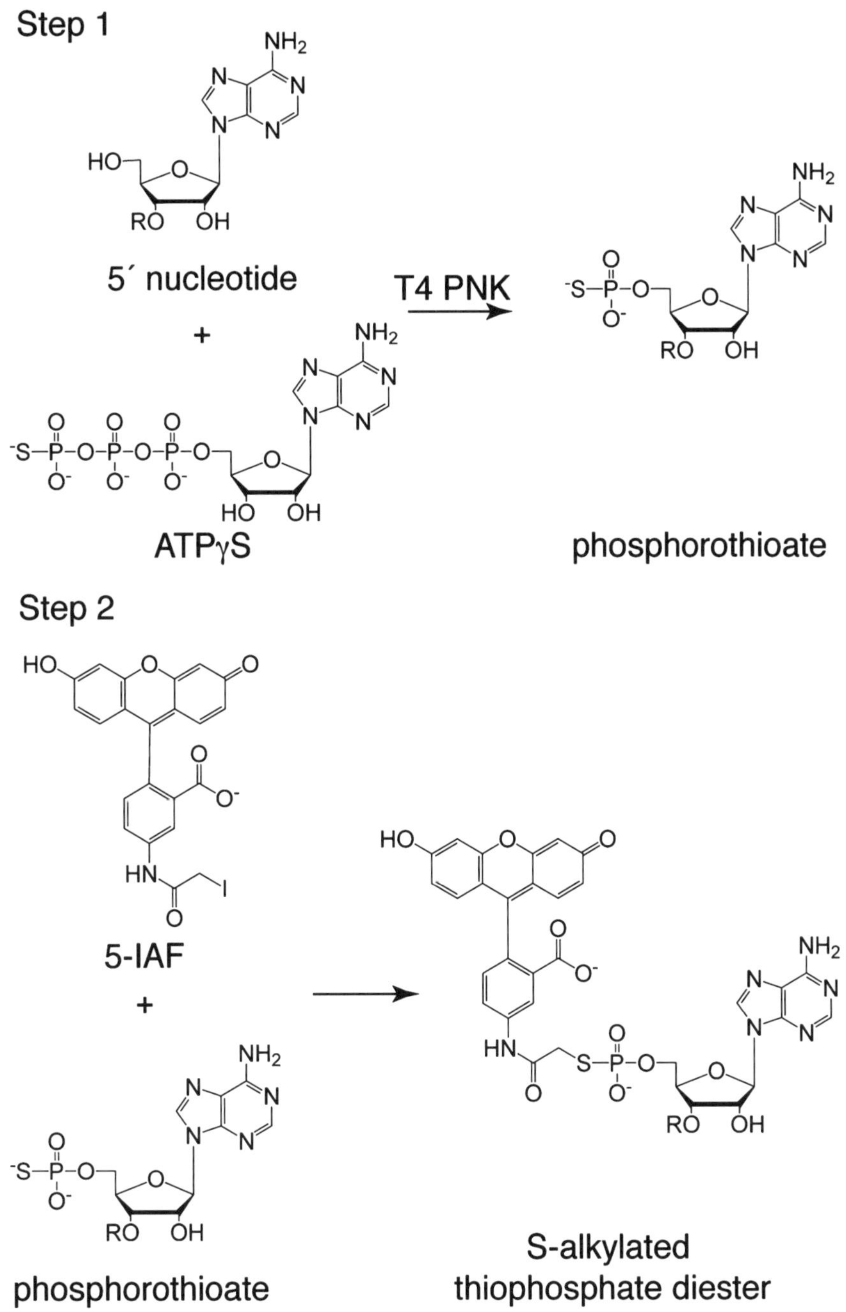

Fig. 1. 5' labeling of DNA and RNA oligonucleotides with fluorescein. Labeling is carried out in two steps. In the *first step*, bacteriophage T4 PNK is used to attach a phosphorothioate from ATPγS to the 5' terminal nucleotide. In the *second step*, the phosphorothioate is reacted with 5-IAF, covalently attaching fluorescein to the oligonucleotide at its 5' end through the unique reactive sulfur. Adenine is used as a representative base in the nucleic acid.

matrix, using adipic-acid dihydrazide-agarose. Both strategies do not require specialized equipment and can be performed on the bench top, adding to the convenience of chemical tags compared to radioactive labels.

Table 1
Commercially available phosphorothioate-reactive iodoacetamides or bromoacetamides that can be used to label the 5′ end of DNA or RNA oligonucleotides

Reagent	Excitation maximum (nm)	Emission maximum (nm)
7-Diethylamino-3-(4-(iodoacetamido)phenyl)-4-methylcoumarin (DCIA)	389	467
Lucifer yellow iodoacetamide	426	531
5-(Iodoacetamido)fluorescein (5-IAF)	492	515
Oregon Green iodoacetamide	496	524
BODIPY FL iodoacetamide	505	513
BIODIPY 507/545 iodoacetamide	507	545
Tetramethyl rhodamine iodoacetamide (TMRIA)	555	580
Texas Red bromoacetamide	595	615
NIR-664 iodoacetamide	664	689

Oligonucleotides with fluorescent labels can easily be detected on modern instruments. Figure 3 shows two examples: an RNA electromobility shift assay conducted with RNA that was labeled at the 3′ end with FTSC and an RT-PCR assay carried out with DNA primers that were labeled at the 5′ end with 5-IAF. In both cases, the gel was scanned while wet on a Fuji Fluorescent Image Analyzer (FLA-5000 or FLA-9000) using a blue laser. In instruments equipped with multiple lasers, capable of specifically exciting a subset of fluorophores with the appropriate excitation spectra, it may be possible to monitor multiple nucleic acids in the same gel, by adjusting the excitation and emission wavelengths used during the scan. The diversity of fluorescent reagents available is a great asset to the development of such techniques.

2. Materials

Throughout the procedure, care should be taken to maintain an RNase-free environment. Gloves should be used at all times. Water should be MilliQ quality or similar and should be filter sterilized through a 0.2 μm filter. Buffers should be prepared with MilliQ water and filter sterilized prior to use. Additionally, all plasticware should be certified RNase-free. We do not find the use of diethylpyrocarbonate to be necessary in a laboratory environment where

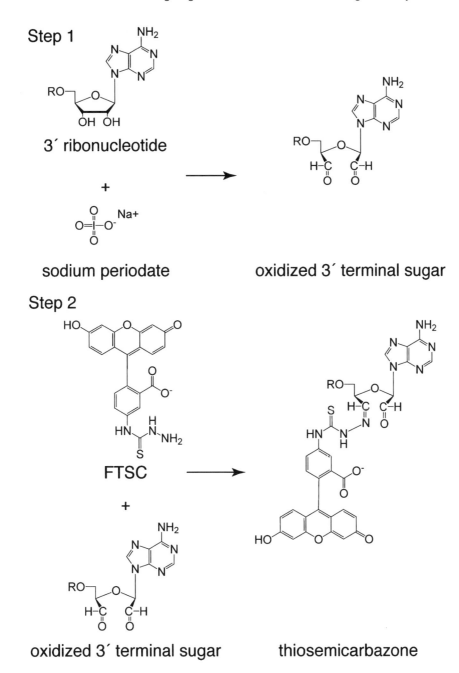

Fig. 2. 3′ labeling of RNA oligonucleotides. Labeling is carried out in two steps. In the *first step*, the vicinal diols of the 3′ terminal sugar are oxidized with sodium periodate, to form reactive aldehydes. In the *second step*, the oxidized nucleic acid is incubated with fluorescein 5-thiosemicarbazide, to form a covalent semicarbazone linkage between fluorescein and the 3′ end of the oligonucleotide. Adenine is used as a representative base in the nucleic acid.

RNase precautions are routinely used. Fluorescent reagents should be shielded from light as often as possible in order to prevent quenching. Individual microcentrifuge tubes and racks can be wrapped in aluminum foil, and fluorescent RNAs should be stored in the dark at −20°C.

Table 2
Commercially available aldehyde-reactive compounds that can be used to selectively label the 3′ end of RNA oligonucleotides

Reagent	Excitation maximum (nm)	Emission maximum (nm)
Alexa Fluor 350 hydrazide	345	445
Fluorescein 5-thiosemicarbazide	492	515
BODIPY FL hydrazide	505	513
Alexa Fluor 568 hydrazide	576	599
Texas Red hydrazide	595	615
Alexa Fluor 647	649	666

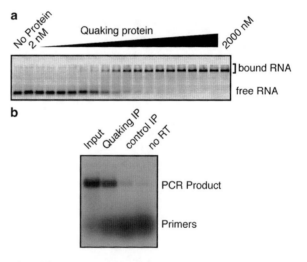

Fig. 3. Examples of fluorescent nucleic acid use. (**a**) An RNA electromobility shift assay. RNA was labeled at the 3′ end with FTSC as described in the accompanying protocol and incubated with the indicated concentration of protein. After incubation, the reaction was loaded onto a native gel and electrophoresed. The gel was scanned while wet on a Fuji FLA-5000 with a blue laser. (**b**) A semiquantitative RT-PCR assay. DNA primers were labeled at the 5′ end as described in the accompanying protocol and used in RT-PCR using a one-step RT-PCR kit, as described by the manufacturer. After thermocycling, the reaction was analyzed on an agarose gel. Immediately after electrophoresis, the gel was scanned on a Fuji FLA-5000 with a blue laser. Note that the signal is proportional to the number of moles of the nucleic acid in each band, rather than the mass. Images reproduced with permission from ref. 6 under the Creative Commons Attribution License.

1. 0.1 mM nucleic acid in an aqueous solution. We routinely use chemically synthesized RNA or DNA oligonucleotides. The resuspension solution can be either water or TE (10 mM Tris–Cl pH 8.0, 1 mM EDTA).
2. 3 M Sodium acetate, pH 5.2.

3. Ethanol, 200 proof.
4. 70% Ethanol in water.
5. 20 mg/ml Glycogen.
6. Incubator or water bath at 37°C.
7. Centrifuges: Microcentrifuge and low-speed centrifuge.
8. −20°C Freezer.
9. Spectrophotometer capable of reading both UV and visible range absorbance.
10. Microcentrifuge tubes.
11. Aluminum foil.
12. Spin columns filled with Sephadex G-25 or another suitable resin. The type of resin should be optimized for the size of the nucleic acid and the particular fluorescent molecule being used (see Note 1).

2.1. Materials Specific for Labeling RNA or DNA at the 5′ End

1. 5-IAF or other fluorescent iodoacetamide (see Note 2; Table 1). 5-IAF is unstable and should be dissolved in DMSO immediately before use (see Note 3). Additionally, it should be stored desiccated at −20°C.
2. 25 mM ATPγS, prepared in MilliQ water immediately prior to use (see Note 3).
3. T4 PNK.
4. 10× T4 PNK Buffer: 700 mM Tris–Cl pH 7.6 and 100 mM $MgCl_2$.
5. 0.1 M Dithiothreitol (DTT).
6. Phenol/chloroform/isoamyl alcohol (25:24:1).
7. 25 mM HEPES, pH 7.4.
8. Dimethyl sulfoxide (DMSO).

2.2. Materials Specific for Labeling RNA at the 3′ End

1. 200 mM FTSC prepared in dimethylformamide (DMF) and stored at −20°C (see Note 2). Alternatively, for biotin labeling, a stock of 25 mg/ml BACH can be prepared in DMSO.
2. 50 mM $NaIO_4$.
3. 5 M NaCl.

3. Methods

3.1. Labeling RNA or DNA at the 5′ End

1. Assemble the phosphorylation reaction, using ATPγS as a substrate for T4 PNK. We typically label 1.5 nmoles of oligonucleotide in a 50 μl volume. The reaction is assembled as described in Table 3, and contains the following final reagent

Table 3
Components of a phosphorylation reaction with ATPγS

Reagent	Volume added	Stock concentration
Water	28.5 µl	NA
T4 PNK buffer	5 µl	10×
DTT	2.5 µl	0.1 M
ATPγS	1 µl	25 mM
Oligonucleotide	11 µl	0.1 mM
T4 PNK	2 µl	10 U/µl

concentrations: 0.03 mM oligonucleotide, 0.5 mM ATPγS, 1× T4 PNK buffer, 5 mM DTT, and 0.4 U/µl T4 PNK. ATPγS should be prepared immediately before use.

2. Incubate overnight at 37°C (see Note 4). Shorter incubation times may be possible, but the reaction is slower with ATPγS compared to ATP.

3. Extract the nucleic acid from the reaction with phenol/chloroform/isoamyl alcohol. To facilitate recovery of the aqueous phase, add 150 µl (3 volumes) of water prior to extraction. Add an equal volume (200 µl) of phenol/chloroform/isoamyl alcohol (25:24:1). Mix until emulsified and centrifuge for 5 min at ≥16,000×g. Carefully remove and save the aqueous supernatant, leaving the interphase behind.

4. Precipitate with ethanol: Add 20 µl (0.1 volume) of 3 M sodium acetate pH 5.2, 1 µl of 20 mg/ml glycogen, and 550 µl (2.5 volumes) of 200 proof ethanol. Mix gently and incubate at −20°C for at least 30 min or on dry ice for 20 min.

5. Centrifuge the tubes at ≥16,000×g for 25 min at 4°C. At the end of the centrifugation, the pellet should be visible as a small 1–2 mm white spot at the bottom of the tube. The carrier glycogen aids in visualizing the pellet.

6. Remove the supernatant and wash the pellet with 1 ml of 70% ethanol. Centrifuge briefly before removing the wash solution (see Note 5).

7. Briefly air-dry, for approximately 1 min, to remove residual ethanol, but do not overdry or the pellet will be difficult to resuspend.

8. Resuspend the pellet in 42.5 µl 25 mM HEPES pH 7.4.

9. Immediately before use, prepare a 10 mM stock of 5-IAF in DMSO. Make a small stock; the unused portion should be discarded at the end of the day.

Table 4
Components of a sodium periodate oxidation reaction

Reagent	Volume	Stock
Water	25 μl	NA
Sodium acetate, pH 5.2	10 μl	0.5 M
RNA oligonucleotide	5 μl	100 μM
NaIO$_4$	10 μl	0.5 mM

Table 5
Components of a fluorescein 5-thiosemicarbazide (FTSC) labeling solution

Reagent	Volume	Stock
Sodium acetate, pH 5.2	80 μl	0.5 M
Fluorescein 5-thiosemicarbazide	3 μl	200 mM (in DMF)
Water	317 μl	NA

10. Add 7.5 μl of the 10 mM 5-IAF solution (vast excess, 50 equivalents) to the phosphorothioate oligonucleotide. The excess reactant helps drive the reaction to completion. Mix gently and incubate for 2–3 h at room temperature in the dark. Proceed to purification (Subheading 3.3).

3.2. Labeling RNA at the 3′ End

1. Prepare a fresh solution of 0.5 mM NaIO$_4$ from a 50 mM stock solution.

2. Assemble the oxidation reaction. We typically label 0.5 nmoles of oligonucleotide in a 50 μl volume. The oxidation reaction is assembled as described in Table 4 and contains the following final reagent concentrations: 100 mM NaOAc pH 5.2, 100 μM NaIO$_4$, and 10 μM RNA.

3. React at room temperature for 90 min.

4. Precipitate the RNA by adding 2.5 μl 5 M NaCl (0.05 volume), 1 μl 20 mg/ml glycogen, and 100 μl of 200 proof ethanol (2 volumes). Incubate at −20°C for 20 min and spin at ≥16,000 × g for 25 min.

5. Meanwhile, prepare a fresh FTSC labeling solution containing 1.5 mM FTSC and 100 mM NaOAc pH 5.2 (see Note 6). See Table 5 for specific amounts. If BACH is used for biotin labeling, use 9 μl of 25 mg/ml BACH and decrease the water to maintain the same final volume.

6. Remove the supernatant from the pelleted RNA, carefully removing the last traces of the ethanol with a 200 μl pipet tip. Air-dry briefly, for approximately 1 min, and resuspend each pellet in 50 μl (vast excess, 150 equivalents in this example) of the FTSC or BACH labeling solution (see Note 5).
7. Incubate the labeling reaction at 4°C overnight in the dark. Proceed to purification (Subheading 3.3).

3.3. Purification of Labeled Nucleic Acids

1. Precipitate the nucleic acid by adding 5 μl of 3 M NaOAc pH 5.2 (0.1 volumes) and 140 μl ethanol (2.5 volumes). Mix and then incubate at −20°C for at least 30 min or on dry ice for 20 min.
2. Centrifuge at ≥16,000×g for 25 min at 4°C to pellet the labeled nucleic acid. If fluorescein is used as the label, at this point, unreacted fluorescein will remain in the supernatant, and the fluorescein-labeled pellet will have a deep yellow color. A white pellet is an indication that the reaction was not successful.
3. Remove the supernatant and wash the pellet by adding 1 ml of 70% ethanol. Briefly centrifuge and remove the wash solution without dislodging the pellet (see Note 5).
4. Resuspend the pellet in 50 μl of 0.1× TE.
5. Prepare a Sephadex G-25 (see Note 1) column by adding 2 ml of a 12.5% slurry of Sephadex G-25 resin to a 2 ml centrifuge column. With the column placed in a 15 ml conical centrifuge tube, centrifuge at 1,100×g for 1 min in a swinging bucket rotor to pack the column. Add 50 μl 0.1× TE to the top of the column and centrifuge again at 1,100×g for 1 min.
6. Place two microcentrifuge tubes with their lids removed inside the bottom of a clean 15 ml conical centrifuge tube. Place the packed column in the tube. The tip of the column should fall near the top of the upper microcentrifuge tube.
7. Add the labeled nucleic acid to the column. Take care to apply the nucleic acid directly to the center of the top of the Sephadex bed. If the sample is applied to the edge, significant amounts of contaminating free fluorescein can pass into the eluate by running between the resin bed and the inner wall of the column (see Note 7).
8. Centrifuge at 1,100×g for 2 min. Keep the flow-through, which should have a pale yellow hue if fluorescein was used as the label.
9. For fluorescein-labeled nucleic acids, determine the labeling efficiency by measuring the absorbance at 260 nm, to obtain the nucleic acid concentration, and at 492 nm, to obtain the fluorescein concentration (see Note 8). The labeling efficiency is the molar ratio of fluorescein to nucleic acid. Typically, labeling efficiencies of 60–70% can be obtained for 5′ labeling and 70–90% for 3′ labeling (see Note 9).

4. Notes

1. For nucleic acids in the range of 10–30 nucleotides, we purify the labeled oligonucleotide with G-25 resin; however, for longer nucleic acids it may be preferable to use G-50, which has a larger pore size and may provide a more efficient separation. Columns can be commercially obtained or can be prepared on site by swelling dry resin in 0.1× TE for at least 3 h, adding 2 ml to an empty 2 ml centrifuge column, spinning for 1 min at $1,100 \times g$, washing one time with 50 µl 0.1× TE, and repeating the centrifugation. Different fluorescent substrates may have different separation characteristics on the resin, and it may be necessary to optimize this step when labeling with fluorophores other than fluorescein.

2. When adapting the protocol for use with fluorophores other than fluorescein, it may be useful to try several fluorophores with the desired excitation and emission spectra. One reason is that interactions between the fluorophore and nearby bases may occur, influencing the fluorescence properties of the labeled nucleic acid. For example, BODIPY GTPγS has been reported to undergo electron-transfer quenching due to an interaction between the BODIPY dye and guanine (11).

3. We find the 5′ labeling procedure to be particularly sensitive to the quality of the reagents. Aged bottles of fluorescein iodoacetamide often have reduced or no reactivity, and freshly prepared ATPγS improves the reaction. If the reaction fails, the cause can almost always be traced to one of these two reagents.

4. Due to the small reaction volume and long incubation time of the T4 PNK reaction in the 5′ labeling procedure, it is helpful to use an air incubator or a thermocycler with a hot bonnet to reduce evaporation.

5. After centrifuging nucleic acids that have been precipitated with ethanol, the pellet frequently becomes detached from the side of the tube, so take care not to discard it. The bulk of the supernatant can be removed by decanting or with a pipet, but either way, it is useful to carefully remove the small amount of residual ethanol solution with a pipet tip while watching to ensure that the pelleted nucleic acids remain in the tube.

6. Note that because FTSC is not soluble in aqueous solution, a significant amount of precipitation will be visible upon dilution of the FTSC stock into the aqueous buffer. This does not appear to inhibit the reaction.

7. It is very important to remove all of the unincorporated fluorescein from the labeled nucleic acid. It is often useful to analyze the labeled RNA on an agarose gel to determine whether a significant amount of free fluorescein remains. The gel need not include ethidium bromide, since the label itself serves as a means of detection. During electrophoresis, the apparatus should be covered with foil to inhibit quenching due to ambient light. The labeled RNA should run as a fairly tight band; if free fluorescein is present, it appears more diffuse than the labeled RNA and is often visible as a second species on the gel. It is useful to run a small amount of the free fluorescein label alongside the nucleic acid to indicate its position under the specific gel conditions used.

8. Concentration can be determined by applying the Beer–Lambert law: $A = \varepsilon l c$, where A is the absorbance; ε is the extinction coefficient for the relevant component in M^{-1} cm^{-1}; l is the path length, usually 1 cm for a standard cuvette; and c is the concentration in M. For the nucleic acid, the extinction coefficient should be individually determined for the specific nucleic acid being labeled. For commercially supplied oligonucleotides, extinction coefficients are often supplied with the accompanying product information. Otherwise, they can be calculated based upon the base content of the oligonucleotide. The extinction coefficient for the fluorophore can be obtained from the manufacturer. For 5-IAF at pH 9, ε_{492} is 78,000 M^{-1} cm^{-1} (Invitrogen). If fluorescent labels other than fluorescein are used, the extinction coefficient and absorbance maximum will need to be adjusted according to the properties of the fluorophore being used.

9. The product of the 3′ labeling reaction between the hydrazide and the aldehyde is chemically reversible. It is therefore possible that labeled oligonucleotides may lose their label over time. We have not observed this phenomenon; however, if a reverse reaction does complicate experimental results, it is possible to reduce the product to a stable form by treatment with sodium cyanoborohydride. This compound is toxic; appropriate safety precautions should be followed during its use.

Acknowledgements

We would like to thank John Pagano, Brian Farley, Bill Flaherty, and Lisa McCoig for their efforts in developing the protocols described in this article. Work in S.P.R.'s lab is supported by NIH grant GM081422.

References

1. Sambrook J, Russell DW (2001) Molecular cloning: a laboratory manual. Cold Spring Harbor Laboratory, Cold Spring Harbor, NY
2. Chao JA et al (2010) ZBP1 recognition of beta-actin zipcode induces RNA looping. Genes Dev 24:148–158
3. Pagano JM, Clingman CC, Ryder SP (2011) Quantitative approaches to monitor protein-nucleic acid interactions using fluorescent probes. RNA 17:14–20
4. Farley BM, Pagano JM, Ryder SP (2008) RNA target specificity of the embryonic cell fate determinant POS-1. RNA 14:2685–2697
5. LeTilly V, Royer CA (1993) Fluorescence anisotropy assays implicate protein-protein interactions in regulating trp repressor DNA binding. Biochemistry 32:7753–7758
6. Zearfoss NR et al (2011) Quaking regulates Hnrnpa1 expression through its 3′ UTR in oligodendrocyte precursor cells. PLoS Genet 7:e1001269
7. Ruby SW et al (1990) Affinity chromatography with biotinylated RNAs. Methods Enzymol 181:97–121
8. Lamed R, Levin Y, Wilchek M (1973) Covalent coupling of nucleotides to agarose for affinity chromatography. Biochim Biophys Acta 304:231–235
9. Czworkowski J, Odom OW, Hardesty B (1991) Fluorescence study of the topology of messenger RNA bound to the 30S ribosomal subunit of Escherichia coli. Biochemistry 30:4821–4830
10. Reines SA, Cantor CR (1974) New fluorescent hydrazide reagents for the oxidized 3′-terminus of RNA. Nucleic Acids Res 1:767–786
11. Korlach J et al (2004) Spontaneous nucleotide exchange in low molecular weight GTPases by fluorescently labeled gamma-phosphate-linked GTP analogs. Proc Natl Acad Sci USA 101:2800–2805

Chapter 15

High-Purity Enzymatic Synthesis of Site-Specifically Modified tRNA

Ya-Ming Hou

Abstract

Transfer RNA (tRNA) molecules play the key role in adapting the genetic code sequences with amino acids. The execution of this key role is highly dependent on the presence of modified nucleotides in tRNA, each of which performs a distinct function. To better understand how individual modifications modulate tRNA function, a method to isolate and purify a site-specifically modified tRNA is essential. This chapter describes an enzymatic method to synthesize a site-specifically modified tRNA, followed by purification of this tRNA away from unmodified tRNA using a selective oligonucleotide-based hybridization approach. This method is broadly applicable to site-specific tRNA modifications that interfere with nucleic-acid base-pairing principles.

Key words: Nucleic acid hybridization, 2′-O-methylation of nucleic acid backbones, RNase H cleavage

1. Introduction

All transfer RNA (tRNA) molecules synthesized in nature are made up of approximately 70–90 nucleotides in length that are folded into a conserved cloverleaf secondary structure and an L-shaped tertiary structure (Fig. 1a, b), consisting of the acceptor stem domain, the D stem-loop domain (D: dihydrouridine), the anti-codon stem-loop domain, the variable loop domain, and the T stem-loop domain (T: thymidine). These domains are arranged such that the 3′ end of each tRNA, carrying the conserved CCA sequence, is localized to one end of the L shape, while the anti-codon triplet complementary to a specific codon in the genetic code is localized to the other end. Amino acid attachment to the terminal ribose of the CCA sequence enables the amino acid to be physically associated with the anticodon triplet in the tRNA, permitting the transfer of the amino acid to the ribosome protein

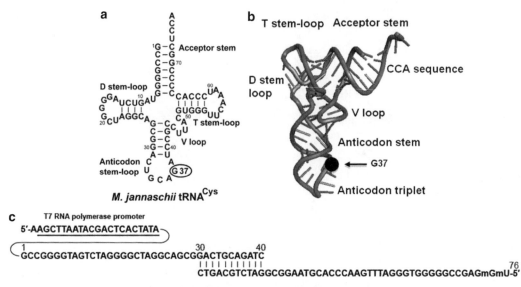

Fig. 1. Sequence of *Methanococcus jannaschii* tRNA^Cys in cloverleaf and tertiary structures. (**a**) The cloverleaf structure, showing the acceptor stem domain, the D stem-loop domain, the anticodon stem-loop domain, the variable loop domain, and the T stem-loop domain. The site of m^1G37 modification catalyzed by *M. jannaschii* Trm5 is circled. The folding of the cloverleaf structure is driven by sequence complementarity among regions of the tRNA. Note that the numbering of nucleotide sequence of *M. jannaschii* tRNA^Cys is based on the standard 76-nucleotide framework of tRNA (38), although the sequence of this tRNA lacks nucleotide 17 and is made up of only 75 nucleotides. (**b**) The L-shaped tRNA tertiary structure, showing the coaxial stacking of the acceptor stem with the T stem-loop to form the horizontal arm of the L and the coaxial stacking of the D stem-loop and the anticodon stem-loop to form the vertical arm of the L. The two arms are joined together in the elbow region through long-range tertiary interactions, positioning the CCA sequence at one end and the anticodon triplet at the other end. The position of G37 is shown as a closed circle. (**c**) The two overlapping primer sequences that form the substrate for primer extension by Sequenase to synthesize the template sequence for transcription of the tRNA. The T7 promoter sequence is underlined. The first primer encodes the promoter sequence (*underlined*) and the tRNA nucleotides from G1 to C40 (based on the standard numbering of nucleotides (38)), while the second primer encodes the complement of the tRNA nucleotides from A76 to G30. The Um and Gm letters in the second primer denote 2'-*O*-methyl backbone for the residues T and G, respectively, which are included to reduce the heterogeneity of T7 RNA polymerase at the terminus (39). The two primers can hybridize to anneal at the tRNA sequence from G30 to C40, allowing for the enzyme Sequenase (32) to fill in the single-stranded portions to create a double-stranded DNA that serves as the template for transcription of tRNA. These oligonucleotide primers need not be gel purified.

synthesis machinery at a codon position complementary to the anticodon. This decoding of nucleic acid sequence into amino acid sequence is essential for cellular survival at all levels. However, theoretical calculations indicate that the free energy provided by three base pairs of natural nucleotides between an anticodon and a codon is simply insufficient to discriminate against incorrect interactions (1, 2). Indeed, tRNAs have evolved with extensive modifications to nucleotide bases and backbones (3–5), many of which are present in or near the anticodon to enhance decoding specificity. Additional modifications are often localized to the elbow region of the L shape, such as the D and T modified bases that help to stabilize tRNA tertiary folding, as well as other modifications that further facilitate tRNA folding in unusual sequence *contexts* (6, 7). While elimination of one modification usually does not give rise to a clear growth phenotype, elimination of additional modifications can lead to synthetic lethality (8, 9). The synergistic growth effect of tRNA modifications, together with the observation that incomplete modifications accelerate tRNA degradation (10–12), supports the notion that the modifications present in a given tRNA sequence serve as a regulatory device to promote cell fitness and growth (13). Indeed, of the over 100 distinct modifications found in natural tRNA, some have been implicated in human disease, such as mitochondrial disorders and cardiomyopathy (14–16), suggesting that an understanding of the functions of these modifications will help to improve human health.

The study of individual tRNA modifications has benefited from the identification and cloning of genes responsible for modifications. These genes encode site-specific enzymes acting on nascent tRNA transcripts. The substantial genome space occupied by these genes in each cellular organism in all three biological domains emphasizes the importance of tRNA modifications to optimize tRNA sequences for function. However, the key to successful elucidation of the function of a specific tRNA modification is to obtain high purity of the site-specifically modified tRNA without the presence of other modifications. This cannot be achieved by isolating the tRNA from natural sources, because elimination of other modifications requires inactivation of multiple enzymes, leading to the problem of synthetic lethality. In the case of inosine (typically present at the wobble position of the anticodon, position 34), for example, incorporation of the modified nucleotide into a short RNA fragment by chemical synthesis is possible, allowing the introduction of the site-specific modification into a tRNA sequence by joining the chemically synthesized short RNA with RNA fragments made up of the remainder of the tRNA sequence. However, the types of modified nucleotides accessible to RNA chemical synthesis are limited and the prices of RNA chemical synthesis can be prohibitively high, even for a short RNA of 10–25 nucleotides in length. In addition, the joining of a chemically modified short RNA with additional RNA fragments (17–19) usually suffers from low yields and the probability of success varies depending on the sequences at the joining site.

A practical and economically reasonable approach to generate a site-specific modification on a tRNA is to perform enzymatic reactions on the site of an unmodified tRNA transcript. This applies to the modifications that can be synthesized by a single enzyme (such as the 2′-*O*-methylation on the ribose) and to those that are synthesized by a series of enzymes in successive reactions, such as wybutosine (20). This approach is most attractive when the appropriate enzymes are known and the enzymatic reactions are well characterized. However, the major obstacle of this approach is the presence of leftover unmodified tRNA (ranging from 50 to 70%), due to incomplete enzymatic reactions (21), even with an excess of enzyme. The reason for the sub-stoichiometry is not clear, possibly due to loss of enzyme activity in some cases, suboptimum reaction conditions, or partial folding of the unmodified tRNA transcript as a substrate in other cases. The incomplete reaction generates a mixture of both modified and unmodified transcripts, which hinders rigorous interpretation of biochemical analysis. Thus it is highly desirable to have a method to separate the modified from the unmodified transcript. However, because the two types of transcripts differ by a single base modification, which may not change the chemical property or molecular weight of the base (e.g., U to Ψ) or represent a small molecular-weight addition such as a methyl group, separation of the two types by the conventional denaturing gel electrophoresis or by high-performance liquid chromatography (HPLC) is usually unsuccessful.

This chapter describes a method of enzymatic synthesis of a site-specifically modified tRNA, followed by a simple and robust purification step to separate the modified tRNA away from the unmodified transcript, leading to a high-purity modified tRNA that can be produced in large quantities for detailed and extensive kinetic analysis. The method is applicable to base modifications that interfere with Watson–Crick base-pairing interactions (22), which account for over 50% of the tRNA modifications found in databases. Such a base modification confers resistance to pairing with complementary oligonucleotides and thus resistance to cleavage by RNase H (22), a ribonuclease that hydrolyzes the RNA strand of an RNA–DNA hybrid (23). In contrast, the unmodified tRNA is accessible to hybridization and is thus sensitive to RNase H cleavage, resulting in tRNA fragments that can be easily separated from the cleavage-resistant modified tRNA transcript by denaturing gel electrophoresis.

The example described here is the high-purity isolation of the m^1G37-modified tRNA^{Cys} transcript of the archaeon *Methanococcus jannaschii*. The m^1G37 modification is catalyzed by the tRNA methyltransferase Trm5 in archaea and eukaryotes and by TrmD in bacteria, both using *S*-adenosyl-L-methionine (AdoMet) as the methyl donor for methyl transfer to the N1 position of G37 adjacent to the 3′ of the anticodon (21). The m^1G37 modification is present in all three domains of life and is essential for growth of several bacteria species (24–26) due to its importance for maintaining the reading frame fidelity during tRNA decoding on the ribosome (26, 27). The archaeon *M. jannaschii* and related organisms have an unusual two-step pathway to synthesize Cys-tRNA^{Cys} for decoding cysteine codons (28), in contrast to all other organisms synthesizing Cys-tRNA^{Cys} using one single enzyme CysRS (Cys-tRNA *synthetase*) (29). In the archaeal two-step pathway, tRNA^{Cys} is first aminoacylated with Sep (where Sep = phosphoserine) by the unusual enzyme SepRS, and the synthesized Sep-tRNA^{Cys} is modified to Cys-tRNA^{Cys} by the downstream enzyme SepCysS.

It has been shown that the efficiency of phosphoserylation of tRNA^{Cys} by SepRS is dependent on the m^{1}G37 base (30), and that in some branches of archaeal methanogens where both the CysRS and SepRS–SepCysS pathways exist, the m^{1}G37 modification is also required for efficient cysteinylation of tRNA^{Cys} by CysRS (31). Notably, the use of the method described here allowed successful purification of the m^{1}G37-tRNA transcript away from the unmodified transcript to demonstrate that, compared to the unmodified transcript, the m^{1}G37 modification specifically promotes the transition state of tRNA aminoacylation (30).

2. Materials

2.1. DNA Template Preparation

Prepare all solutions using analytical grade reagents and autoclaved double-deionized water.

1. Sequenase, a T7 DNA polymerase lacking the editing domain. This enzyme can be purchased or purified from an overproducer strain (32).
2. DNA oligonucleotides for construction of transcription templates, synthesized by a commercial supplier and used directly without further purification.
3. Sequenase buffer (5×): 12.5 mM DTT, 250 mM NaCl, 100 mM MgCl$_2$, and 200 mM Tris–HCl, pH 7.5.
4. 25 mM each dNTPs.
5. TE buffer: 10 mM Tris–HCl, pH 8.0, and 1 mM EDTA.
6. 3 M ammonium acetate.
7. Ethanol, absolute and 70%.
8. Speedvac system.

2.2. tRNA In Vitro Transcription and Purification

1. DNA template from Subheading 3.1 or a restriction-enzyme linearized plasmid encoding the sequence of a tRNA gene.
2. T7 RNA polymerase, purified from an over-expression clone such as pAR1219 in BL21(DE3) (33).
3. 1 M Tris–HCl, pH 8.0.
4. 1 M MgCl$_2$.
5. 0.1 M spermidine.
6. 0.5 M DTT.
7. 0.5% Triton-X100.
8. 50 mM each of ATP, CTP, GTP, and UTP, pH 8.0.
9. 200 mM GMP, pH 8.0.
10. 0.5 M EDTA, pH 8.0.

11. Items 5–7 from Subheading 2.1.
12. RNA loading dye solution: 7 M urea, 0.05% xylene cyanol, and 0.05% bromophenol blue in 1× TBE buffer.
13. A handheld UV lamp.

2.3. Denaturing Polyacrylamide Gel Analysis

1. 20× TBE buffer: Dissolve 486.6 g of Tris-base, 37.2 g of EDTA (disodium salt), and 220 g of boric acid in water and to a final volume of 2 L.
2. Stock solution of 12% acrylamide gel solution with 7 M urea (12% PAGE/7 M urea): Mix 200 g of acrylamide:bis-acrylamide (29:1), 700 g of urea, 83.25 mL 20× TBE, and water to 1,665 L. Stir to dissolve all components at room temperature overnight. Adjust the final volume to 2 L with additional water, filter the solution through a 0.22 μm filtering unit, and store in a dark brown bottle at room temperature.
3. 1× TBE buffer: 89 mM Tris–HCl, pH 8.0, 89 mM boric acid, and 2 mM EDTA. Dilute 20× TBE 19:1 with water.
4. Mini gel electrophoresis system.
5. Preparative gel electrophoresis system with plates of dimensions ~400 × 200 mm and 2.0 mm spacers and comb. Depending on your system, heavy packaging tape and metal binder clips may be required to seal the plates when pouring the gel.
6. 10% ammonium persulfate (APS).
7. N,N,N',N'-tetramethyl-ethane-1,2-diamine (TEMED).

2.4. Enzymatic tRNA Modification and Isolation of the Modified tRNA

1. Site-specific modification enzyme, such as *M. jannaschii* Trm5 used as the example here (21), purified from a suitable overexpression clone. A suitable buffer for the modification enzyme (determined empirically) at 5× concentration.
2. Modification substrates and cofactors, such as AdoMet for the Trm5-dependent synthesis of m^1G37-tRNA^{Cys}.
3. ^{3}H-AdoMet with a specific activity of ~60 Ci/mmol (8.7 μM) and 0.55 μCi/μL.
4. TE buffer.
5. 1 M Tris–HCl, pH 8.0.
6. 2 M KCl.
7. 1 M $MgCl_2$.
8. 0.5 M DTT.
9. 50 mM EDTA.
10. 10 mg/ml bovine serum albumin (BSA).
11. Heat–cool buffer: 10 mM Tris–HCl, pH 8.0, and 20 mM $MgCl_2$.
12. Whatman 3 MM filter pads.

13. 5% trichloroacetic acid (TCA).
14. 95% ethanol.
15. Ether.
16. A liquid scintillation counter.
17. Quick spin column, e.g., Centri Spin 20 column (Princeton Separations).
18. RNase H. This enzyme can be purchased or purified in-house from a suitable over-expression clone (see (23) and Chapter 2).
19. 10× RNase H buffer: 750 mM KCl, 500 mM Tris–HCl, pH 8.3, 30 mM $MgCl_2$, and 100 mM DTT.
20. DNA oligonucleotide with 2′-O-methyl backbone for RNase H reaction, purchased from a commercial source.

3. Methods

3.1. Preparation of Template Sequence for Transcription of M. jannaschii tRNA^{Cys}

1. Design two DNA oligonucleotide primers that together encompass the sequence of a T7 RNA polymerase promoter and the coding sequence of *M. jannaschii* tRNA^{Cys} (Fig. 1c).
2. Mix the two primers at a final concentration of 4 µM each in a final volume of 1 mL. Add 200 µL of a 5× Sequenase buffer and water to bring the volume to 970 µL.
3. Divide the solution containing the two primers into two equal volumes. Incubate for 2.5 min at 80°C to denature any secondary structures of the primers. Remember to secure the top of each tube with a plastic clamp.
4. Spin the tubes briefly in a microfuge and place them in an ice bath to allow the two primers to anneal. Reserve one aliquot of 3.0 µL for use as controls for subsequent electrophoretic analysis of the Sequenase reaction.
5. Add 10 µL of 25 mM dNTPs and 2.5–10 µL of Sequenase to each solution at 37°C. The amount of Sequenase to use is determined empirically by adding graded amounts of the enzyme to 100 µL reactions, followed by analysis for product formation on a mini-size 12% PAGE/7 M urea gel for 30–40 min at 200 V in 1× TBE. The extension of primers by Sequenase will synthesize a double-stranded DNA that migrates slower than either of the two starting primers.
6. Incubate the rest of the Sequenase reaction overnight at 37°C. Check for completion of the reaction by analysis of a 3 µL aliquot of one of the reactions on a mini-size 12% PAGE/7 M urea gel (see Note 1).
7. Divide the total 1 mL reaction into 3 × 333 µL aliquots in separate tubes.

8. Add 33 μL of 3 M ammonium acetate (1/10 volume) and cold 1.0 mL ethanol (3 volumes) to each tube. Keep the solution at –20°C for 30 min and then spin for 15 min at maximum speed in a refrigerated microfuge. Pour off the ethanol supernatant and wash the pellets with 1.0 mL cold 70% ethanol. Dry pellets for 5 min in a Speedvac.

9. Dissolve each set of pellets in 100 μL of TE buffer.

10. Determine the concentration of the DNA by measuring the absorbance at 260 nm (OD_{260}: 1 unit = 50 μg/mL), which is usually in the range of 25 μM.

11. Store the DNA template at –20°C, which should be stable for several months. For each transcription reaction, a 40 μL aliquot of the synthesized template is used for 1 mL of T7 transcription reaction.

3.2. Synthesis of M. jannaschii tRNA^{Cys} by In Vitro Transcription

1. In a 1 mL T7 RNA polymerase transcription reaction, add the following reagents in order:

	Stock concentration	Volume	Final concentration
DNA template	25 μM	40 μL	1.0 μM
Tris–HCl, pH 8.0	1 M	40 μL	40 mM
$MgCl_2$	1 M	24 μL	24 mM
Spermidine	0.1 M	10 μL	1 mM
DTT	0.5 M	10 μL	5 mM
Triton X-100	0.5%	10 μL	0.005%
ATP	50 mM	150 μL	7.5 mM
CTP	50 mM	150 μL	7.5 mM
GTP	50 mM	150 μL	7.5 mM
UTP	50 mM	150 μL	7.5 mM
GMP	200 mM	150 μL	30 mM
T7 RNA polymerase (see Note 2)		10 μL	
H_2O		To 1000 μL	

2. Allow the transcription to continue for 3–5 h at 37°C.

3. Spin down pyrophosphates that have formed for 10 min in a microfuge at the maximum speed. Transfer the supernatant containing the tRNA transcript to a new tube.

4. Adjust the solution by adding EDTA to a final concentration of 0.1 M and ammonium acetate to a final concentration of 0.3 M. Add two volumes of cold ethanol and precipitate the tRNA transcript at –20°C for 15 min.

5. Spin in a microfuge at the maximum speed for 15 min at 4°C. Resuspend the pellet in 100 μL TE at 37°C for 10 min. Not all of the pyrophosphate precipitation will go into solution.

6. Add 100 μL RNA loading dye to the resuspended pellet. The sample is ready for gel isolation of the tRNA transcript.

3.3. Isolation of tRNA Transcript from the Transcription Reaction

1. Make a large preparative 12% PAGE/7 M urea gel by assembling two glass plates and spacers.

2. Seal the short-edge side of the glass plates with heavy packaging tape, and clamp along the two long-edge sides with metal binder clips.

3. Mix a 10 mL solution of 12% PAGE/7 M urea with 120 μL of 10% APS and 6 μL of TEMED and pour the solution to the bottom of the assembled glass plates.

4. Upon solidification, the 10 mL gel serves as a seal at the bottom.

5. Mix 160 mL of 12% PAGE/7 M urea with 960 μL of 10% APS and 48 μL of TEMED and pour the gel solution to fill the rest of the assembled glass plates. Insert combs or spacers to form the sample-loading wells.

6. After 10–20 min, the gel should be solidified and ready to use. Remove the combs, clamps, and tape from the glass plates, and place the gel in an appropriate electrophoresis apparatus. Fill both the top and bottom chambers with 1× TBE buffer.

7. Make sure that each well on the 12% PAGE/7 M urea gel is cleared of urea by washing it with 1× TBE buffer several times and then immediately load the 200 μL solution of tRNA in RNA loading dye solution (from Subheading 3.2, step 6). Run the gel at 700 V for 15 h until xylene cyanol is about 8 cm above the bottom of the gel.

8. Remove the glass plates from the apparatus, transfer the gel to a Saran Wrap, and place the gel and Saran Wrap on top of a silica gel fluorescent TLC plate.

9. Use a handheld UV lamp to localize a UV shadow, indicating the site of migration of the tRNA transcript. Cut off the portion of the gel that exhibits UV shadow and crush the gel into pieces using a sterile glass rod.

10. Add 5 mL TE to the crushed gel pieces and shake the suspension on a rotator shaker at room temperature for 4–6 h to elute the tRNA.

11. Spin down gel pieces using a tabletop centrifuge. Remove the supernatant to a clean tube.

12. Add more TE back to the gel solution and continue elution for another 4–6 h. Again, spin and keep the supernatant.

13. Combine the two supernatants and precipitate the tRNA transcript by adding 1/10 volume of 3 M ammonium acetate and 3 volumes of ethanol.
14. Spin down the tRNA transcript from ethanol precipitation and wash the pellet two times with 70% ethanol.
15. Dry the pellet and resuspsend the tRNA in 100 μL of TE buffer. Determine the tRNA concentration by measuring the absorbance at 260 nm (OD_{260}: one unit for tRNA is 40 μg/mL).

3.4. Small-Scale Enzymatic m^1G37 Modification of M. jannaschii tRNA^{Cys} Transcript

1. Take an aliquot of the unmodified transcript of *M. jannaschii* tRNA^{Cys} (500 pmol) and adjust the volume with TE to 17.5 μL.
2. Heat the tRNA solution for 3 min at 80°C, a temperature that is above the estimated melting temperature of the tRNA transcript.
3. Quickly spin the solution and add 20 μL of the heat–cool buffer. Anneal the tRNA at 37°C for 15 min.
4. Prepare a 5× reaction buffer as below:

Component	Volume	5× Concentration	1× Concentration
1 M Tris–HCl, pH 8.0	50.0 μL	0.5 M	0.1 M
2 M KCl	25.0 μL	0.5 M	0.1 M
1 M $MgCl_2$	3.0 μL	30 mM	6 mM
0.5 M DTT	4.0 μL	20 mM	4 mM
50 mM EDTA	1.0 μL	0.5 mM	0.1 mM
10 mg/mL BSA	1.2 μL	0.12 mg/mL	0.024 mg/mL
Water	15.8 μL		
Total	100 μL		

5. Add to the tRNA solution the following reagents in order:

Methylation reaction:	Volume	Final concentration
tRNA in heat–cool buffer	30.7 μL	10 μM
5× reaction buffer	10.0 μL	1×
AdoMet (1 mM)	2.5 μL	50 μM
^{3}H-AdoMet (8.7 μM)	1.8 μL	0.31 μM
Enzyme, e.g., Trm5 (25 μM)	5.0 μL	2.5 μL
Total	50 μL	

6. Incubate the reaction at 55°C (a temperature below the growth temperature of *M. jannaschii* of 83°C but sufficiently high to

allow the reaction to take place). Remove a 5 μL aliquot at an appropriate time interval (e.g., 2, 5, 10 min, etc.) onto a Whatman 3 MM filter pad and drop the filter pad into a beaker containing 100–200 mL cold 5% TCA. Estimate the volume of TCA as 5 mL per filter pad.

7. After all pads are spotted and in TCA, shake the solution for 10 min at 4°C to wash off unincorporated AdoMet, while allowing the m^{1}G37-tRNA to precipitate on filter pads in TCA.

8. Decant and repeat the 5% TCA wash.

9. Wash the filter pads with 95% ethanol by shaking for 10 min at 4°C in the beaker. Repeat the ethanol wash one more time.

10. Wash the filter pads with ether. Agitate gently by hand and let the ether solution sit at room temperature for 5 min under a fume hood. Decant off the either and dry the filter pads under the fume hood for 15 min.

11. Transfer each filter pad to a scintillation solution in a scintillation vial. Measure the amount of radioactivity of ^{3}H-tRNA^{Cys} using a liquid scintillation counter.

12. Calculate the amount of ^{3}H-tRNA^{Cys} based on the specific activity of the reaction as shown below:

    Total concentration of ^{3}H-AdoMet in the reaction: 0.31 μM.

    Total concentration of unlabeled AdoMet in the reaction: 50 μM.

    Combined concentration of AdoMet: 50.31 μM.

    Total μCi in the reaction: 0.55 μCi/μL × 1.8 μL = 0.99 μCi.

    Specific activity in dpm/pmol: $(0.99 \, \mu Ci \times (2.2 \times 10^6 \, dpm/\mu Ci))/(50.31 \, pmole/\mu L \times (50 \, \mu M)) = 865$ dpm/pmol (see Note 3).

13. Correct the ^{3}H counting by measuring the quenching factor using the following procedure: Take a 5 μL aliquot at the final time point and pass it through a quick spin column to remove unincorporated ^{3}H-AdoMet. Directly transfer the eluate 5 μL (which contains counts only associated with the methylated tRNA) into the liquid scintillation fluid and measure the counts. The ratio of the direct measurement of this count value over the count value on the TCA precipitated filter pad at the same time point reveals the quenching factor, which should be used to correct the fraction of methylation (see Note 3).

3.5. Large-Scale m^{1}G37 Modification and Removal of Unmodified Transcripts

1. Scale up the reaction of Subheading 3.4, by tenfold or to the desired amount, while eliminating ^{3}H-AdoMet from the reaction. A tenfold scale-up reaction should generate ~5 nmol of tRNA.

2. Design a hybridization oligonucleotide that targets the modified base in the middle region of the sequence (see Fig. 2 and Notes 4–6).

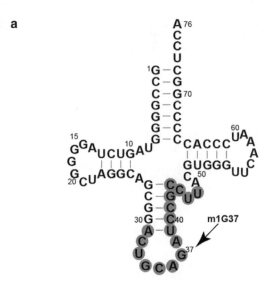

M. jannaschii tRNA^{Cys} (75-mer)

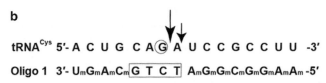

Fig. 2. Design of the hybridization oligonucleotide targeting *Methanococcus jannaschii* tRNA^{Cys}. (a) The tRNA cloverleaf structure showing the sequence that is targeted by the hybridization oligonucleotide in *grey*. (b) The hybrid region between the oligonucleotide (Oligo 1) and the targeting sequence in the tRNA, indicating the primary and secondary sites of RNase H cleavage by *long* and *short arrows*, respectively.

3. Mix the hybridization oligonucleotide with an equal amount of the tRNA in the Trm5 reaction (e.g., 5 nmol each of the oligonucleotide and the tRNA). Note that the tRNA after the Trm5 reaction exists both in the unmodified form and in the m^{1}G37-modified form in a volume of 8 µL of TE buffer. Heat the mixture at 85°C for 10 min. Spin briefly and add 1 µL of a 10× RNase H buffer and incubate at 37°C for 10 min (see Note 5).

4. Add an appropriate amount of RNase H to a final volume of 10 µL. Incubate the reaction at 37°C while removing aliquots of 1 µL at different time points (e.g., 0, 20, 40 min, etc.) and adding to 1 µL of RNA loading dye (see Note 7).

5. Analyze the RNase H-dependent cleavage by denaturing 12% PAGE/7 M urea gel using a mini gel system. Run the gel at 200 V in 1× TBE for ~50 min until bromophenol blue runs to the bottom. Stain the gel with ethidium bromide and visualize the tRNA bands under UV light (Fig. 3). The m^{1}G37-modified tRNA is resistant to cleavage, while the unmodified tRNA is completely cleaved by RNase H (see Notes 8–10).

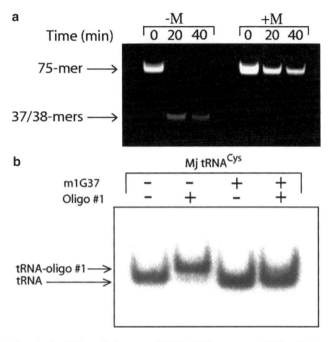

Fig. 3. Gel analysis of RNase H cleavage of tRNA. (a) Time course of RNase H cleavage of *Methanococcus jannaschii* tRNA^{Cys} transcript unmodified (−M) and m^{1}G37-modified (+M). The full-length tRNA consists of 75 nucleotides in length (75-mer) and is cleaved into two fragments (37-mer and 38-mer, respectively) by RNase H. (b) Native gel and phosphorimager analysis of tRNA hybridization to the oligonucleotide shown in Fig. 2b (indicated as Oligo #1). The transcript of *M. jannaschii* tRNA^{Cys} with or without m^{1}G37 is indicated as "+" or "−," respectively. The hybridization leads to a mobility shift of the tRNA, which is observed only when the tRNA is unmodified.

6. Cut out the piece of the gel that contains the m^{1}G37-modified tRNA transcript. Crush the gel into pieces and soak the pieces in TE buffer overnight for elution of tRNA.

7. Recover the eluted tRNA by ethanol precipitation and resuspension in TE. This tRNA can be used for biochemical analysis (see Notes 11 and 12).

4. Notes

1. In the Sequenase reaction, some of the overlapping primers are extended to completion in only 2–3 h while others take longer time. Overnight incubation should assure complete reaction.

2. In the tRNA transcription reaction, if T7 RNA polymerase is purified from an overproducer strain (32), it should be titrated to the level where 10 μL of the enzyme would give visible precipitation of pyrophosphate that forms aggregates with Mg^{+2} in less than 1 h at 37°C. The pyrophosphate is released from

NTP due to incorporation of NMP during active transcription. The observation of such precipitation is usually a good indication of strong transcription. If no precipitation is observed in more than 1 h, then add more T7 RNA polymerase to the transcription reaction.

3. Based on the amount of ^{3}H-tRNA^{Cys} synthesized (after correction for the quenching factor) relative to the amount of the input tRNA (500 pmol), determine the fraction of the tRNA transcript that has been converted to m^{1}G37-tRNA. This fraction is usually 75% for Trm5 but can vary for other enzymes. If the fraction of conversion is lower than 20%, increase the enzyme and reaction time.

4. In this design, the oligonucleotide contains 2'-O-methyl backbones throughout the sequence except for the middle four nucleotides, where the base that targets m^{1}G37 is the second from the 5' end. The presence of the 2'-O-methyl backbones is to improve the accessibility of the oligonucleotide to the tRNA target, which has a high propensity to fold into a compact L shape structure. The tRNA–oligonucleotide hybrid leaves the targeting region of the oligonucleotide as a DNA backbone, allowing RNase H to cleave the tRNA substrate in the hybrid. The cleavage by RNase H may occur at a primary site at the 3' phosphodiester linkage of the target base and a secondary site one nucleotide after the target base at the 3' linkage (Fig. 2b) (34).

5. For some modifications in tRNA, such as the m^{1}G37 modification, it has been shown that the presence of the modification prevents the accessibility of the oligonucleotide to hybridize to the tRNA (Fig. 3b) (22). The hybridization analysis is performed with ^{32}P-labeled tRNA (either by body labeling during T7 transcription or by end labeling using polynucleotide kinase at the 5' end or the CCA enzyme at the 3' end (35)). The ^{32}P-labeled tRNA is purified away from the free ^{32}P label by a Centricon-20 spin column and then annealed with the oligonucleotide under the conditions described in Subheading 3.5, step 3. Hybridization is then analyzed by running the tRNA samples (with 8% glycerol in 1× TBE, 0.05% xylene cyanol, and 0.05% bromophenol blue) on native 12% PAGE (1× TBE and 10 mM MgCl$_2$) in a mini-gel system at 100 V for 90 min at room temperature. The gel is dried and analyzed using a phosphorimager. This analysis should show that the unmodified tRNA transcript forms a hybrid complex, thus migrating slower, whereas the m^{1}G37-modified tRNA transcript is not accessible to hybridization, thus migrating faster. However, because hybridization is an equilibrium process and can be reversible, it is unable to completely separate the modified from the unmodified tRNA transcripts. For complete separation, the RNase H cleavage reaction is recommended.

6. Successful design of the hybridization oligonucleotide for a specific modification should take into account the flanking sequence context to allow the formation of stable hybrid with unmodified transcripts at 37°C. This can be determined in a heat–cool process, followed by gel shift analysis as shown in Fig. 3. For GC-rich sequences, such as *M. jannaschii* tRNA^{Cys} and tRNA^{Pro}, a 17-mer hybridization oligonucleotide should be sufficient, whereas for AU-rich sequences, such as mitochondrial tRNA, longer oligonucleotides may be necessary.

7. The design of the hybridization oligonucleotide is important for the protection of the modified tRNA from cleavage. Even if the modified tRNA can form a hybrid with the oligonucleotide, a proper design of the oligonucleotide can protect the modified tRNA from RNase H cleavage. According to the crystal structure of RNase H bound to an RNA–DNA hybrid (23), the enzyme stabilizes the RNA substrate for cleavage by making direct interactions with two backbone 2′-OH groups on the 5′ side of the scissile phosphate and two backbone 2′-OH groups on the 3′ side. These four continuous 2′-OH groups are necessary for cleavage. The design of the oligonucleotide to target m^{1}G37 places the scissile phosphate in the middle of the 4-base-pair region of an RNA–DNA hybrid (Fig. 2b), which would destroy the required continuity of four 2′-OH groups along the active site of RNase H for cleavage.

8. Gel analysis of RNase H cleavage in Fig. 3 reveals that, while the unmodified transcript is completely cleaved in 20 min, a significant fraction of the modified transcript is resistant to cleavage up to 40 min. This fraction is ~60% in 40 min, consistent with the extent of the m^{1}G37 modification as determined by measuring the synthesis of ^{3}H-m^{1}G37-tRNA. The cleavage-resistant fraction remains constant in 40–60 min, even with addition of more RNase H, indicating that the cleavage is complete and that little of the unmodified transcript is left. However, if the extent of cleavage increases with time, this indicates that more RNase H should be used.

9. The RNase H cleavage is dependent on the accessibility of the modified region of the target tRNA to the hybridization oligonucleotide. While the G37 position in the anticodon loop is easily accessible to hybridization and has been successfully verified in several tRNA sequence contexts (including *M. jannaschii* tRNA^{Cys} and tRNA^{Pro}, and *E. coli* tRNA^{Leu}), other sites in tRNA have also been shown to be accessible (22). For example, the A58 site in the T loop is also accessible, permitting the use of RNase H cleavage to separate an unmodified tRNA transcript from an m^{1}A58-modified tRNA transcript, catalyzed by the enzyme TrmI (36).

10. However, some other modification sites may not be readily accessible. An example is the G9 site, which is localized at the junction between the acceptor stem and D stem. A frequent modification is m^1G9, catalyzed by the enzyme Trm10 (37). Analysis by the RNase H cleavage reveals that the cleavage at the target site is incomplete, due to the poor accessibility, but that longer incubation with RNase H results in cleavage at a second site that exhibits partial complementarity to the central portion of the targeting oligonucleotide. This example emphasizes that the specificity of cleavage requires that the site of modification does not resemble other sequences in the target tRNA.

11. In scale-up reactions to prepare large quantities of m^1G37-tRNA transcript, it is feasible to apply 5–10 nmol of tRNA into just one lane of the mini-gel apparatus and use UV shadowing to identify the intact tRNA band.

12. Broader application of the method to other modified tRNA transcripts requires the availability of the modification enzymes and the type of the base modifications that disrupt conventional Watson–Crick base pairing. Because each modification is distinct in chemical nature and in the ability to disrupt base pairing, the condition of hybridization and RNase H cleavage needs to be identified empirically.

Acknowledgement

This work was supported by NIH grant R01GM81601 to Y.M.H. The author thanks Dr. Cuiping Liu, Dr. Reiko Sakaguchi, and Dr. Howard Gamper for preparation of figures.

References

1. Rodnina MV, Wintermeyer W (2001) Ribosome fidelity: tRNA discrimination, proofreading and induced fit. Trends Biochem Sci 26: 124–130
2. Ogle JM, Carter AP, Ramakrishnan V (2003) Insights into the decoding mechanism from recent ribosome structures. Trends Biochem Sci 28:259–266
3. Bjork GR (1995) Genetic dissection of synthesis and function of modified nucleosides in bacterial transfer RNA. Prog Nucleic Acid Res Mol Biol 50:263–338
4. Agris PF (2004) Decoding the genome: a modified view. Nucleic Acids Res 32:223–238
5. Cantara WA, Crain PF, Rozenski J, McCloskey JA, Harris KA, Zhang X, Vendeix FA, Fabris D, Agris PF (2011) The RNA modification database, RNAMDB: 2011 update. Nucleic Acids Res 39:D195–D201
6. Helm M, Brule H, Degoul F, Cepanec C, Leroux JP, Giege R, Florentz C (1998) The presence of modified nucleotides is required for cloverleaf folding of a human mitochondrial tRNA. Nucleic Acids Res 26:1636–1643
7. Helm M, Giege R, Florentz C (1999) A Watson-Crick base-pair-disrupting methyl group (m1A9) is sufficient for cloverleaf folding of human mitochondrial tRNALys. Biochemistry 38:13338–13346
8. Persson BC, Jager G, Gustafsson C (1997) The spoU gene of Escherichia coli, the fourth gene of the spoT operon, is essential for tRNA

(Gm18) 2′-O-methyltransferase activity. Nucleic Acids Res 25:4093–4097
9. Urbonavicius J, Durand JM, Bjork GR (2002) Three modifications in the D and T arms of tRNA influence translation in Escherichia coli and expression of virulence genes in Shigella flexneri. J Bacteriol 184:5348–5357
10. Alexandrov A, Martzen MR, Phizicky EM (2002) Two proteins that form a complex are required for 7-methylguanosine modification of yeast tRNA. RNA 8:1253–1266
11. Chernyakov I, Baker MA, Grayhack EJ, Phizicky EM (2008) Identification and analysis of tRNAs that are degraded in Saccharomyces cerevisiae due to lack of modifications. Methods Enzymol 449:221–237, Chapter 11
12. Chernyakov I, Whipple JM, Kotelawala L, Grayhack EJ, Phizicky EM (2008) Degradation of several hypomodified mature tRNA species in Saccharomyces cerevisiae is mediated by Met22 and the 5′-3′ exonucleases Rat1 and Xrn1. Genes Dev 22:1369–1380
13. Persson BC (1993) Modification of tRNA as a regulatory device. Mol Microbiol 8:1011–1016
14. Yasukawa T, Suzuki T, Ishii N, Ohta S, Watanabe K (2001) Wobble modification defect in tRNA disturbs codon-anticodon interaction in a mitochondrial disease. EMBO J 20:4794–4802
15. Yasukawa T, Kirino Y, Ishii N, Holt IJ, Jacobs HT, Makifuchi T, Fukuhara N, Ohta S, Suzuki T, Watanabe K (2005) Wobble modification deficiency in mutant tRNAs in patients with mitochondrial diseases. FEBS Lett 579:2948–2952
16. Kirino Y, Goto Y, Campos Y, Arenas J, Suzuki T (2005) Specific correlation between the wobble modification deficiency in mutant tRNAs and the clinical features of a human mitochondrial disease. Proc Natl Acad Sci U S A 102:7127–7132
17. Shitivelband S, Hou YM (2005) Breaking the stereo barrier of amino acid attachment to tRNA by a single nucleotide. J Mol Biol 348:513–521
18. Sherlin LD, Bullock TL, Nissan TA, Perona JJ, Lariviere FJ, Uhlenbeck OC, Scaringe SA (2001) Chemical and enzymatic synthesis of tRNAs for high-throughput crystallization. RNA 7:1671–1678
19. Moore MJ, Query CC (2000) Joining of RNAs by splinted ligation. Methods Enzymol 317:109–123
20. Noma A, Kirino Y, Ikeuchi Y, Suzuki T (2006) Biosynthesis of wybutosine, a hyper-modified nucleoside in eukaryotic phenylalanine tRNA. EMBO J 25:2142–2154
21. Christian T, Evilia C, Williams S, Hou YM (2004) Distinct origins of tRNA(m^{1}G37) methyltransferase. J Mol Biol 339:707–719
22. Hou YM, Li Z, Gamper H (2006) Isolation of a site-specifically modified RNA from an unmodified transcript. Nucleic Acids Res 34:e21
23. Nowotny M, Gaidamakov SA, Crouch RJ, Yang W (2005) Crystal structures of RNase H bound to an RNA/DNA hybrid: substrate specificity and metal-dependent catalysis. Cell 121:1005–1016
24. Baba T, Ara T, Hasegawa M, Takai Y, Okumura Y, Baba M, Datsenko KA, Tomita M, Wanner BL, Mori H (2006) Construction of Escherichia coli K-12 in-frame, single-gene knockout mutants: the Keio collection. Mol Syst Biol 2(2006):0008
25. O'Dwyer K, Watts JM, Biswas S, Ambrad J, Barber M, Brule H, Petit C, Holmes DJ, Zalacain M, Holmes WM (2004) Characterization of Streptococcus pneumoniae TrmD, a tRNA methyltransferase essential for growth. J Bacteriol 186:2346–2354
26. Bjork GR, Wikstrom PM, Bystrom AS (1989) Prevention of translational frameshifting by the modified nucleoside 1-methylguanosine. Science 244:986–989
27. Bjork GR, Jacobsson K, Nilsson K, Johansson MJ, Bystrom AS, Persson OP (2001) A primordial tRNA modification required for the evolution of life? EMBO J 20:231–239
28. Sauerwald A, Zhu W, Major TA, Roy H, Palioura S, Jahn D, Whitman WB, Yates JR 3rd, Ibba M, Soll D (2005) RNA-dependent cysteine biosynthesis in archaea. Science 307:1969–1972
29. Hou YM, Perona JJ (2005) Cysteinyl-tRNA synthetase. In: Ibba M, Francklyn C, Cusack S (eds) The aminoacyl-tRNA synthetases. Landes Bioscience, Georgetown, pp 12–23
30. Zhang CM, Liu C, Slater S, Hou YM (2008) Aminoacylation of tRNA with phosphoserine for synthesis of cysteinyl-tRNA(Cys). Nat Struct Mol Biol 15:507–514
31. Hauenstein SI, Hou YM, Perona JJ (2008) The homotetrameric phosphoseryl-tRNA synthetase from Methanosarcina mazei exhibits half-of-the-sites activity. J Biol Chem 283:21997–22006
32. Tabor S, Huber HE, Richardson CC (1987) Escherichia coli thioredoxin confers processivity on the DNA polymerase activity of the gene 5 protein of bacteriophage T7. J Biol Chem 262:16212–16223

33. Grodberg J, Dunn JJ (1988) ompT encodes the Escherichia coli outer membrane protease that cleaves T7 RNA polymerase during purification. J Bacteriol 170:1245–1253
34. Lapham J, Yu YT, Shu MD, Steitz JA, Crothers DM (1997) The position of site-directed cleavage of RNA using RNase H and 2′-O-methyl oligonucleotides is dependent on the enzyme source. RNA 3:950–951
35. Francis TA, Ehrenfeld GM, Gregory MR, Hecht SM (1983) Transfer RNA pyrophosphorolysis with CTP(ATP):tRNA nucleotidyltransferase. A direct route to tRNAs modified at the 3′ terminus. J Biol Chem 258: 4279–4284
36. Roovers M, Wouters J, Bujnicki JM, Tricot C, Stalon V, Grosjean H, Droogmans L (2004) A primordial RNA modification enzyme: the case of tRNA (m1A) methyltransferase. Nucleic Acids Res 32:465–476
37. Jackman JE, Montange RK, Malik HS, Phizicky EM (2003) Identification of the yeast gene encoding the tRNA m^{1}G methyltransferase responsible for modification at position 9. RNA 9:574–585
38. Sprinzl M, Horn C, Brown M, Ioudovitch A, Steinberg S (1998) Compilation of tRNA sequences and sequences of tRNA genes. Nucleic Acids Res 26:148–153
39. Kao C, Zheng M, Rudisser S (1999) A simple and efficient method to reduce nontemplated nucleotide addition at the 3 terminus of RNAs transcribed by T7 RNA polymerase. RNA 5:1268–1272

Chapter 16

Se-Derivatized RNAs for X-ray Crystallography

Lina Lin and Zhen Huang

Abstract

Selenium derivatization of RNA is an important strategy for crystal structure determination and functional studies of noncoding RNAs and protein–RNA interactions. We describe here the synthesis of nucleoside 5′-(α-P-seleno)-triphosphate analogs (Se-NTPs) and their use in vitro transcription and purification of Se-derivatized RNA samples (phosphoroselenoate RNA, PSe-RNA).

Key words: Selenium-derivatized nucleoside triphosphates, Se-derivatized RNA, Selenium nucleic acid, Transcription, Crystallography

1. Introduction

The phase problem has been one of the long-standing challenges for RNA crystallography (1). To solve the phase problem through the MAD phasing technique, RNA has to be derivatized by heavy atoms, such as selenium, either through indirect derivatization where the RNA binds seleno-protein (2–4) or through direct derivatization with Se covalently incorporated into the RNA itself (5, 6). Although the indirect derivatization technique, for example using Se-Met U1A protein (an RNA binding protein), has successfully been used to solve several RNA structures, it is labor-intensive because it requires preparing numerous RNA constructs for derivatization. Direct Se-derivatized nucleic acids have been found to be stable and do not cause significant structure perturbation (5, 7–13). Selenium can be directly introduced into RNA through solid-phase synthesis or enzymatic transcription (5, 6). However, due to the relatively high cost of solid-phase synthesis, RNA in vitro transcription is still more accessible and affordable for most molecular and structural biology laboratories. Thus, we developed the synthesis of nucleoside 5′-(α-P-seleno)-triphosphate analogs (Se-NTP; Fig. 1) to prepare PSe-RNA through enzymatic transcription (14, 15).

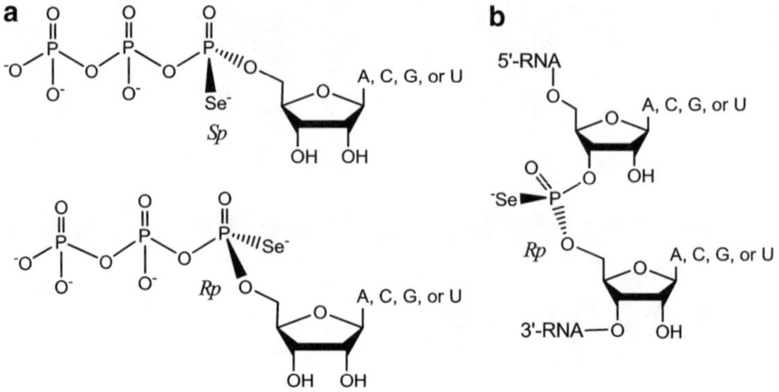

Fig. 1. Chemical structures of the Se-derivatized nucleotides. (**a**) Nucleoside 5′-(α-P-seleno)-triphosphates (Se-NTP, Sp and Rp). (**b**) Phosphoroselenoate RNA (PSe-RNA, Rp).

2. Materials

2.1. BTSe Synthesis

1. 2,2′-Dithiosalicylic acid (1.5 g).
2. Triphenylphosphine selenide (5.1 g).
3. 1,4-Dioxane (ACS grade).
4. 100 mL round bottom flask.
5. Reflux condenser.
6. Clamps.
7. Heating mantle.
8. Stir bar.
9. Magnetic stirrer.
10. Septa.
11. Balloon filled with argon gas.
12. Syringe needle.
13. Thin layer chromatography (TLC) plate, 250 μm.
14. Petroleum ether.
15. Dichloromethane.
16. UV lamp for monitoring TLC.
17. Rotary evaporator.
18. Ethyl acetate.
19. Silica gel column.
20. Ethanol.
21. Filter paper.
22. Funnel.

2.2. Se-NTP Synthesis

1. Individual ribonucleosides.
2. Tributylammonium pyrophosphate.
3. 2-Chloro-4*H*-1,3,2-benzodioxaphosphorin-4-one.
4. 3*H*-1,2-Benzothaselenol-3-one (BTSe; from Subheading 3.1).
5. Dimethylformamide (DMF), anhydrous.
6. Dimethyl sulfoxide (DMSO), anhydrous.
7. Tributylamine (TBA).
8. 1,4-Dioxane, anhydrous.
9. 10 mL round-bottom flasks.
10. Stir bars.
11. Parafilm.
12. Septa.
13. Syringe needles.
14. Syringes.
15. Oil vacuum pump.
16. Balloons filled with argon gas.
17. Magnetic stirrer.
18. Clamps.
19. 1 M dithiothreitol (DTT).
20. 3 M NaCl.
21. Ethanol.
22. Ammonium hydroxide.
23. Isopropanol.
24. −80°C freezer.
25. Preparative centrifuge, rotor and 50 mL high-speed centrifuge tubes.
26. TLC plate, 250 μm.
27. UV lamp.
28. Reverse-phase HPLC system with C18 column.
29. HPLC Buffer A: 20 mM triethylamine–acetic acid (TEAAc) buffer in deionized water, pH 7.
30. HPLC Buffer B: 20 mM TEAAc buffer in 50% acetonitrile and deionized water (v/v), pH 7.
31. Lyophilizer.

2.3. PSe-RNA Transcription

1. T7 RNA polymerase. This enzyme is commercially available and should be supplied with reaction buffer (we use enzyme and 10× buffer from New England Biolabs®). If transcription kit is preferred, we recommend AmpliScribe™ T7-Flash™ Transcription kit from Epicentre®.

2. 10× T7 Transcription Buffer: 400 mM Tris–HCl, pH 7.9, 60 mM $MgCl_2$, 100 mM DTT, and 20 mM spermidine.
3. 100 mM $MgCl_2$.
4. 100 mM $MnCl_2$.
5. 100 mM solutions of each rNTP except the one(s) being substituted for the Se-rNTP analog.
6. 100 mM DTT.
7. DNA template solution: Single-stranded template and promoter DNA (10 μM), PCR template 200 ng/μL, or plasmid template 500 ng/μL.
8. 25× Inorganic pyrophosphatase stock solution: 0.1 unit/μL.
9. 10× Gel loading dye: 0.21% Bromophenol Blue, 0.21% Xylene Cyanol FF, 0.2 M EDTA, pH 8.0, and 50% glycerol.
10. RNase-free water.
11. Sterile 0.5 mL tube.
12. A heating block or a water bath.
13. Pipettes and pipettes tips.

2.4. Purification of PSe-RNA by Polyacrylamide Gel Electrophoresis

1. 0.5 M EDTA: Weigh out 9.31 g EDTA disodium salt. Dissolve in 40 mL deionized water and adjust the pH with NaOH until all EDTA is dissolved (approximately a pH of 8.0). Bring final volume to 50 mL by adding deionized water.
2. 5× TBE stock solution: 1.1 M Tris base, 900 mM boric acid, and 25 mM EDTA, pH 8.3. Weigh out 108 g Tris base and 55 g boric acid and transfer them to an Erlenmeyer flask. Add 40 mL of 0.5 M EDTA solution and 1,900 mL of deionized water to the flask. Adjust pH to 8.3 by adding concentrated HCl. Bring the final volume to 2 L by adding deionized water.
3. 40% (w/v) Acrylamide/bis-acrylamide (19:1) solution stock solution. Weigh out 380 g acrylamide and 20 g bis-acrylamide and bring the final volume to 1 L by adding deionized water. Alternatively, premixed solutions are commercially available. Store at 4°C.
4. 10% ammonium persulfate solution in water. Store at 4°C.
5. N,N,N,N-tetramethyl-ethylenediamine (TEMED). Store at 4°C.
6. Polyacrylamide gel electrophoresis (PAGE) apparatus.
7. 0.2 μm nylon syringe filter.
8. Preparative centrifuge, rotor, and 50 mL high-speed centrifuge tubes.
9. Tube rotator.
10. 4°C refrigerator.

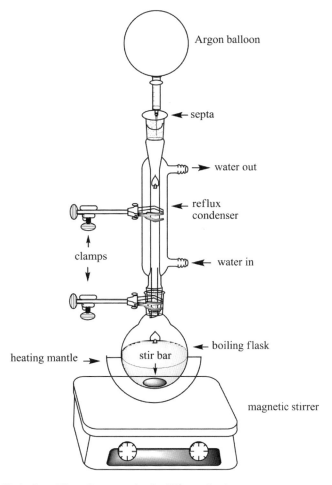

Fig. 2. Illustration of the reflux apparatus for BTSe synthesis.

3. Methods

3.1. 3H-1,2-Benzothaselenol-3-One Synthesis

1. Dissolve the 2,2′-dithiosalicylic acid (1.5 g, 5 mmol) and triphenylphosphine selenide (5.1 g, 15 mmol) in 1,4-dioxane (50 mL) in a 100-mL round bottom flask.
2. Reflux (see Fig. 2 for setup) the reaction for 3 days and monitor the generation of the product by TLC under a UV lamp using petroleum ether:dichloromethane (3:1) as eluent (see Note 1 and Fig. 3 for a sample TLC result).
3. Evaporate the solvent using a rotary evaporator (see Note 2).
4. Redissolve and purify the solid residue on a silica gel column with a step gradient of ethyl acetate in petroleum ether (0–10%) as eluent. Monitor the eluates by TLC as before and pool the appropriate fractions together.
5. Evaporate the solvent from the BTSe-containing fractions in a round bottom flask using a rotary evaporator.

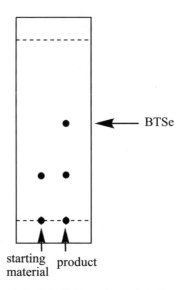

Fig. 3. Example of TLC analysis of the BTSe product and starting material.

6. Recrystallize solid residue from ethanol by dissolving the solid residue in a minimum amount of hot ethanol. Filter the hot solution to remove the insoluble impurities. Slowly cool down the solution to recrystallize the BTSe (a bright orange colored compound). Filter the solution again to collect the BTSE solid.

7. The reaction yield is approximately 70%. Check ^{1}H-NMR for purity. See Note 3 for BTSe NMR data (16).

3.2. Se-NTP Synthesis and Purification

The following procedure should be performed under argon with stirring. All organic solvents required for this experiment must be anhydrous and all other solutions should be purged with argon before use (see Note 4).

1. Weigh out the individual nucleoside (compound 1, Fig. 4; 0.45 mmol), tributylammonium pyrophosphate (compound 3, Fig. 4; 426 mg, 0.9 mmol, 2 eq.), and 3H-1,2-benzothaselenol-3-one (BTSe, from Subheading 3.1, Fig. 4; 195 mg, 0.9 mmol, 2 eq.) and place separate 10 mL round bottom flasks.

2. Put a stir bar into each of the flasks with pyrophosphate and individual nucleoside. Seal all flasks with septa and wrap the septa with parafilm (see Note 5).

3. Dry each compound under high vacuum (created by an oil pump) via a needle connected with vacuum hose for 1 h.

4. Remove the tributylammonium pyrophosphate (compound 3, Fig. 4) flask from the vacuum and quickly attach a balloon inflated with argon to it via a needle. See Fig. 5 for setup of reaction apparatus.

5. Inject DMF (0.6 mL) to dissolve the pyrophosphate, followed by the addition of TBA (1.2 mL).

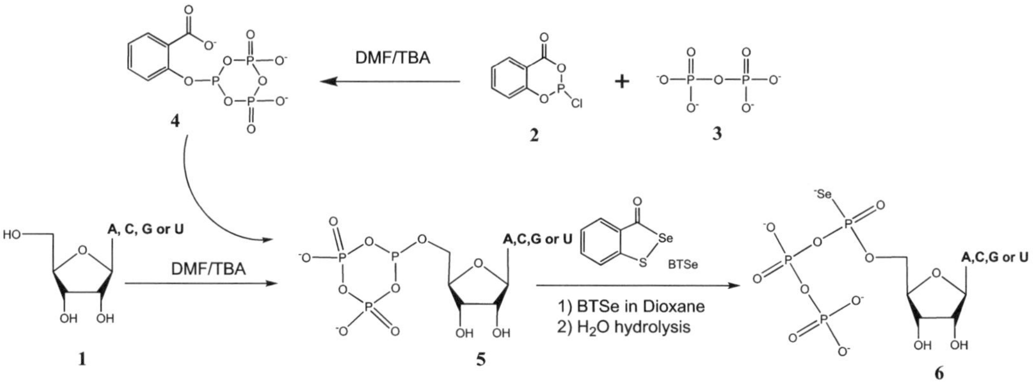

Fig. 4. Facile synthesis of the Se-NTP analogs. *DMF* dimethylformamide, *TBA* tributylamine.

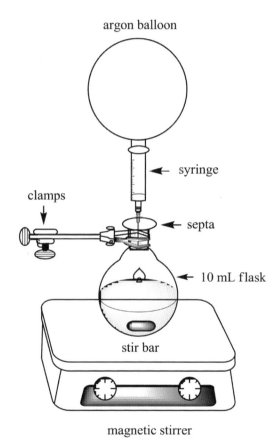

Fig. 5. Illustration of the apparatus for the Se-NTP synthesis.

6. Weigh out and dry 2-chloro-4*H*-1,3,2-benzodioxaphosphorin-4-one (compound 2, Fig. 4; 109 mg, 0.54 mmol, 1.2 eq.) in a flask under vacuum for 15 min.

7. Take the flask off vacuum and quickly attach a balloon inflated with argon to it via a needle.

8. Inject DMF (1.2 mL) to dissolve the 2-chloro-4H-1,3,2-benzodioxaphosphorin-4-one (compound 2, Fig. 4) and then inject this solution into the flask containing the tributylammonium pyrophosphate (compound 3, Fig. 4) from step 5.
9. Stir the reaction mixture at room temperature for 30 min.
10. Remove the flask containing the nucleoside (compound 1, Fig. 4) from the vacuum and quickly attach a balloon inflated with argon to it via a needle at the same time.
11. Dissolve the nucleoside (compound 1, Fig. 4) by injecting: DMF (0.45 mL) for cytidine and uridine; a mixture of DMF (0.32 mL) and DMSO (0.13 mL) for adenosine; or a mixture of DMF (0.23 mL) and DMSO (0.22 mL) for guanosine.
12. Transfer the in situ generated reagent (compound 4, Fig. 4) from step 9 into the nucleoside flask using a syringe and stir the reaction at room temperature for 1 h.
13. Remove the flask containing the BTSe from the vacuum and quickly attach a balloon inflated with argon to it via a needle.
14. Dissolve the BTSe in 1.5 mL 1,4-dioxane (anhydrous) and inject the BTSe solution into the flask containing the cyclic phosphite (compound 5, Fig. 4) generated in step 12. Stir at room temperature for 1 h.
15. Inject 10 mL of water to the reaction flask to initiate the final hydrolysis step (Fig. 4), and stir at room temperature for 2 h (see Note 6).
16. Open the flask and transfer the hydrolyzed Se-NTP into a clean 50 mL centrifuge tube.
17. Add 1 mL of 3 M NaCl, 50 μL of 1 M DTT, and 30 mL of ethanol to the Se-NTP. Seal the tube with a cap and shake to mix thoroughly.
18. Place the tube into a –80°C freezer to chill for 30 min. Collect the Se-NTP product by centrifugation at >8,000 × g for 30 min at 4°C.
19. Remove the supernatant and redissolve the Se-NTP pellet in a minimum amount of water (~100 μL; see Note 7).
20. Check the concentration of Se-NTP by collecting a UV–vis spectrum. The Se-NTPs have the same UV extinction constants as their unmodified equivalents (17) (see Table 1).
21. Take a Se-NTP sample, adjust the concentration to 10 mM and perform a TLC with the corresponding NTP as a control. The eluent for this TLC is isopropanol/ammonium hydroxide/water (5:3:2). TLC analysis will take 45 min to 1 h to finish (an example is shown in Fig. 6).
22. Analyze the synthesized Se-NTPs (compound 6, Fig. 4) by HPLC using a C18 column. We suggest using a linear gradient

Table 1
UV absorption of RNA nucleoside-5′-monophosphates

MTP	ε_{260}	ε_{max}	λ_{max} (nm)
A	15.02	15.04	259
C	7.07	8.74	271
G	12.08	14.09	252
U	9.66	9.78	262

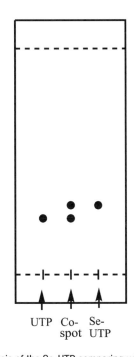

Fig. 6. Example of TLC analysis of the Se-UTP comparing with the native UTP.

from Buffer A (20 mM triethylammonium acetate (TEAAc), pH 7.0) to 12.5% Buffer B (50% acetonitrile in water, 20 mM TEAAc, pH 7.0) over 20 min.

This synthesis method generates both Se-NTP diastereomers. Only the first diastereomer eluted by HPLC is accepted by T7 RNA polymerase while the second one is neither a substrate nor an inhibitor of T7 RNA polymerase. The Se-NTPs can be purified on the HPLC using a similar linear gradient as in **step 22** above, but on a preparative HPLC column. The fractions of the Se-NTP diastereomeric peaks from HPLC should be combined, followed by lyophilization to remove water. RNase-free water (200 µL) is added to rinse the tube and redissolve the Se-NTP. Another NaCl/ethanol precipitation in the presence of DTT is performed (as in **steps 16–19**) for the redissolved Se-NTP before transcription.

The final concentration of Se-NTP is determined by a UV–vis analysis and adjusted to 100 mM for RNA transcription. The crude product can be purified for transcription without separation of diastereomers, such as using boronate affinity column (18, 19). These two NTP-Se diastereomers have an approximately 50:50 ratio. If the mixture of diastereomers is used for transcription, double the amount of the purified NTP-Se should be used.

3.3. PSe-RNA Transcription

1. Set a heating block or a water bath at 37°C.
2. Combine the following reaction components in a 1.5 mL tube at room temperature in the given order. Any one of the standard (commercial) NTPs can be substituted with the corresponding Se-NTP in one 100 μL transcription reaction (see Note 8).

RNase-free water to a final volume of 100 μL	24 μL
PCR DNA template, 200 ng/μL	10 μL
10× T7 Transcription buffer	10 μL
100 mM DTT	10 μL
100 mM ATP/SeATP	4 μL
100 mM CTP/SeCTP	4 μL
100 mM GTP/SeGTP	4 μL
100 mM UTP/SeUTP	4 μL
Inorganic pyrophosphatase (0.1 U/μL)	4 μL
100 mM $MgCl_2$	14 μL
100 mM $MnCl_2$	2 μL
T7 RNA polymerase (50 U/μL)	10 μL

3. Mix well by pipetting.
4. Put the transcription tube in a water bath (37°C) or a heating block. Incubate for 3 h.
5. Add 10 μL 10× gel loading dye to quench the reaction.

3.4. Gel Purification of PSe-RNA

1. Purify PSe-RNA by denaturing PAGE. Load PSe-RNA mixed with gel loading dye on a preparative gel (see Note 9).
2. After the gel electrophoresis is finished, remove one glass plate and place a layer of plastic wrap on the top of the PAGE gel. Place a fluorescent TLC plate on the top of the plastic wrap (with the coated side towards the plastic wrap) and flip over the whole assembly so that the glass plate is on the top. Carefully separate the PAGE gel from the remaining glass plate with a spatula.
3. Shine UV light on the gel to visualize the RNA band (see Fig. 7).

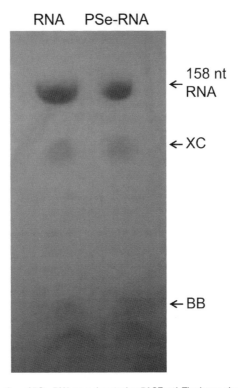

Fig. 7. UV visualization of PSe-RNA on a denaturing PAGE gel. The lanes show 158 nucleotide RNA transcribed with all native NTPs ("RNA"; a positive control) and transcribed with Se-CTP and three other native NTPs ("PSe-RNA"). XC and BP indicate positions of the dyes xylene cyanol FF and bromophenol blue, respectively.

4. Cut the RNA band from the gel, transfer the gel to a clean tube, and crush it with a clean (RNase-free) spatula.

5. Add RNase-free water (two gel volumes) to the crushed gel and add DTT (final concentration 1 mM) to the soaking solution in order to prevent oxidization (or deselenization). Soak the gel debris for 5 h with rotation at 4°C (see Note 10).

6. Centrifuge the gel soaking suspension at $1,000 \times g$ at 4°C for 5–10 min to pellet the gel fragments.

7. Transfer the supernatant to a fresh tube and add RNase-free water (one gel volume) to wash the gel debris.

8. Centrifuge the suspension again at $1,000 \times g$ at 4°C for 5–10 min to pellet the gel debris.

9. Repeat the gel washing step twice.

10. Combine all collected supernatants and filter through a 0.2 or 0.4 μm nylon syringe filter. The sample can be lyophilized to reduce the solution volume, if desired.

11. Perform an NaCl/ethanol precipitation as described in Subheading 3.2 (steps 16–19) to precipitate the PSe-RNA.

12. Redissolve the PSe-RNA pellet in water. Determine the transcription yield of PSe-RNA by UV absorption at 260 nm. Recheck the quality of PSe-RNA on an analytical PAGE if necessary.
13. Store the purified PSe-RNA in a −80°C freezer for future use.

4. Notes

1. The reaction may take a longer time to finish and should be monitored daily by TLC. Check the TLC for the new spot corresponding to product and monitor the ratio of the starting material and product.
2. Solids may be present in the suspension and a filtration step can be helpful before proceeding to the column purification.
3. The ^{1}H NMR spectrum of BTSe clearly indicated four characterized protons in the aromatic area: 7.35 (m, 1H), 7.65 (m, 2H), 7.94 (d, J=8 Hz, 1H). The starting material will have more than four and the spectrum will be much more complicated.
4. For a simple argon purge setup, immerse a syringe needle that is connected with argon tubing into the sample solution. Adjust the argon air flow and make the bubble come out at rate of 1–2 per second. The recommended time is 1 min/mL of solution.
5. A good seal is very important for the reaction, which needs to be anhydrous.
6. After the hydrolysis step is complete argon is no longer needed.
7. The insoluble materials can be removed by centrifugation. The synthesized Se-NTP dissolves in water very well.
8. According to the protocol from New England Biolabs, Mg^{2+} concentration has to be 4 mM higher than the NTP concentration. From our experience, an additional 2 mM Mn^{2+} in the transcription buffer will enhance the transcription yield of PSe-RNA.
9. Make sure everything that contacts the PSe-RNA is RNase-free.
10. If the PSe-RNA transcription and purification cannot be finished in 1 day then the sample should be kept in a −80°C freezer overnight.

Acknowledgments

This work was financially supported by NIH (GM095086) and the Georgia Cancer Coalition (GCC) Distinguished Cancer Clinicians and Scientists.

References

1. Ke A, Doudna JA (2004) Crystallization of RNA and RNA-protein complexes. Methods 34(3):408–414
2. Ferre-D'Amare AR, Zhou K, Doudna JA (1998) Crystal structure of a hepatitis delta virus ribozyme. Nature 395(6702): 567–574
3. Rupert PB, Ferre-D'Amare AR (2001) Crystal structure of a hairpin ribozyme-inhibitor complex with implications for catalysis. Nature 410(6830):780–786
4. Ferre-D'Amare AR (2010) Use of the spliceosomal protein U1A to facilitate crystallization and structure determination of complex RNAs. Methods 52(2):159–167
5. Caton-Williams J, Huang Z (2008) Biochemistry of selenium-derivatized naturally occurring and unnatural nucleic acids. Chem Biodivers 5(3):396–407
6. Sheng J, Huang Z (2010) Selenium derivatization of nucleic acids for X-ray crystal-structure and function studies. Chem Biodivers 7(4): 753–785
7. Jiang J et al (2007) Selenium derivatization of nucleic acids for crystallography. Nucleic Acids Res 35(2):477–485
8. Salon J et al (2007) Oxygen replacement with selenium at the thymidine 4-position for the Se base pairing and crystal structure studies. J Am Chem Soc 129(16):4862–4863
9. Sheng J et al (2007) Synthesis of a 2′-Se-thymidine phosphoramidite and its incorporation into oligonucleotides for crystal structure study. Org Lett 9(5):749–752
10. Olieric V et al (2009) A fast selenium derivatization strategy for crystallization and phasing of RNA structures. RNA 15(4):707–715
11. Sheng J et al (2010) Synthesis and crystal structure study of 2′-se-adenosine-derivatized DNA. Sci China Chem 53:78–85
12. Hassan AE et al (2010) High fidelity of base pairing by 2-selenothymidine in DNA. J Am Chem Soc 132(7):2120–2121
13. Salon J et al (2010) Synthesis and crystal structure of 2′-se-modified guanosine containing DNA. J Org Chem 75(3):637–641
14. Carrasco N et al (2005) Efficient enzymatic synthesis of phosphoroselenoate RNA by using adenosine 5′-(alpha-P-seleno)-triphosphate. Angew Chem Int Ed Engl 45(1):94–97
15. Brandt G, Carrasco N, Huang Z (2006) Efficient substrate cleavage catalyzed by hammerhead ribozymes derivatized with selenium for X-ray crystallography. Biochemistry 45(29): 8972–8977
16. Stawinski J, Thelin M (1994) Nucleoside H-phosphonates. 14. Synthesis of nucleoside phosphoroselenoates and phosphorothioselenoates via stereospecific selenization of the corresponding H-phosphonate and H-phosphonothioate diesters with the aid of new selenium-transfer reagent, 3 H-1,2-benzothiaselenol-3-one. J Org Chem 59:130–136
17. Cavaluzzi MJ, Borer PN (2004) Revised UV extinction coefficients for nucleoside-5′-monophosphates and unpaired DNA and RNA. Nucleic Acids Res 32(1):e13
18. Liu XC, Scouten WH (2000) Boronate affinity chromatography. Methods Mol Biol 147: 119–128
19. Batey RT et al (1992) Preparation of isotopically labeled ribonucleotides for multidimensional NMR spectroscopy of RNA. Nucleic Acids Res 20(17):4515–4523

Chapter 17

Biosynthetic Preparation of ^{13}C/^{15}N-Labeled rNTPs for High-Resolution NMR Studies of RNAs

Luigi Martino and Maria R. Conte

Abstract

High-resolution investigations of the structure and dynamics of RNA molecules by nuclear magnetic resonance (NMR) methodologies require the production of ^{13}C/^{15}N-isotopically labeled samples. A common strategy entails the preparation of ^{13}C/^{15}N-enriched ribonucleoside 5′-triphosphates (rNTPs) to be incorporated into RNA oligomers by in vitro transcription. Here, we describe the methods to obtain isotopically labeled rNTP in a uniform or selective fashion from bacterial cultures, using common and versatile *E. coli* strains. This chapter also covers procedures for extraction and digestion of the total RNA from bacterial cells, purification of the ribonucleoside 5′-monophosphates and their enzymatic phosphorylation to rNTPs.

Key words: RNA, ^{13}C/^{15}N-labeled rNTPs, NMR, Site-specific labeling, Isotopic labeling, *E. coli* strains

1. Introduction

Nuclear magnetic resonance (NMR) spectroscopy is a valuable tool for investigating structure and dynamics of nucleic acids (and their complexes) in solution. One of the challenges for NMR investigations of RNA molecules is the requirement for milligram quantities of ^{13}C, ^{15}N and, in some instances ^{2}H labeled samples, brought about by the poor chemical shift dispersion, lower proton density and increased resonance linewidths exhibited by RNAs compared to proteins. Uniform ^{13}C/^{15}N-isotopic labeling of RNA oligos, however, has now become routine (1–10). Most RNAs for NMR studies are prepared by T7 RNA polymerase in vitro transcription, using either commercially available ^{13}C- ^{15}N- and/or ^{2}H-labeled ribonucleoside 5′-triphosphates (rNTPs) or in-house isotopically labeled rNTPs obtained from bacteria cultures. For the latter, *Escherichia coli* (*E. coli*) strains are typically grown on minimal media supplemented with ^{15}N- and ^{13}C-sources; labels may be introduced in a uniform or selective manner according to the desired ^{13}C-incorporation (see below). The total RNA, extracted from the bacterial cells following lysis, is enzymatically degraded to ribonucleoside 5′-monophosphates (rNMPs). rNMPs are separated from the deoxyribonucleoside 5′-monophosphates (dNMPs) and enzymatically converted to rNTPs, which are then utilized as building blocks to generate RNA oligomers (1, 11). Here we describe the protocol, depicted in Fig. 1, to obtain biosynthetically pure isotopically labeled rNTPs ready to use in T7 polymerase in vitro transcriptions. This method is general and could be adapted for the production of in-house unlabeled rNTPs; furthermore bespoke variations have been introduced for the preparation of ^{13}C/^{15}N-dNTPs (12). Modifications of the method also include purification of individual ^{13}C/^{15}N-enriched rNTPs (steps indicated with dotted lines in Fig. 1; (7, 9, 11, 13) and see Chapter 18). This may be desirable for the production of RNA samples only containing a subset of isotopically labeled nucleotides.

The benefits of the alternate specific labeling are twofold: first, the simplification of the resonance assignments, even more a problem for larger RNA molecules, and second the removal of the strong ^{13}C–^{13}C J-couplings and the one bond ^{13}C–^{13}C dipolar couplings, thereby simplifying the analysis of ^{13}C relaxation data (2, 3, 14). This enables a more comprehensive analysis of the conformational dynamics of RNA molecules over a wide range of timescales, to investigate the relative amplitude of internal motions including base pair opening, base flipping, ribose-pucker conformational averaging, secondary structure fluctuations, etc. (3, 15, 16).

For larger RNAs, where the adverse effects of the ^{1}H dipolar relaxation become very severe, perdeuteration of non-exchangeable sites has proved useful to enhance the sensitivity of NOE-based experiments between exchangeable protons (17). The procedure to obtain uniformly ^{15}N/^{2}H-labeled rNTPs is described by Nikonowicz et al. (17). The most attractive strategy however entails specific deuteration, where selected sites on the RNA are labeled with ^{2}H. Methods have been developed to obtain ribose rings differentially labeled with ^{2}H, using a number of enzymatic reactions to convert unlabeled glucose to rNTPs (reviewed in refs. 18, 19); nevertheless, as several of the required enzymes are not yet commercially available, this will not be covered in this chapter.

Various methods exist to biosynthetically produce ^{13}C/^{15}N-labeled rNTPs. Although in the past decade the relative cost of ^{13}C-labeled sources propelled the use of *Methylophilus methylotropus* grown on ^{13}C-methanol containing media, this has now been superseded by *E. coli* grown on other ^{13}C-labeled carbon sources to produce labeled rNTPs (2, 3, 11, 19). In this chapter, the methods to obtain rNTPs with uniform or alternate site-specific ^{13}C-labeling are described. The latter involves appropriate combinations

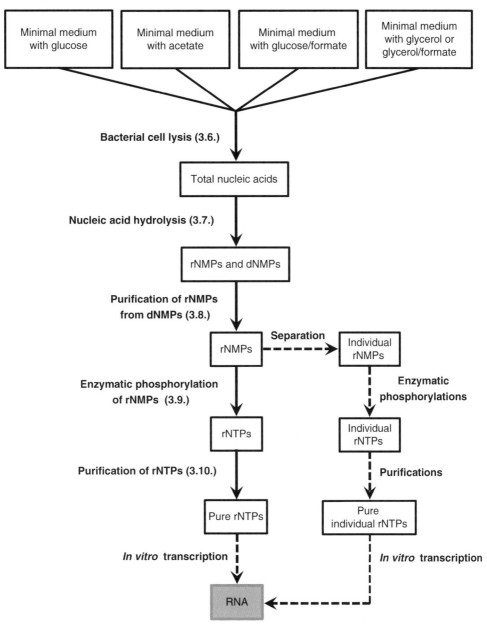

Fig. 1. Flowchart showing the general procedure for the biosynthetic production of $^{13}C/^{15}N$-labeled rNTPs for RNA in vitro transcription. The steps indicated by *solid arrows* represent the protocols described in this chapter. The steps indicated with a *broken arrow* are not dealt with in this chapter (*see* text for details).

of selectively ^{13}C-labeled carbon sources and bacterial strains, including routinely used *E. coli* types and strains carrying metabolic gene mutations (13, 19, 20). In particular, these consist of DL323, deficient in two tricarboxylic acid (TCA) cycle enzymes (succinate dehydrogenase, *sdh*, and malate dehydrogenase, *mdg*), and K10-1516, lacking in glucose-6-phosphate dehydrogenase (G6PDH) enzyme (13, 20). Table 1 summarizes the different permutations described here and the resultant site-specific isotopic labeled patterns.

2. Materials

2.1. Bacterial Strains

1. *E. coli* strains routinely used, including the JM series, BL21 series, and K12 (see Note 1).
2. *E. coli* mutant strain DL323, genotype: F- *sdh-1*, λ-, *mdh-2*, *rph-1*. DL3212 can be obtained from the Yale Coli Genetic Stock Centre (#7538).
3. *E. coli* mutant strain K10-1516, genotype: HFr *fhuA22*, *zwf-2*, *relA1*, *T2R*, *pfk-10*. K10-1516 can be obtained from the Yale Coli Genetic Stock Centre (#4858).
4. LB-agar plates to streak out cells prior to culture growth.

2.2. Media for Bacterial Growth: Minimal Medium

1. Minimal medium base solution (see Note 2): 7 g of Na_2HPO_4, 3 g of KH_2PO_4, 1 g of $^{15}NH_4Cl$, and 0.5 g of NaCl. Dissolve the solids in 0.8 L of distilled water, adjust the pH to 7.0, make up to 1 L final volume with additional water and autoclave.
2. Using distilled water, prepare the following individual stock solutions:
   (a) 1 M $MgSO_4$.
   (b) 0.1 M $CaCl_2$.
   (c) 1 M thiamine.
   (d) *E. coli* trace elements: 5 g of EDTA, 0.5 g of $FeCl_3$, 0.05 g of $ZnCl_2$, 0.01 g of $CuCl_2$, 0.01 g of $CoCl_2 \cdot 6H_2O$, and 0.01 g of H_3BO_3 dissolved in 1.0 L distilled water. First dissolve the EDTA in 0.8 L of water and adjust to pH 7.0 with concentrated HCl. Next, add the other reagents in order returning to pH 7 after each component and finally bring the solution to a final volume of 1 L with distilled water.

   Filter sterilize each of the stock solutions, and wrap the *E. coli* trace elements and thiamine solution in aluminum foil. Store at 25°C until use (see Note 3).
3. 10 mL stock solution of the required ^{13}C-labeled carbon source to achieve the desired rNTP labeling pattern (see Table 1 for amounts and Note 4).
4. 1 mL stock solution of the correspondent unlabeled carbon (^{12}C) source.

Table 1
Experimental conditions using minimal or Studier medium correlating *E. coli* strain, ^{13}C-labeling source and their resultant ^{13}C-labeling pattern for biosynthetically produced rNTPs

Cells	^{13}C source	Amount per L (g)	Medium	Labeling pattern		References
E. coli	^{13}C-glucose	2	Minimal	–	Uniform	
E. coli	^{13}CH$_3$^{13}COOH	1.5	Minimal	–	Uniform	
E. coli	^{13}CH$_3$COOH	1.5	Minimal	Ribose	>80% C2'; >90% C1', C4', C5'	(23)
				Purine	>95% C2, C5 and C8	
				Pyrimidine	>90% C5 and C6	
E. coli	CH$_3$^{13}COOH	1.5	Minimal	Ribose	>75% C3'	(23)
				Purine	>90% C4 and C6	
				Pyrimidine	>95% C2 and C4	
E. coli	^{12}C-glucose/^{13}C-formate	2/0.2	Minimal	Ribose	–	(3)
				Purine	>85% C8	
				Pyrimidine	–	
E. coli	4-^{13}C-glucose	1	Minimal	Ribose	C3'	(13)
				Purine	–	
				Pyrimidine	–	
DL323	1,3-^{13}C$_2$-glycerol	1–2	Minimal	Ribose	Mixture of C2'/C3'/C5' (55%) and C1'/C3'/C5' (25%)	(13)
				Purine	–	
				Pyrimidine	90% C5	

(continued)

Table 1 (continued)

Cells	^{13}C source	Amount per L (g)	Medium	Labeling pattern		References
DL323	2-^{13}C-glycerol	1–2	Minimal	Ribose	Mixture of C1'/C4' (55%) and C2'/C4' (30%)	(13)
				Purine	–	
				Pyrimidine	90% C6	
K10-1516	2-^{13}C-glycerol	2	Minimal/ Studier	Ribose	>80% C2' and C4'	(13, 20)
				Purine	–	
				Pyrimidine	~50% C5 and C6	
K10-1516	2-^{13}C-glycerol/^{13}C-formate	2/0.2	Studier	Ribose	>80% C2' and C4'	(20)
				Purine	40% C8; 26% C2	
				Pyrimidine	~50% C5 and C6	

5. Prepare the final minimal medium by adding the following to the minimal medium base solution after it has cooled after autoclaving: 1 mL of $MgSO_4$, 1 mL of $CaCl_2$, 1 mL of thiamine, 10 mL of *E. coli* trace elements, and the 10 mL stock solution of ^{13}C-labeled carbon source.

6. Per liter of final minimal medium with ^{13}C-labeled carbon source (item 5, above), prepare 100 mL of the same medium by scaling the quantities of reagents appropriately and using the 1 mL stock solution of unlabeled carbon (^{12}C) source. This unlabeled medium is used for initial culture steps.

2.3. Media for Bacterial Growth: Studier Medium

1. Studier medium base solution: 6.8 g of KH_2PO_4, 7.1 g of Na_2HPO_4, and 3.3 g of $(^{15}NH_4)_2SO_4$. Dissolve the solids in 0.8 L of distilled water, adjust the pH to 7.0, make up to 1 L with distilled water and autoclave.

2. Using distilled water, prepare the following stock solutions (21):
   (a) 1 M $MgSO_4$
   (b) 0.1 M $FeCl_3$, dissolve in 0.1 M HCl
   (c) 1 M $CaCl_2$
   (d) 1 M $MnCl_2$
   (e) 1 M $ZnSO_4$
   (f) 0.2 M $CoCl_2$
   (g) 0.1 M $CuCl_2$
   (h) 0.2 M $NiCl_2$
   (i) 0.1 M Na_2MnO_4
   (j) 0.1 M Na_2SeO_3
   (k) 0.1 M H_3BO_3

   Filter sterilize the stock solutions, wrap them in aluminum foil and store at 25°C until use.

3. 10 mL stock solution of the required ^{13}C-labeled carbon source to achieve the desired rNTP labeling pattern (see Table 1 and Note 4).

4. 1 mL stock solution of the correspondent unlabeled carbon (^{12}C) source.

5. Prepare 1 L Studier medium by adding the following to the Studier medium base solution after it has cooled after autoclaving: 2 mL of $MgSO_4$, 5 mL of $FeCl_3$, 0.2 mL of $CaCl_2$, 0.1 mL of $MnCl_2$, 0.1 mL of $ZnSO_4$, 0.1 mL of $CoCl_2$, 0.2 mL of $CuCl_2$, 0.1 mL of $NiCl_2$, 0.2 mL of Na_2MnO_4, 0.2 mL of Na_2SeO_3, 0.2 mL of H_3BO_3, and the 10 mL stock solution of ^{13}C-labeled carbon source.

6. Per liter of final Studier medium with ^{13}C-labeled carbon source (item 5, above), prepare 100 mL of the same medium by scaling the quantities of reagents appropriately and using the 1 mL stock solution of unlabeled carbon (^{12}C) source. This unlabeled medium is used for initial culture steps.

2.4. Isotopes

^{13}C- and ^{15}N-labeled compounds at 99% enrichment are available from Cambridge Isotopes Laboratories or Isotec-Sigma Aldrich.

2.5. Bacterial Cell Lysis

1. Sodium Tris EDTA (STE) buffer: 10 mM Tris–HCl, 100 mM NaCl, 1 mM EDTA, pH 8.0.
2. 10% w/v sodium dodecyl sulfate (SDS), pH 7.2.
3. Phenol:chloroform:isoamyl alcohol solution (25:24:1) (see Note 5).
4. Chloroform.
5. 3 M sodium acetate, pH 5.2.
6. Isopropyl alcohol.
7. Polypropylene tube(s) with cap (50–250 mL) and appropriate centrifuge/rotor to spin the tubes at $12,000 \times g$.

2.6. Nucleic Acid Hydrolysis

1. Nuclease P1 (Sigma-Aldrich).
2. 3 M sodium acetate, pH 5.2.
3. 40 mM $ZnSO_4$.

2.7. Purification of rNMPs from dNMPs

1. Tris-EDTA (TE) Buffer: 10 mM Tris–HCl, pH 8.0, 1 mM EDTA.
2. 1 M triethylammonium bicarbonate (TEABC), pH 9.5. Prepared by passing CO_2 gas into a 1 M aqueous solution of triethylamine at 5°C (see Note 6).
3. Acidified water at pH 4–5 (see Note 7).
4. Affi-gel boronate-derivatized polyacrylamide gel (Bio-Rad).
5. 20×2.5 cm glass column with FPLC end adaptors.
6. Automated FPLC system refrigerated at 4°C and equipped with UV detector and fraction collector.

2.8. Enzymatic Phosphorylation of rNMPs

1. Phosphoenolpyruvate (PEP; VWR International).
2. Myokinase (MK) from rabbit muscle (Sigma-Aldrich).
3. Pyruvate kinase (PK) from rabbit muscle (Sigma-Aldrich).
4. Guanylate kinase (GK) from porcine brain (Sigma-Aldrich).
5. Nucleoside monophosphate kinase (NMP) from beef liver (Roche).
6. Three-necked round bottom flask (50–100 mL).
7. Nitrogen gas line.

8. Reaction buffer: 140 mM Tris–HCl, 80 mM KCl, 80 mM MgCl$_2$, 400 mM PEP, and 0.8 mM ATP, pH 7.5.
9. 0.1 M dithiothreitol (DTT).
10. 0.5 M HCl.

2.9. Purification of rNTPs

All reagents described for purification of rNMPs from dNMPs (Subheading 2.7) are also required for the final purification of rNTPs.

1. Centrifugal microconcentrators, 10 kDa molecular weight cut-off.
2. Appropriate centrifuge and rotor to spin microconcentrators at $2,000 \times g$.

3. Methods

Carry out all procedures at room temperature unless otherwise specified. The protocol described here refers to 1 L of bacterial culture but can be scaled up as necessary (see Note 8). Bacterial culture in isotopically labeled minimal media (Subheadings 3.1–3.4) or Studier medium (Subheading 3.5) is performed in three stages: an unlabeled 5 mL starter culture, a labeled 50 mL culture, and a labeled 1 L culture split into two 500 mL aliquots. At all stages during this procedure, take care that the cultures do not reach saturation, measured by reading the optical density at 600 nm.

3.1. Bacterial Cell Growth on Minimal Medium and Glucose

1. Streak *E. coli* from a glycerol stock on an LB plate without antibiotic and incubate overnight at 37°C (see Note 9).
2. Prepare the starting culture medium with unlabeled glucose as described in Subheading 2.2.
3. Prepare the minimal medium as described in Subheading 2.2 using the appropriate labeled glucose as carbon source (see Table 1).
4. With an individual colony inoculate a 5 mL starting culture in the minimal medium with unlabeled glucose and leave it to grow for 12–16 h with shaking (220–270 rpm) at 37°C.
5. Centrifuge the culture at $6,000 \times g$ for 5 min and wash the resultant pellet twice with minimal medium with unlabeled carbon source.
6. Resuspend the pellet in 50 mL of minimal medium with ^{13}C-labeled carbon source.
7. Grow with shaking at 37°C for approximately 12 h. Split this culture in half to inoculate each of the two 500 mL aliquots of minimal medium with ^{13}C-labeled carbon source.

8. Incubate the 500 mL cultures at 37°C with agitation for approximately 12–16 h.
9. Harvest the cells by centrifugation at $6{,}400 \times g$ for 15–20 min and store the pellet at –80°C.

3.2. Bacterial Cell Growth on Minimal Medium and Acetate

1. Streak *E. coli* from a glycerol stock on an LB-agar plate without antibiotic and incubate overnight at 37°C (see Note 9).
2. Prepare the starting culture medium with unlabeled glucose as described in Subheading 2.2.
3. Prepare the 50 mL and 1 L minimal medium as described in Subheading 2.2 using the appropriate labeled acetate as carbon source for the desired labeling pattern (see Table 1 and Note 10).
4. Conduct the bacterial cultures in three stages as described in Subheading 3.1 (steps 4–9). The initial 5 mL overnight cell culture is conducted in medium containing unlabeled glucose as before. Use this to inoculate the labeled sodium acetate medium (see Note 11).

3.3. Bacterial Cell Growth on Minimal Media and Glucose/Formate

1. Streak *E. coli* from a glycerol stock on an LB-agar plate without antibiotic and incubate overnight at 37°C (see Note 9).
2. Prepare the starting culture with unlabeled glucose as described in Subheading 2.2.
3. Prepare the 50 mL and 1 L minimal medium as described in Subheading 2.2 using ^{12}C-glucose and ^{13}C-formate as carbon source for the desired labeling pattern (see Table 1 and Note 12).
4. Conduct the bacterial cultures in three stages as described in Subheading 3.1 (steps 4–9). The initial 5 mL overnight cell culture is conducted in medium containing unlabeled *glucose* as before. Use this to inoculate the labeled glucose/formate medium.

3.4. Bacterial Cell Growth on Minimal Media and Glycerol or Glycerol/Formate

1. Streak *E. coli* from a glycerol stock on an LB-agar plate without antibiotic and incubate overnight at 37°C (see Note 9).
2. Prepare the starting culture with unlabeled glucose as described in Subheading 2.2.
3. Prepare the 50 mL and 1 L minimal medium as described in Subheading 2.2 using one of the following sources of carbon: 1,3-^{13}C-glycerol; 2-^{13}C-glycerol; or 2-^{13}C-glycerol/^{13}C-formate.
4. Conduct the bacterial cultures in three stages as described in Subheading 3.1 (steps 4–9) using glycerol or glycerol/formate as source of carbon and mutant *E. coli* strains in the appropriate combination according to the required ^{13}C-incorporation (see Table 1 and Note 13).

3.5. Bacterial Cell Growth on Studier Medium

1. Streak K10-1516 cells from a glycerol stock on an LB plate without antibiotic and incubate overnight at 37°C (see Note 9).

2. Prepare the starting culture with unlabeled glycerol as described in Subheading 2.2.

3. Prepare the Studier medium as described in Subheading 2.3 (step 4) using the appropriate ^{13}C-labeled carbon source (see Table 1 and Note 14).

4. With a single colony inoculate a 5 mL starting culture of Studier medium with the corresponding unlabeled carbon source, and incubate for 12–16 h with shaking (220–270 rpm) at 37°C.

5. Centrifuge the sample at $6,000 \times g$ for 5 min and wash twice the pellet with medium with unlabeled carbon source.

6. Resuspend the pellet in 5 mL of Studier medium with unlabeled carbon source, and incubate at 37°C for 12–14 h with shaking (270 rpm), taking care that cells do not reach stationary phase.

7. Centrifuge the sample at $6,000 \times g$ for 5 min and wash the resultant pellet in unlabeled medium before resuspending it in 50 mL of Studier medium without any carbon source.

8. Add 5 mL of this suspension to each of the two 500 mL Studier medium containing ^{13}C-labeled carbon source, and incubate with shaking at 37°C for 12 h.

9. Harvest the cells by centrifugation at $6,400 \times g$ for 15–20 min and store the pellet at −80°C.

3.6. Bacterial Cell Lysis

This procedure is reported per liter of culture, corresponding to approximately 4 g of wet cell pellet (see Note 15). With this procedure the total cellular nucleic acid content is extracted, therefore requiring a subsequent purification of ribonucleotides from deoxyribonucleotides (Subheading 3.8; see Note 16).

1. Resuspend the cell pellet in 100 mL of STE buffer. Ensure that no clumps remain in the suspension.

2. At 37°C, add 5 mL of 10% SDS solution to the cell suspension (to a final SDS concentration of 0.5% w/v) and keep the sample under vigorous stirring for 15 min for a complete cell lysis.

3. Transfer the cells to a polypropylene tube with cap and add 100 mL of phenol:chloroform:isoamyl alcohol (25:24:1) solution at room temperature (see Note 5). Mix briefly until an emulsion forms (see Note 17).

4. Separate the emulsion by centrifugation at $12,000 \times g$ for 3–5 min at room temperature. Collect the upper aqueous layer (which contains the nucleic acids), transfer it to a new tube and discard the lower organic layer (see Note 18).

5. Repeat steps 3 and 4 on the retained aqueous phase three times or until the proteins are no longer visible at the interface (indicating that all they have been removed; see Note 18).

6. Mix the aqueous phase with an equal volume of chloroform in order to remove any residual phenol. The two phases will separate without centrifugation. Remove the upper aqueous phase and transfer to a new tube.

7. To the aqueous phase add the required volume of 3 M sodium acetate to reach a final concentration of 300 mM. Mix the resulting solution with an equal volume of isopropyl alcohol and incubate overnight at −20°C. This will cause the precipitation of the nucleic acids.

8. Separate the precipitated nucleic acids from the supernatant by centrifugation at $12,000 \times g$ for 30 min. The liquid is discarded and the pellet is stored at −20°C.

3.7. Nucleic Acid Hydrolysis

This protocol applies to the nucleic acid pellet obtained in Subheading 3.6 from 1 L of bacterial culture (approximately 3,250–3,500 A_{260} units; see Note 19). Adjust the scale if necessary.

1. Resuspend the nucleic acid pellet from the lysis procedure in 25 mL of STE buffer. Heat the suspension in a water bath at 95°C for 5–6 min.

2. Cool the solution on ice and add 125 μl of 3 M sodium acetate and 62.5 μl of 40 mM $ZnSO_4$, to reach final concentrations of 15 mM sodium acetate and 0.1 mM $ZnSO_4$, respectively.

3. Hydrolyse the nucleic acids by adding six to ten units of nuclease P1 and incubate for 1–2 h at 55°C (see Note 20).

3.8. Purification of rNMPs from dNMPs

The chromatographic procedure described here is conducted at 4°C to ensure optimal rNMP separation (see Note 21) and also removes salts and other impurities. This step can be omitted if an alternative strategy was used during lysis that removes DNA (see Note 16). An alternative method using Ion-Pair Reverse-Phase HPLC is described in Chapter 18.

1. Hydrate 5 g of Affi-gel Boronate gel with TE buffer. Pack the resin in the glass column, connect the column to an FPLC system and equilibrate it with 1 M TEABC at 4°C (see Note 22).

2. Lyophilize the nucleotide solution from the nuclease P1 digestion (Subheading 3.7) and resuspend it in 10 mL of 1 M TEABC buffer.

3. Load the nucleotide solution onto the column and wash with 1 M TEABC at 4°C until the UV absorbance returns to baseline. The rNMPs bind to the boronate column in these conditions, whereas the dNMPs, which do not interact with the boronate

gel, are washed out in the flow through, together with salts and other impurities.

4. Elute the rNMPs with acidified water at pH 4–5 at 4°C, collecting fractions until the A_{260} drops below 0.1 (see Note 23).

5. Pool together the fractions containing the rNMPs and lyophilize the solution to remove the volatile TEABC. Resuspend the rNMPs in 5 mL of water (see Note 24).

3.9. Enzymatic Phosphorylation of rNMPs

This procedure is a modification of the method developed by Whitesides and coworkers (22) and is carried out in a three-necked round bottom flask flushed with N_2 gas (see Note 25). The protocol described here involves the phosphorylation of the four rNMPs simultaneously, but enzymatic phosphorylation could be carried out on each individual rNMP if required (see Note 26).

1. Dilute the 5 mL solution from the boronate purification step (Subheading 3.8) containing the rNMPs into the reaction buffer to give a final rNMP concentration of 100 mM (see Note 27). Adjust the pH of the solution to 7.5.

2. Deaerate the solution with N_2 for 30–40 min and add DTT to a final concentration of 2.5 mM.

3. Add 2 units of GK, 800 units of MK, 80 units of PK, and 6.5 units of NMPK and stir the reaction at 37°C for 14 h under positive pressure of N_2. Adjust the pH during the course of the reaction every 2 h by adding the appropriate amount of 0.5 M HCl.

4. After completion (see Note 28), store the reaction mixture at −20°C.

3.10. Purification of rNTPs

This step is carried out to eliminate any salt and high molecular weight impurities (enzymes, etc.; see Note 29).

1. Lyophilize the phosphorylation reaction mixture containing the rNTPs (Subheading 3.9) and resuspend in 10 mL of cold 1 M TEABC buffer, pH 9.5.

2. Load the rNTP solution onto a boronate affinity column and carry out the wash and elution steps as described in Subheading 3.8 (steps 3–4).

3. Collect, pool, and lyophilize the fractions containing the rNTPs.

4. Resuspend the pellet in 2 mL of distilled water and place it in a centrifugal microconcentrator with a 10 kDa molecular weight cut-off membrane. Pass the solution through the centrifugal membrane by centrifugation at $2,000 \times g$ and collect the filtrate, containing the pure rNTPs (see Note 30).

5. The concentration of rNTPs is measured by UV absorbance at 260 nm (see Note 27).

4. Notes

1. In several reports the exact strain of *E. coli* used is not specified and strains such as BL21, BL21(DE3), JM109 have been used interchangeably.
2. There are several largely equivalent versions of minimal media described in literature. The amount of $^{15}NH_4Cl$ varies between 0.7 and 2 g/L and could also be replaced by $(^{15}NH_4)_2SO_4$ in the same amounts (1, 3, 19, 23). The recipes are given here per liter of media but they can be directly scaled up for larger cultures.
3. We find that it is best to prepare the stock solutions fresh each time. The *E. coli* trace element solution in our hands lasts up to 6 months if properly stored (sterile filtered, wrapped in aluminum foil and at temperatures around or below 25°C).
4. Production of labeled nucleotides has been optimized for a number of *E. coli* strains using different ^{13}C sources, in different amounts and/or different media. For details, refer to ref. (19).
5. The phenol:chloroform:isoamyl alcohol solution (25:24:1) mixture can be purchased from a commercial supplier or prepared from components. It is made of three components: TE buffer-saturated phenol (obtained by equilibrating solid phenol against 10 mM Tris–HCl, pH 8.0 and 1 mM EDTA), chloroform and isoamyl alcohol in a ratio of 25:24:1. It is stored at 2–8°C for up to 2 years. Since the phenol is a toxic and caustic chemical, users are required to wear appropriate laboratory clothing.
6. As described in detail by Batey et al. (11), to prepare this solution at pH 9.5, CO_2 is bubbled through 1 M triethylamine for 2–4 h using a glass pipette. The volatility of TEABC makes it easy to remove subsequently from the nucleotide sample after purification.
7. Acidified water can be easily prepared by bubbling CO_2 into distilled water through a glass Pasteur pipette.
8. Because of the cost of ^{13}C-labeled sources, it may be advisable to try the protocol for the first time using the corresponding unlabeled compounds.
9. A good sterile working practice is required here, especially because no antibiotic is used in the growth.
10. A sample prepared using $^{13}CH_3COOH$ is enriched at all ribose carbons with the exception of C3′ and exhibits >90% labeling efficiency for pyrimidine C5 and C6, and purine C2, C5, and C8 carbon positions (Table 1). These are all positions useful for proton-detected NMR experiments, although this labeling pattern does not alleviate the problem of strong ^{13}C-^{13}C J- and

dipolar couplings (23). Growing cells on media containing $CH_3^{13}COOH$ leads to >90% ^{13}C-incorporation at positions C2 and C4 for pyrimidines and C4 and C6 for purines, and higher than 75% labeling efficiency for ribose C3' position (23) (see Table 1). Some of these positions are, however, not useful for proton-detected NMR.

11. Cell growth rates on media containing sodium acetate are reduced compared to media containing an equal mass of glucose, with a typical 3 h doubling time compared to 45 min (23).

12. The combination of ^{13}C-formate and unlabeled glucose leads to >85% labeling efficiency solely at position C8 of purine rings, simplifying the NMR spectra and eliminating the ^{13}C-^{13}C J-couplings to C4 and C5 carbons (3).

13. Note that DL323 strains grow on glycerol minimal media slower than *E. coli* K12, whereas K10-1516 cells are indistinguishable (13). DL323 grown on 2-^{13}C-glycerol yields a mixture of ribose isotopic isomers partially labeled at C1'/C4' positions (55%) or C2'/C4' (30%), and gives ~90% ^{13}C-label only at position C6 of pyrimidine rings (13) (Table 1). The same DL323 cells grown on 1,3-$^{13}C_2$-glycerol exhibit 90% ^{13}C incorporation only at position C5 of pyrimidines and generate a mixture of isotopomeric ribose species partially labeled at C2'/C3'/C5' (55%) or C1'/C3'/C5' positions (25%) (13) (see Table 1). K10-1516 cells grown on 2-^{13}C-glycerol provide high and selective labeling efficiency (>80%) to positions C2' and C4' for the ribose, and roughly 50% of each C5 and C6 sites of pyrimidine rings (13) (see Table 1). For K10-1516 grown on media supplemented with 2-^{13}C-glycerol in the presence of 0.2 g of ^{13}C formate, the labeling levels at positions C5 and C6 of pyrimidines remain unchanged, but significant isotopic enrichment of the C8 (40%) and C2 (26%) positions of the purines is observed (20) (see Table 1). The alternate site labeling of rNTPs capable of removing ^{13}C-^{13}C couplings provide the ideal system for NMR relaxation studies (14).

14. Growth on Studier medium compared with an M9 type of minimal medium has advantages (faster growth, higher yield of rNMPs) especially for some bacterial strains and some ^{13}C-labeled sources (19).

15. The bacterial growth protocols described here using 2×500 mL cultures will typically yield 4 g of wet cell pellet when using glucose-containing minimal medium. However, the amount of wet cell pellet depends on both the growth medium and the ^{13}C-labeling source used. This has been found to vary between 3 and 6 g/L of culture (19); outside of this range, scale the protocols appropriately.

16. The cell lysis can be conducted with an alternative protocol to the one described in Subheading 3.6, where the DNA is

precipitated in the organic layer, yielding only RNA in the aqueous phase (7). Additional cell lysis methods have also been reported, as summarized by Batey et al. (11). In these cases, the steps of Subheading 3.8 are not required.

17. This operation can be done splitting the sample in several 50 mL polypropylene tubes if required.

18. Remove the upper aqueous layer using a pipette. It is important not to disturb the interface between the aqueous phase and lower organic layer. This interface typically appears as an opaque disc and contains the denatured proteins.

19. The amount of nucleic acids obtained per g of frozen pellet depends on the bacterial growth conditions (see Note 15). RNA is estimated to amount to 20% of the cellular biomass content of *E. coli* cells growing exponentially in aerobic conditions at 37°C on glucose minimal media (for a complete definition see ref. (24)).

20. Completeness of the hydrolysis reaction could be assessed by Thin Layer Chromatography (TLC) (8) or analytical HPLC (11). Refer to Batey et al. for exemplary HPLC chomatogram profiles (11).

21. The boronate chromatography is a cis-diol affinity method exploiting the different affinity of dNMPs and rNMPs for the boronate-derivatized polyacrylamide gel. In particular, the former do not interact with the resin whereas the latter have a high affinity for it at low temperature (4–5°C). Hence, it is essential to carry out this purification step at low temperature.

22. Take care that your glass column has the right specification and adaptors to be connected to an FPLC system. A wide column is necessary here to ensure good flow rates throughout the purification, where significant changes of resin volume occur with pH and ionic strength. Such typical behavior experienced by the boronate resin during the purification is described in more detail by Batey et al. (11).

23. This procedure needs to be performed carefully. Do not overload the column: maximum 200 mg of rNMPs (6,000 A_{260}) per purification on 5 g of resin. Overloading the column will result in loss of rNMP material. Representative chromatographic traces can be found in ref. (11).

24. This solution contains a mixture of the 4 rNMPs that will undergo enzymatic phosphorylation as described in Subheading 3.9. Nevertheless, it may be required to separate the rNMP into individual fractions containing rAMP, rCMP, rGMP and rUMP respectively. Ion-exchange chromatographic procedures, following the boronate affinity column, have been successfully utilized to accomplish this (Fig. 1). Please refer to

additional separation protocols discussed elsewhere if this is required (7, 9, 11, 13) and Chapter 18.

25. Note that a 50-mL screw-cap conical tube could be used instead of a three-neck round bottom flask, following the procedure described in ref. (8). Here the solution is degassed by passing nitrogen for 30 min, the reaction is started at a lower pH (6.8–6.9) and no stirring or pH adjustment is carried out during the course of the reaction (8).

26. Variations on the enzymatic phosphorylation method have been reported by several groups. This particularly applies if the enzymatic conversion of individual rNMPs is required (Fig. 1). Please refer to protocols described in detail elsewhere (7, 8, 10, 11). Some of the protocols include the in situ preparation of Phosphoenolpyruvate (PEP), a thermodynamically strong phosphoryl donor, from d-(−)-3-phosphoglyreric acid (3-PGA) as the cost of the commercially available PEP was prohibitive in the past (22). The reaction described in Subheading 3.9 could be scaled up to phosphorylate large amounts of rNMPs, by increasing the volumes and keeping concentration of the components constant.

27. Note that at this stage some variability in rNMP yield could be expected. For a general protocol it is therefore advised to dilute the 5 mL solution obtained from the boronate step accordingly to obtain a final concentration of rNMPs of 100 mM. The composition of the rNMP mixture obtained here, and the final rNTPs, reflects the relative prevalence of the bases in *E. coli* RNA, where the G:A:U:C molar ratio is estimated at approximately 1.6:1.3:1.1:1 (1, 10). To measure the concentration of the rNMP mixture, an average extinction coefficient is used, equivalent to 10,950 cm^{-1} M^{-1} (individual rNMP extinction coefficients were taken from ref. 25). Notably, this is very similar to the weighted average (taking into account the exact base composition), calculated at 11,110 cm^{-1} M^{-1}. This also applies to the rNTPs as the presence of phosphates has no detectable influence on the nucleotides' molar extinction coefficients (26).

28. If desired, the reaction can be monitored by TLC and HPLC (10, 11).

29. The purification of rNTPs at this stage may not be strictly required. According to an alternative protocol, following completion of the phosphorylation reaction, rNTPs are precipitated by an equal volume of ethanol and pelleted by centrifugation. This material is then used in the transcription reactions without further purification (7).

30. This step allows the removal of any remaining high molecular weight contaminant coming from the enzymatic reaction.

Acknowledgements

MRC is indebted to the Wellcome Trust. LM acknowledges the European Molecular Biology Organization (EMBO) for a long-term fellowship.

References

1. Batey RT, Inada M, Kujawinski E, Puglisi JD, Williamson JR. Preparation of isotopically labeled ribonucleotides for multidimensional NMR spectroscopy of RNA. Nucleic Acids Res. 1992;20:4515–23.
2. Dayie KT. Key labeling technologies to tackle sizeable problems in RNA structural biology. Int J Mol Sci. 2008;9:1214–40.
3. Latham MP, Brown DJ, McCallum SA, Pardi A. NMR methods for studying the structure and dynamics of RNA. Chembiochem. 2005;6:1492–505.
4. Nozinovic S, Furtig B, Jonker HR, Richter C, Schwalbe H. High-resolution NMR structure of an RNA model system: the 14-mer cUUCGg tetraloop hairpin RNA. Nucleic Acids Res. 2010;38:683–94.
5. Scott LG, Hennig M. RNA structure determination by NMR. Methods Mol Biol. 2008;452:29–61.
6. Lu K, Miyazaki Y, Summers MF. Isotope labeling strategies for NMR studies of RNA. J Biomol NMR. 2010;46:113–25.
7. Hines JV, Landry SM, Varani G, Tinoco I. Carbon-proton scalar couplings in RNA: 3D heteronuclear and 2D isotope-edited NMR of a 13C-labeled extra stable hairpin. J Am Chem Soc. 1994;116:5823–31.
8. Nikonowicz EP, Sirr A, Legault P, Jucker FM, Baer LM, Pardi A. Preparation of 13C and 15N labelled RNAs for heteronuclear multi-dimensional NMR studies. Nucleic Acids Res. 1992;20:4507–13.
9. Polson AG, Crain PF, Pomerantz SC, McCloskey JA, Bass BL. The mechanism of adenosine to inosine conversion by the double-stranded RNA unwinding/modifying activity: a high-performance liquid chromatography-mass spectrometry analysis. Biochemistry. 1991;30:11507–14.
10. Michnicka MJ, Harper JW, King GC. Selective isotopic enrichment of synthetic RNA: application to the HIV-1 TAR element. Biochemistry. 1993;32:395–400.
11. Batey RT, Battiste JL, Williamson JR. Preparation of isotopically enriched RNAs for heteronuclear NMR. Methods Enzymol. 1995;261:300–22.
12. Zimmer DP, Crothers DM. NMR of enzymatically synthesized uniformly 13C15N-labeled DNA oligonucleotides. Proc Natl Acad Sci USA. 1995;92:3091–5.
13. Johnson Jr JE, Julien KR, Hoogstraten CG. Alternate-site isotopic labeling of ribonucleotides for NMR studies of ribose conformational dynamics in RNA. J Biomol NMR. 2006;35:261–74.
14. Hoogstraten CG, Johnson Jr JE. Metabolic labeling: taking advantage of bacterial pathways to prepare spectroscopically useful isotope patterns in proteins and nucleic acids. Concepts Magn Reson Part A. 2008;32A:34–55.
15. Akke M, Fiala R, Jiang F, Patel D, Palmer 3rd AG. Base dynamics in a UUCG tetraloop RNA hairpin characterized by 15 N spin relaxation: correlations with structure and stability. RNA. 1997;3:702–9.
16. Hoogstraten CG, Wank JR, Pardi A. Active site dynamics in the lead-dependent ribozyme. Biochemistry. 2000;39:9951–8.
17. Nikonowicz EP, Michnicka M, Kalurachchi K, DeJong E. Preparation and characterization of a uniformly 2 H/15 N-labeled RNA oligonucleotide for NMR studies. Nucleic Acids Res. 1997;25:1390–6.
18. Scott LG, Tolbert TJ, Williamson JR. Preparation of specifically 2H- and 13C-labeled ribonucleotides. Methods Enzymol. 2000;317:18–38.
19. Thakur CS, Brown ME, Sama JN, Jackson ME, Dayie TK. Growth of wildtype and mutant E. coli strains in minimal media for optimal production of nucleic acids for preparing labeled nucleotides. Appl Microbiol Biotechnol. 2010;88:771–9.
20. Dayie TK, Thakur CS. Site-specific labeling of nucleotides for making RNA for high resolution NMR studies using an E. coli strain disabled

in the oxidative pentose phosphate pathway. J Biomol NMR. 2010;47:19–31.
21. Tyler RC, Sreenath HK, Singh S, Aceti DJ, Bingman CA, Markley JL, Fox BG. Auto-induction medium for the production of (U-15N)- and (U-13C, U-15N)-labeled proteins for NMR screening and structure determination. Protein Expr Purif. 2005;40:268–78.
22. Simon ES, Grabowski S, Whitesides GM. Convenient syntheses of cytidine 5′-triphosphate, guanosine 5′-triphosphate and uridine 5′-triphosphate and their use in the preparation of UDP-glucose, UDP-glucuronic acid amd GDP-mannose. J Org Chem. 1990;55:1834–47.
23. Hoffman DW, Holland JA. Preparation of carbon-13 labeled ribonucleotides using acetate as an isotope source. Nucleic Acids Res. 1995;23:3361–2.
24. Feist AM, Henry CS, Reed JL, Krummenacker M, Joyce AR, Karp PD, Broadbelt LJ, Hatzimanikatis V, Palsson BO. A genome-scale metabolic reconstruction for Escherichia coli K-12 MG1655 that accounts for 1260 ORFs and thermodynamic information. Mol Syst Biol. 2007;3:121.
25. Cavaluzzi MJ, Borer PN. Revised UV extinction coefficients for nucleoside-5′-monophosphates and unpaired DNA and RNA. Nucleic Acids Res. 2004;32:e13.
26. Cantor CR, Schimmel PR. Biophysical chemistry. San Francisco: W. H. Freeman and Company; 1980. p. 349–408.

Chapter 18

Preparative Separation of Ribonucleoside Monophosphates by Ion-Pair Reverse-Phase HPLC

Pierre Dagenais and Pascale Legault

Abstract

Structural and dynamic investigations of RNA by nuclear magnetic resonance (NMR) spectroscopy strongly benefit from isotopic-labeling strategies. Among these, nucleotide-specific and site-specific labeling methods can help tremendously in simplifying complex NMR data, while providing unique opportunities for structural investigation of larger RNAs. Such methods generally require separation of individual isotopically labeled ribonucleoside monophosphates prior to their conversion into nucleoside triphosphates and selective incorporation of these nucleoside triphosphates into the RNA. This chapter provides the experimental details for preparative separation of ribonucleoside monophosphates by ion-pair reverse-phase HPLC. It also describes a quick procedure for clean-up and quality control of the individual ribonucleoside monophosphates.

Key words: Ribonucleoside monophosphates (NMPs), NMP separation, Ion-pair reverse-phase HPLC, RNA in vitro transcription, Isotopic-labeling, Nucleotide-specific labeling, Site-specific labeling

1. Introduction

Structural and dynamic studies of RNA by nuclear magnetic resonance (NMR) spectroscopy tremendously benefit from isotopic-labeling ($^{13}C/^{15}N/^{2}H$) in combination with heteronuclear multidimensional experiments (1, 2). Uniform $^{13}C/^{15}N$-labeling of RNA is now a standard approach for structural and dynamic studies of small RNAs (<35 nt; (3–8)). In addition, several isotopic-labeling strategies have been developed to reduce spectral crowding and resonance linewidths and, thereby, allow NMR studies of larger RNA molecules (9–20). Among these strategies, nucleotide-specific (10, 14, 18) and site-specific labeling (13, 16) methods can help tremendously in reducing the number of observable resonances of otherwise complex NMR data. Since RNA molecules investigated by NMR spectroscopy are generally prepared by in vitro transcription using the bacteriophage T7 RNA polymerase, these labeling strategies depend on the availability of individual isotopically labeled ribonucleoside 5′-triphosphates (NTPs). These isotopically labeled NTPs can be either purchased from commercial sources or prepared from bacterial cells grown on isotopically enriched media (3–6, 8, 20). In the latter case, the crucial step in the process is the separation of the individual NMPs generated from nuclease digestion of bacterial RNA. Given their chemical stabilities, it is preferable to separate the individual NMPs prior to their conversion into NTPs.

Several chromatographic methods have been developed for separation of NMPs, which are generally derived from early reports for analytical separation by anion-exchange (21), reverse-phase (22) and ion-pair reverse phase methods (23, 24). For NMR applications, large quantities of isotopically labeled NMPs can be quickly purified using preparative HPLC methods (6, 8, 10). However, to our knowledge, only a single detailed protocol for preparative HPLC separation of NMPs has been reported, which uses an anion-exchange polyethyleneimine resin (8). Given the potential of preparative HPLC for the separation of large quantities of NMPs, additional protocols that rely on other types of resins could provide valuable alternatives to the existing methodology.

In this chapter, we describe a detailed protocol for preparative separation of individual NMPs from an isotopically labeled ribosomal RNA (rRNA) hydrolysate by ion-pair reverse-phase HPLC. To achieve optimal separation of isotopically labeled NMPs, the RNA hydrolysis is performed with the S1 Nuclease in formate buffer (6). Using this ion-pair reverse-phase HPLC protocol, approximately 400–500 mg of isotopically labeled NMPs are separated quickly in 8–10 HPLC injections on a preparative C_{18} column. Subsequently, the individual NMPs are further purified by reverse-phase HPLC on a preparative C_{18} column and tested to ensure compatibility with in vitro transcription using T7 RNA polymerase. The separated NMPs can then be converted to NTPs using established procedures (25).

2. Materials

Sterilize all solutions either by autoclaving or filtering (0.22-μm filter). Store all reagents at room temperature, unless indicated otherwise, and follow proper disposal regulations when disposing of waste materials.

2.1. Preparation of the Isotopically Labeled NMP Mixture

1. Isotopically labeled rRNA prepared from bacterial cells stored at –20°C (4).
2. Concentrated formic acid solution.

3. 10 mM $ZnCl_2$.
4. S1 Nuclease (332 U/μL) stored at −20°C.
5. 0.5 M EDTA, pH 8.0.
6. PEI-cellulose plates (with vertical length of ~12.5 cm) for thin-layer chromatography (TLC) stored at 4°C.
7. LiCl solutions (0.3, 1.0, and 1.6 M).
8. TLC developing tank with lid.
9. Heat gun, if available.
10. Ultraviolet (UV) lamp.
11. UV/Vis spectrophotometer with a quartz cuvette.

2.2. Reverse-Phase HPLC Separation and Clean-Up of NMPs

All solutions are degassed under vacuum and filtered through a 0.22-μm filter membrane prior to usage to avoid the introduction of gas and undesirable impurities in the HPLC system.

1. Stock solutions of commercial unlabeled 5′-NMPs: 100 mM adenosine 5′-monophosphate sodium salt (5′-AMP); 100 mM cytidine 5′-monophosphate disodium salt (5′-CMP); 100 mM guanosine 5′-monophosphate disodium salt (5′-GMP), and 100 mM uridine 5′-monophosphate disodium salt (5′-UMP). Prepare each NMP by dissolution in water. Store at −20°C.
2. Isotopically labeled NMP mixture (see Subheading 3.1).
3. Concentrated formic acid solution.
4. Ion-Pair Solvent A: 5 mM tetrabutylammonium (TBA) hydroxide adjusted to pH 2.3 with formic acid.
5. Ion-Pair Solvent B: 5 mM TBA hydroxide adjusted to pH 2.3 with formic acid and 25% (v/v) methanol.
6. Clean-Up Solvent A: sterile water.
7. Clean-Up Solvent B: 50% (v/v) methanol.
8. 0.22-μm vacuum filter system.
9. HPLC system equipped with a multi-wavelength detector and a 5-mL injection loop.
10. Preparative C_{18} HPLC column, e.g., Prep Nova-Pak HR C_{18} Column, 6 μm, 19 × 300 mm (Waters Corporation).
11. Sterile screw-cap conical tubes.
12. Autoclaved glassware (e.g. 1-L bottles or Erlenmeyer flasks) for HPLC fraction collection.
13. Rotary evaporator.
14. Round-bottom flask (1 L) for solvent evaporation.
15. 1 M NaOH.

2.3. Quality Control

1. HPLC-purified CMP, AMP, GMP, and UMP (see Subheading 3.2).
2. 400 mM HEPES pH 8.0.
3. 1 M DTT prepared fresh.
4. 1% Triton X-100.
5. 25 mM Spermidine stored at −20°C.
6. 0.5 M $MgCl_2$.
7. Nucleotide solutions: 100 mM ATP, 100 mM CTP, 100 mM GTP, and 100 mM UTP. Prepare NTP solutions on ice and adjust to pH 8.0 using NaOH. Store at −20°C.
8. Transcription buffer: 40 mM HEPES pH 8.0, 50 mM DTT, 0.1% Triton X-100, 1 mM spermidine, 25 mM $MgCl_2$, 4 mM ATP, 4 mM CTP, 4 mM GTP, and 4 mM UTP. Prepare just before use.
9. Linearized plasmid DNA template (~1.5 mg/mL) stored at 4°C.
10. His-tagged T7 RNA polymerase (~6 mg/mL); prepared in-house and stored at −20°C.
11. Temperature-controlled water bath.
12. Gel loading buffer: 20 mg of bromophenol blue, 20 mg of xylene cyanol, 5 mL of 0.5 M EDTA pH 8.0 and 95 mL of formamide.
13. TBE buffer: 50 mM Tris-Base, 50 mM boric acid, and 1 mM EDTA. Prepare as a 10× stock solution.
14. 10% gel solution: 10% acrylamide:bisacrylamide (19:1), 7 M urea in TBE buffer. Store at 4°C. Caution: unpolymerized acrylamide and bisacrylamide are strong neurotoxins. Protective equipment (gloves, mask, laboratory coat, and glasses) should be worn and care should be taken when handling acrylamide powder and solutions.
15. 10% analytical denaturing polyacrylamide gel: mix 40 mL of 10% gel solution with 200 μL of ammonium persulfate 10% (w/v) and 40 μL of TEMED. Immediately pour in a glass plate assembly using 20 × 20 cm glass plates and 0.7 mm thick comb and spacers.
16. High-voltage power supply, e.g., Thermo EC600-90.
17. SYBR Gold staining solution: a fresh 1:10,000 dilution of SYBR Gold nucleic acid gel stain in TBE buffer is prepared daily.
18. Molecular Imager and analysis software. Here, we use a Molecular Imager FX densitometer and ImageLab software version 3.0 (Bio-Rad).
19. 0.5 M EDTA pH 8.0.

3. Methods

All procedures are carried out at room temperature unless specified otherwise.

3.1. RNA Hydrolysis with the S1 Nuclease

To achieve optimal HPLC separation of isotopically labeled NMPs, hydrolysis of rRNA is first performed with the S1 Nuclease at a low pH adjusted with formic acid (see Note 1). Isotopically labeled rRNA is prepared from bacterial cells, as previously described ((4, 26), see Note 2).

1. Combine ~400 mg of isotopically labeled rRNA with 0.2 mM $ZnCl_2$ in a total volume of 30 mL. Adjust pH to 4.4 with formic acid. Take a 5-µL aliquot and add 8,000 U of S1 Nuclease (20 U/mg rRNA; see Note 3).

2. Incubate 1 h 30 min at 45°C. Take a 5-µL aliquot to check reaction completion before stopping it.

3. Check completion of the reaction by TLC. First, spot 3-µL samples (or 3 times 1 µL for better resolution) from the hydrolysis reaction aliquots on a TLC plate. Allow samples to migrate by placing TLC plate in a developing tank with 0.3 M LiCl for 20 s; 1.0 M LiCl for 1 min; and 1.6 M LiCl for 25 min. Dry TLC plate with a heat gun, if available, and view reaction products with a UV lamp. The reaction is completed when all the detected compounds migrate away from the loading spot (retention factor should be at least 0.4).

4. Stop the reaction by adding EDTA pH 8.0 to a final concentration of 0.4 mM and heat the solution to 90°C for 2 min to denature the S1 Nuclease. Transfer to 4°C.

5. Determine the concentration of the NMP mixture by UV spectroscopy (see Note 4). Proceed to HPLC separation or store at −80°C.

3.2. Reverse-Phase HPLC Separation and Clean-Up of NMPs

The following protocol describes the separation of isotopically labeled NMPs prepared from bacterial cells (see Subheading 3.1). As a control, the method can also be tested with a mixture of NMPs obtained from a commercial source (see Fig. 1).

3.2.1. Ion-Pair Reverse-Phase HPLC Separation of Individual NMPs

1. Prior to the first injection, adjust NMP mixture to pH 2.8 with formic acid and dilute to 30 mM total NMP concentration. In addition, equilibrate a preparative C_{18} HPLC column with 0% Ion-Pair Solvent B (100% Ion-Pair Solvent A) over 50 mL at a flow rate of 10 mL/min.

2. Inject NMP mixture in 5-mL aliquots (~50 mg NMPs) onto the column at 10 mL/min.

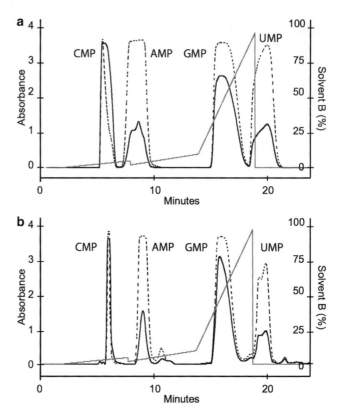

Fig. 1. Separation of NMP mixtures by ion-pair reverse-phase HPLC. Elution profiles following injection of (**a**) an NMP mixture prepared by mixing individual NMPs obtained from a commercial source (~60 mg or 5 mL of a 35 mM solution) and (**b**) an ^{15}N-labeled rRNA hydrolysate (~50 mg or 5 mL of a 30 mM solution; see Subheading 3.1) on a Nova-Pak HR C$_{18}$ Preparative Column (Waters Corporation). A gradient elution (% Solvent B, *solid gray line*) was performed with Solvent A (5 mM TBA adjusted to pH 2.3 with formic acid) and Solvent B (Solvent A supplemented with 25% (v/v) methanol) using a flow rate of 10 mL/min. Absorbance was recorded at 254 nm (*dashed black line*) and 280 nm (*solid black line*).

3. Elute using a multi-linear gradient with Ion-Pair Solvents A and B at 10 mL/min and UV detection at 254 and 280 nm: (a) 0–5% Solvent B over 60 mL; (b) 2–10% Solvent B over 60 mL; (c) 10–100% Solvent B over 50 mL; and (d) 0% Solvent B over 50 mL (see Fig. 1; Notes 5 and 6).

4. For each HPLC run, collect fractions corresponding to each NMP into individual 50-mL screw-cap conical tubes. After each run, transfer eluted fractions to individual 1-L autoclaved glass bottles and store at 4°C.

5. Once the entire NMP mixture is separated, transfer individual NMP samples to a round-bottom flask and concentrate on a rotary evaporator until dryness (see Note 7).

3.2.2. Reverse-Phase HPLC Clean-Up of Individual NMPs

After the separation, a reverse-phase HPLC step is performed to purify individual NMPs from the remaining TBA salts (see Note 8).

1. Prior to the first injection, determine the concentration of the individual NMPs by UV spectroscopy (see Note 4) and adjust their concentration to 10 mM CMP, 20 mM AMP, 20 mM GMP, and 10 mM UMP. In addition, equilibrate a preparative C_{18} HPLC column with 4% Clean-Up Solvent B over 50 mL at a flow rate of 10 mL/min.

2. Inject an individual NMP sample in 5-mL aliquots (~34 mg for AMP and GMP; ~17 mg for CMP and UMP) onto a preparative C_{18} HPLC column at 10 mL/min.

3. Elute using a multi-linear gradient with Clean-Up Solvents A and B at 10 mL/min and UV detection at 254 and 280 nm: (a) 4% Solvent B over 60 mL; (b) 4–100% Solvent B over 60 mL; (c) 100% Solvent B over 60 mL; and (d) 4% Solvent B over 50 mL (see Note 5).

4. For each HPLC run, collect NMP fractions directly into a 1-L autoclaved glass bottle pre-cooled at 4°C.

5. Concentrate each individual NMP sample using a rotary evaporator. Evaporate solvent to dryness and wash the round-bottom flask with 30 mL of sterile water. Repeat these last two steps (evaporation and wash) twice to remove all trace methanol. The final sample volume should be minimal (2–3 mL), in order to obtain a final NMP concentration greater than 40 mM.

6. Adjust NMP samples to pH 8.0 with 1 M NaOH.

7. Determine the concentration of the NMP samples by UV spectroscopy (see Note 4) and adjust the final concentration between 40 and 100 mM.

8. Store purified NMP samples at −20°C.

3.2.3. Quality Control

A quality control step may be performed before conversion of the purified NMPs into NTPs (25). This step consists of performing transcription reactions supplemented with each purified NMP to insure that each is free of contaminants that could inhibit a transcription reaction. One should use the transcription reaction of the RNA of interest for this test.

1. Set up small-scale transcription reactions, typically five transcription reactions of 100 μL. The standard reaction contains 1× transcription buffer, 8 μg of linearized plasmid DNA, and 1 μL of T7 RNA polymerase at 6 mg/mL. The other transcription reactions are as the standard reaction except that 4 mM purified NMP (CMP, AMP, GMP, or UMP; see Subheading 3.2.2) is added (see Note 9).

2. Incubate 3 h at 37°C.

3. Stop the transcription reaction by adding EDTA pH 8.0 to a final concentration of 25 mM. Store at −20°C or immediately proceed to analysis by gel electrophoresis.

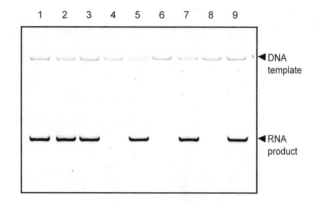

Fig. 2. Quality control of the individual ^{15}N-labeled NMPs after their separation by ion-pair reverse-phase HPLC. Individual ^{15}N-labeled NMPs were added at a concentration of 4 mM to small-scale transcription reactions of an RNA of interest (TL-let-7 g-ARiBo1 RNA; (28)), and these reactions were analyzed on a 10% denaturing polyacrylamide gel stained with SYBR Gold. *Lane 1*: no added NMP; *Lanes 2, 4, 6,* and *8*: addition of 4 mM of ^{15}N-labeled CMP (*lane 2*), AMP (*lane 4*), GMP (*lane 6*), and UMP (*lane 8*) obtained before the HPLC clean-up step; *Lanes 3, 5, 7,* and *9*: addition of 4 mM of ^{15}N-labeled CMP (*lane 3*), AMP (*lane 5*), GMP (*lane 7*), and UMP (*lane 9*) obtained after the HPLC clean-up step. Bands corresponding to the DNA template and the main RNA product are identified on the right of the gel.

4. Analyze samples (1.25 µL of a 1:100 dilution) on an analytical 10% denaturing polyacrylamide gel (375 V for 2 h 45 min) stained with SYBR Gold (see Fig. 2).

5. Scan on a Molecular Imager and quantify band intensities. The intensity of the main product should be similar for all transcriptions, indicating that the purified NMP is free of contaminants that could inhibit the transcription reaction.

4. Notes

1. The hydrolysis of isotopically labeled rRNA obtained from bacterial cells is typically performed with the P1 Nuclease or the S1 Nuclease in sodium acetate buffer (3–8). However, we have found that the acetate buffer interferes with optimal separation of NMPs by ion-pair reverse-phase HPLC.

2. Isotopically labeled NMPs can also be obtained by extracting total nucleic acids from bacterial cells (5). Hydrolysis of such a mixture requires further separation of NMPs from dNMPs on a boronate affinity column. After this purification step, the NMP mixture should be sufficiently pure for separation by ion-pair reverse-phase HPLC (see Subheading 3.2).

3. Alternatively, the S1 Nuclease reaction can be performed overnight using a smaller amount of S1 Nuclease. To achieve this,

combine ~400 mg of isotopically labeled rRNA with 0.2 mM $ZnCl_2$ in a total volume of 30 mL. Adjust pH to 4.4 with formic acid. Take a 5-μL aliquot and add 340 U of S1 Nuclease (0.8-1 U/mg RNA). Incubate at 45°C overnight (~15 h).

4. NMP absorptions are measured at $\lambda = 260$ nm and concentrations are calculated using the following UV extinction coefficients (ε_{260}): 10,960 M^{-1} cm^{-1} for the NMP mixture; 7,070 M^{-1} cm^{-1} for CMP; 15,020 M^{-1} cm^{-1} for AMP; 12,080 M^{-1} cm^{-1} for GMP; and 9,660 M^{-1} cm^{-1} for UMP (27).

5. Subsequent 5-mL aliquots can be injected onto the HPLC column immediately after using this elution profile; no additional wash step is required.

6. The absorbance ratio (A_{254}/A_{280}) can be used to distinguish individual peaks on the elution profile (see Fig. 1).

7. At this step, the evaporation of solvents may produce a small oil-like liquid (<5 mL) in the flask. In this case, stop the evaporation process. Resuspend individual NMPs with a minimal volume of water (~5 mL) and transfer to a 50-mL screw-cap tube. Rinse the round-bottom flask with an additional small volume of water (~5 mL) and transfer to the same 50-mL tube.

8. This HPLC clean-up step is optional for CMP samples (see Fig. 2).

9. For Fig. 2, we performed additional transcription reactions, in which we added the individual NMPs obtained before the HPLC clean-up step to demonstrate the usefulness of this clean-up step.

Acknowledgments

We thank Dominique Chaussé for technical assistance, Geneviève Di Tomasso, and James G. Omichinski for critical reading of the manuscript. This work was supported by a grant from the Canadian Institutes for Health Research (CIHR; MOP-86502) to P. Legault and a M.Sc. scholarship from CIHR to P.D. P. Legault holds a Canada Research Chair in Structural Biology and Engineering of RNA.

References

1. Latham MP, Brown DJ, McCallum SA, Pardi A (2005) NMR methods for studying the structure and dynamics of RNA. Chembiochem 6:1492–1505
2. Lu K, Miyazaki Y, Summers MF (2010) Isotope labeling strategies for NMR studies of RNA. J Biomol NMR 46:113–125
3. Polson AG, Crain PF, Pomerantz SC, McCloskey JA, Bass BL (1991) The mechanism of adenosine to inosine conversion by the double-stranded RNA unwinding/modifying activity: a high-performance liquid chromatography-mass spectrometry analysis. Biochemistry 30:11507–11514

4. Nikonowicz EP, Sirr A, Legault P, Jucker FM, Baer LM, Pardi A (1992) Preparation of ^{13}C and ^{15}N labelled RNAs for heteronuclear multidimensional NMR studies. Nucleic Acids Res 20:4507–4513

5. Batey RT, Inada M, Kujawinski E, Puglisi JD, Williamson JR (1992) Preparation of isotopically labeled ribonucleotides for multidimensional NMR spectroscopy of RNA. Nucleic Acids Res 20:4515–4523

6. Michnicka MJ, Harper JW, King GC (1993) Selective isotopic enrichment of synthetic RNA: application to the HIV-1 TAR element. Biochemistry 32:395–400

7. Hines JV, Landry SM, Varani G, Tinoco IJ (1994) Carbon-proton scale couplings in RNA: 3D heteronuclear and 2D isotope-edited NMR of a ^{13}C-labeled extra-stable hairpin. J Am Chem Soc 116:5823–5831

8. Batey RT, Battiste JL, Williamson JR (1995) Preparation of isotopically enriched RNAs for heteronuclear NMR. Methods Enzymol 261:300–322

9. Batey RT, Cloutier N, Mao H, Williamson JR (1996) Improved large scale culture of Methylophilus methylotrophus for ^{13}C/^{15}N labeling and random fractional deuteration of ribonucleotides. Nucleic Acids Res 24:4836–4837

10. Dieckmann T, Suzuki E, Nakamura GK, Feigon J (1996) Solution structure of an ATP-binding RNA aptamer reveals a novel fold. RNA 2:628–640

11. Nikonowicz EP, Michnicka M, Kalurachchi K, DeJong E (1997) Preparation and characterization of a uniformly ^{2}H/^{15}N labeled RNA oligonucleotide for NMR studies. Nucleic Acids Res 25:1390–1396

12. Dayie KT, Tolbert TJ, Williamson JR (1998) 3D C(CC)H TOCSY experiment for assigning protons and carbons in uniformly ^{13}C- and selectively ^{2}H-labeled RNA. J Magn Reson 130:97–101

13. Ohtsuki T, Kawai G, Watanabe K (1998) Stable isotope-edited NMR analysis of Ascaris suum mitochondrial tRNAMet having a TV-replacement loop. J Biochem 124:28–34

14. Mao H, Williamson JR (1999) Assignment of the L30-mRNA complex using selective isotopic labeling and RNA mutants. Nucleic Acids Res 27:4059–4070

15. Scott LG, Tolbert TJ, Williamson JR (2000) Preparation of specifically ^{2}H- and ^{13}C-labeled ribonucleotides. Methods Enzymol 317:18–38

16. Kurata S, Ohtsuki T, Suzuki T, Watanabe K (2003) Quick two-step RNA ligation employing periodate oxidation. Nucleic Acids Res 31:e145

17. Johnson JE Jr, Julien KR, Hoogstraten CG (2006) Alternate-site isotopic labeling of ribonucleotides for NMR studies of ribose conformational dynamics in RNA. J Biomol NMR 35:261–274

18. Nelissen FH, van Gammeren AJ, Tessari M, Girard FC, Heus HA, Wijmenga SS (2008) Multiple segmental and selective isotope labeling of large RNA for NMR structural studies. Nucleic Acids Res 36:e89

19. Dayie TK, Thakur CS (2010) Site-specific labeling of nucleotides for making RNA for high resolution NMR studies using an E. coli strain disabled in the oxidative pentose phosphate pathway. J Biomol NMR 47:19–31

20. Martino L, Conte MR (2012) Biosynthetic preparation of ^{13}C/^{15}N-labelled rNTPs for high-resolution NMR studies of RNAs. Methods Mol Biol 941:227–245

21. Cohn WE (1950) The anion-exchange separation of ribonucleotides. J Am Chem Soc 72:1471–1478

22. Krstulovic AM, Brown PR, Rosie DM (1977) Identification of nucleosides and bases in serum and plasma samples by reverse-phase high performance liquid chromatography. Anal Chem 49:2237–2241

23. Hoffman NE, Liao JC (1977) Reversed phase high performance liquid chromatographic separations of nucleotides in the presence of solvophobic ions. Anal Chem 49:2231–2234

24. Walseth TF, Graff G, Moos MC Jr, Goldberg ND (1980) Separation of 5′-ribonucleoside monophosphates by ion-pair reverse-phase high-performance liquid chromatography. Anal Biochem 107:240–245

25. Simon ES, Grabowski S, Whitesides GM (1990) Convenient syntheses of cytidine 5′-triphosphate, guanosine 5′-triphosphate, and uridine 5′-triphosphate and their use in the preparation of UDP-glucose, UDP-glucuronic acid, and GDP-mannose. J Org Chem 55:1834–1841

26. Legault P (1995) Structural studies of ribozymes by heteronuclear NMR spectroscopy. University of Colorado at Boulder, Boulder

27. Cavaluzzi MJ, Borer PN (2004) Revised UV extinction coefficients for nucleoside-5′-monophosphates and unpaired DNA and RNA. Nucleic Acids Res 32:e13

28. Di Tomasso G, Dagenais P, Desjardins A, Rompré-Brodeur A, Delfosse V, Legault P (2012) Affinity purification of RNA using an ARiBo tag. Methods Mol Biol 941:137–155

Chapter 19

Splint Ligation of RNA with T4 DNA Ligase

Christopher J. Kershaw and Raymond T. O'Keefe

Abstract

Splint ligation of RNA, whereby specific RNA molecules are ligated together, can be carried out using T4 DNA ligase and a bridging DNA oligonucleotide complementary to the RNAs. This method takes advantage of the property of T4 DNA ligase to join RNA molecules when they are in an RNA:DNA hybrid. Splint ligation is a useful tool for the introduction of modified nucleotides into RNA molecules, insertion of a radiolabel into a specific position within an RNA and for the assembly of smaller synthetic RNAs into longer RNA molecules. Such modifications enable a wide range of experiments to be carried out with the modified RNA including structural studies, co-immunoprecipitations, and the ability to map sites of RNA:RNA and RNA:protein interactions.

Key words: RNA modification, RNA ligation, T7 RNA polymerase, in vitro transcription, RNA purification, T4 DNA ligase

1. Introduction

It is becoming increasing clear that RNAs contribute to a diverse range of biological processes. These RNAs exist in ribonuclear protein particles such as the ribosome and spliceosome. Structural probing of these RNAs is difficult and most of the advances into the structure of these RNAs have been made by inserting modified nucleotides into these RNAs. Due to size limitation, and the high cost, of synthesizing large RNA molecules containing modified nucleotides, methods of RNA ligation have been developed.

The method described here, using T4 DNA ligase, is based on the method developed by Moore and Sharp (1). Originally this method was used to create a nuclear pre-messenger RNA substrate where the 2'-hydroxyl group at either splice site was substituted for a single hydrogen or O-methyl group (1). The authors used this pre-mRNA substrate to show that the 2'-hydroxyl at the 3' splice site is important for the second step of splicing. Subsequently this ligation method has been widely used to investigate all aspects of RNA biology including the spliceosome (2) and ribosome (3). Our experience in RNA ligation has evolved from studying the RNAs associated with the spliceosome. By inserting photo-crosslinkable groups at specific positions into the pre-mRNA or snRNAs the RNA:RNA or protein:RNA interactions within the spliceosome can be probed (2–8). RNA ligation can also be a useful tool for NMR spectroscopy. Producing segmentally labeled full-length RNA from one modified and one unmodified RNA can help in structural determination by NMR (9). Preparation of isotopically labeled rNTPs is described in Chapters 17 and 18.

The method described here utilizes T4 DNA ligase to ligate the 3' end of one RNA to the 5' end of another. The RNA ligase ability of T4 bacteriophage DNA ligase has been extensively investigated (10–12) and has several advantages in comparison to RNA ligase of T4 Bacteriophage. RNA ligase is not as efficient as T4 DNA ligase, it is capable of circularizing RNA and producing RNA oligomers, both of which would be undesirable side products to the RNA ligation reaction. A DNA oligonucleotide bridge complementary to the RNAs either side of the site of ligation is required to facilitate the process of ligation with T4 DNA ligase. This bridging DNA oligonucleotide is hybridized to the RNAs prior to ligation to tether them in the correct orientation and form a double-stranded nucleic acid molecule for the T4 DNA ligase to act on. When using T4 DNA ligase the bridging DNA oligonucleotide specifically designates the site of ligation and prevents the production of undesirable ligation products. This specificity of ligation is also useful as in vitro transcribed RNA produced using T7 RNA polymerase will have a population of 3' ends with additional nucleotides. These +1 transcripts would be ligated by T4 RNA ligase but not by the T4 DNA ligase method removing the requirement for 3' end processing by a ribozyme. Once ligated the RNA is purified by polyacrylaminde gel electrophoresis and recovered from the gel fragment.

2. Materials

As RNA is susceptible to degradation all solutions must be RNase free. It is also advisable to use filter tips when working with both RNA and radiolabeled nucleotides. In vitro transcription requires a DNA template and certain considerations must be taken into account when designing the DNA template. DNA templates can either be plasmid DNA or DNA produced by PCR. For plasmid DNA templates the sequence to be transcribed must be cloned into a plasmid downstream of a phage RNA polymerase promoter like the T3 or T7 promoter. Once cloned into a plasmid, the plasmid DNA must then be cleaved completely with a restriction enzyme that leaves a blunt end or 5′ overhang to allow for run-off transcription. A more convenient and controllable method for producing specific DNA templates of any sequence cloned in a plasmid is PCR. A forward primer is designed that incorporates a phage RNA polymerase promoter, like T7, upstream of the first 18–20 nucleotides of sequence to be transcribed. The only restriction is that the first nucleotide to be transcribed must be a G. A back primer is then designed that will produce the specific 3′ end of the DNA template required (Fig. 1). Production of DNA templates by PCR obviates the need for cloning to produce plasmid DNA templates.

2.1. In Vitro Transcription of RNA Components

1. RNase-free water. This can be achieved by filtering deionized water through a cellulose nitrate filter with a 2 μm pore size or treatment with diethylpyrocarbonate (DEPC), which is also called diethyl dicarbonate. To treat water with DEPC, add to a final concentration of 0.1% v/v, stir overnight on a stir plate at room temperature and autoclave to degrade the DEPC.

2. Transcription buffer (5×): 200 mM Tris–HCl pH 8.0, 10 mM spermidine, 50 mM dithiothreitol (DTT), and 100 mM $MgCl_2$. This can be made by mixing 400 μl of 0.5 M Tris–Cl pH 8, 100 μl of 1 M spermidine, 50 μl of 1 M DTT, 100 μl of 1 M $MgCl_2$, and 350 μl of RNase-free water. Alternatively the 5× transcription buffer and DTT supplied with a commercial T7 RNA polymerase can be used.

3. DNA template, either PCR product or digested plasmid, at a final concentration of 0.05 μg/μl.

4. Nucleotide triphosphate (NTP) mixes (5×): 5 mM of each of ATP, CTP, GTP, and UTP. For incorporation of XpG dinucleotide, GMP or guanosine as the first nucleotide, use NTP mix with GTP adjusted to 2 mM.

5. 50 mM of ApG, GMP or 200 mM guanosine for priming transcription. Guanosine is not soluble in water and must be dissolved in 0.33 M sodium hydroxide (NaOH). The 0.33 M NaOH is made by dissolving 0.132 g of NaOH in 10 ml RNase-free water. The 200 mM guanosine stock is then made by adding 0.17 g of guanosine to 3 ml of 0.33 M NaOH.

6. T7 RNA polymerase (at least 18 units/μl).

7. Ribonuclease inhibitor, e.g., RNasin (Promega), 40 units/μl.

8. RNase-free DNase.

9. 0.5 M disodium ethylenediamine tetraacetate (EDTA) pH 8. Made by dissolving 93.06 g of EDTA in 350 ml of water and altering the pH to 8 using sodium hydroxide pellets. Once the pH is adjusted to 8 bring the total volume of the solution to 500 ml.

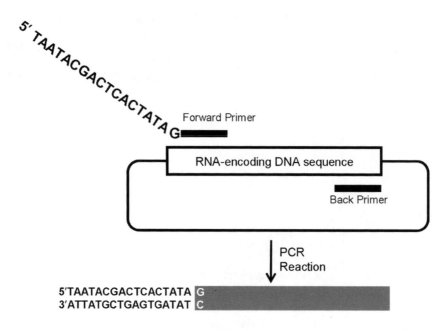

Fig. 1. Production of transcription template DNA by PCR amplification of a specific sequence from any gene cloned into a plasmid. Two PCR primers are designed, a forward primer that contains a T7 RNA polymerase promoter and a back primer. The resulting PCR transcription template will contain a T7 promoter and be used for run-off transcription.

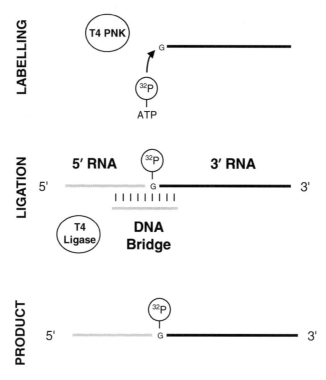

Fig. 2. Diagram of a typical splint ligation with two RNA molecules. A 3′ RNA is first labeled at its 5′ end with ^{32}P by T4 polynucleotide kinase (PNK). The labeled 3′ RNA is then mixed with a 5′ RNA and hybridized to a bridging DNA oligonucleotide. T4 DNA ligase can then catalyze the ligation of the two RNAs in the RNA:DNA hybrid. Finally the ligation product is purified from the other molecules in the reaction.

10. Sodium acetate buffered phenol:chloroform:isoamyl alcohol (25:24:1) made by mixing 25 ml of sodium acetate buffered phenol, 24 ml of chloroform, and 1 ml of isoamyl alcohol.

11. 5 M ammonium acetate in water made by dissolving 77.085 g of ammonium acetate in 200 ml of RNase-free water.

12. 3 M sodium acetate pH 5.3 in water is made by dissolving 24.609 g of sodium acetate in 80 ml of RNase-free water, adjusting the pH to 5.3 and bringing solution to a final volume of 100 ml.

13. Absolute ethanol.

2.2. Purification of In Vitro Transcribed RNA and Synthetic RNA by Polyacrylamide Gel Electrophoresis

Synthetic RNAs can be obtained commercially from several companies.

1. Formamide gel loading dye: 80%v/v formamide, 10 mM EDTA pH 8, 1 mg/ml bromophenol blue, and 1 mg/ml xylene cyanol.

2. Urea.

3. Sequencing grade 40% acrylamide solution (19:1 acrylamide:bis-acrylamide mixture), alternatively premixed polyacrylamide denaturing gel solutions are commercially available.

4. RNase-free water (see Subheading 2.1).

5. N,N,N,N'-Tetramethyl-ethylenediamine (TEMED). Store at 4°C.

6. Ammonium persulfate 25% in water (see Note 1).

7. Tris-borate EDTA buffer (TBE; 5×): 0.45 M Tris-borate and 100 mM EDTA, pH 8. Made by dissolving 54 g of Tris and 27.5 g of orthoboric acid in 980 ml water and adding 20 ml of 0.5 M EDTA pH 8. This stock is then diluted to 1× TBE prior to use.

8. Polyacrylamide gel running apparatus (e.g., Cambridge Scientific): front and back gel plates measuring 185 × 200 mm, 0.5 mm spacers, Tesa 4120 UPVC packaging tape, Repelcote VS water repellent, a 50:50 water/ethanol solution, bulldog clips and a gel tank of sufficient dimensions.

9. Passive elution solution: 300 mM sodium acetate pH 5.3 and 1 mM EDTA pH 8. Made by mixing 898 μl of RNase-free water, 100 μl of 3 M sodium acetate pH 5.3 and 2 μl of 0.5 M EDTA pH 8. *Alternative*: electroelution using Schleicher and Schuell Elutrap electro-preparation system (Whatman).

10. Absolute ethanol.

11. 3 M sodium acetate pH 5.3.

12. 1 mg/ml glycogen.

2.3. End Labeling and Ligation of RNA Components

1. 20 µM solutions of the 3′ RNA and 5′ RNA (in vitro or synthetic).
2. 25 µM solution of DNA bridge oligonucleotide. The DNA must have at least 20 bp complementarity to each RNA, resulting in an double-stranded RNA/DNA hybridization region of at least 40 bp in length.
3. Polynucleotide kinase buffer (10×): 700 mM Tris–HCl (pH 7.6), 100 mM $MgCl_2$, and 50 mM DTT.
4. $\gamma\text{-}^{32}P$-ATP (3,000 Ci/mmol).
5. T4 polynucleotide kinase (T4 PNK).
6. Ligase buffer (5×): 250 mM Tris–HCl (pH 7.6), 50 mM $MgCl_2$, 50 mM DTT, and 5 mM ATP.
7. High concentration T4 DNA ligase (2,000,000 units/ml).
8. RNasin (at least 40 units/µl).
9. RNase-free water.
10. 0.5 M EDTA pH 8.
11. Phenol:chloroform:isoamyl alcohol (25:24:1).
12. 5 M ammonium acetate.
13. 10 mg/ml tRNA or 10 mg/ml glycogen.
14. Absolute ethanol.

2.4. Purification of Ligated RNA Product

1. Formamide loading dye (see Subheading 2.2).
2. Urea.
3. Sequencing grade 40% acrylamide solution (see Subheading 2.2).
4. RNase-free water (see Subheading 2.1).
5. N,N,N,N'-Tetramethyl-ethylenediamine (TEMED). Store at 4°C.
6. 25% ammonium persulfate in water (see Note 1).
7. TBE buffer (1×; see Subheading 2.2).
8. Saran Wrap.
9. Glogos II Autorad Markers (Stratagene/Agilent).
10. Passive elution solution or electroelution system (see Subheading 2.2).

3. Methods

Warning: When working with radioactivity the local rules on safe practice, recording the use of and disposal of radioactive materials must be followed.

3.1. In Vitro Transcription of 5′ or 3′ RNA with Initiation of RNA Transcript with GTP, XpG, GMP, or Guanosine

Depending upon the downstream use of the in vitro transcribed RNA, initiators may need to be incorporated during the in vitro transcription reaction to provide the correct 5′ end of RNA transcript to allow ligation and/or end labeling. When transcribing the 5′ RNA, GTP can be used in equimolar amounts (a final concentration of 1 mM) with ATP, CTP, and UTP. However, to enable the ligation to the 3′ end of an RNA requires that the 3′ RNA possess a single phosphate at its 5′ end. Therefore, when transcribing the 3′ RNA it must be primed with GMP, or either XpG or guanosine, which will allow the addition of a ^{32}P or cold phosphate. In these three cases an NTP mix with reduced (a final concentration of 0.4 mM) GTP concentration must be used to favor incorporation of either GMP, XpG, or guanosine at the beginning of the transcript.

1. In vitro transcribe RNA from the DNA template using one of the following three options depending on the desired target:

   Option A. To produce 5′ RNA without priming: mix 40 μl of 5× transcription buffer with 86 μl of RNase-free water, 40 μl of 5× NTPs and 24 μl of DNA template in a microcentrifuge tube. Then add 5 μl (200 units) of RNasin and 5 μl (90 units) of T7 RNA polymerase. Incubate at 37°C for 3 h.

   Option B. To produce RNA primed with either XpG or GMP: mix 40 μl of 5× transcription buffer with 78 μl of RNase-free water, 40 μl of 5× NTPs with 2 mM of GTP, 8 μl of 50 mM XpG or GMP, and 24 μl of DNA template in a microcentrifuge tube. Then add 5 μl (200 units) of RNasin and 5 μl (90 units) of T7 RNA polymerase. Incubate at 37°C for 3 h.

   Option C. To produce RNA primed with guanosine: mix 40 μl of 5× transcription buffer with 66 μl of RNase-free water, 40 μl of 5× NTPs with 2 mM of GTP, 20 μl of 200 mM guanosine, and 24 μl of DNA template in a microcentrifuge tube. Then add 5 μl (200 units) of RNasin and 5 μl (90 units) of T7 RNA polymerase. Incubate at 37°C for 3 h.

2. Add 10 μl (10 units) of RNase-free DNase to the reaction and incubate at 37°C for 15 min to digest the DNA template.

3. After the DNase incubation the RNA must be purified. To the reaction add 20 μl of 0.5 M EDTA pH 8 (see Note 2) and 220 μl of phenol:chloroform:isoamyl alcohol. Phenol extract the reaction by vortexing for 2 min and centrifugation in a bench-top microcentrifuge for 2 min at maximum rpm. Remove 200 μl of the upper aqueous layer to a new microcentrifuge tube and add 40 μl of 5 M ammonium acetate and 600 μl of absolute ethanol then mix by vortexing.

4. Precipitate the RNA for at least 30 min at –20°C.

5. Centrifuge for 5 min at maximum speed in a bench-top centrifuge, carefully remove the ethanol and discard leaving the small

Table 1
Solutions for acrylamide gels to resolve RNAs. Dissolve 10.5 g of urea in 5 ml of 5× TBE, 40% acrylamide, and RNase-free water

Gel percentage	40% Acrylamide (xml)	RNase free water (xml)	Size separation	Xylene cyanol (light blue dye)	Bromophenol blue (dark blue dye)
6%	3.9	8.6	100 or above	~106	~26
12%	7.8	4.7	40–100	~40	~15
15%	9.8	2.7	25–40	~30	~9–10
19%	12.5	0	25 or less	~22	~6

white pellet of RNA behind (see Note 3). Resuspend this RNA pellet in 10 µl of RNase-free water and 20 µl of formamide loading dye.

3.2. Purification of In Vitro Transcribed and Synthetic RNAs

In vitro transcribed and synthetic RNAs should be gel purified to obtain RNA of the desired size. This is performed by purifying the RNA in a denaturing acrylamide gel, excising the full-length RNA and eluting the RNA from the gel.

1. Assemble the gel casting apparatus. First, coat one gel plate (usually the notched plate) with Repelcote VS water repellent to encourage the gel to stick to the opposite gel plate when the gel plates are separated in step 5. Remove all excess repellent with a 50:50 water/ethanol solution. Ensure the gel plates are clean and then, after placing the spacers between the glass plates, surround the bottom and the sides of the plates with Tesa 4120 UPVC packaging tape or equivalent product.

2. Pour the RNA purification gel:
   (a) *For in vitro transcribed RNA*: make 20 ml of 6% polyacrylamide gel solution (see Table 1 for gel constituents), add 40 µl TEMED and 40 µl 25% ammonium persulfate. Act quickly to transfer the gel solution into the gel plates taking care not to introduce bubbles into the gel solution (see Note 4). Insert the comb and hold the gel together with bulldog clips. Remove the excess gel solution from around the top of the gel and allow the gel to polymerize for at least 30 min.
   (b) *For synthetic RNAs*: resuspend the RNA in RNase-free water and add equal volume of formamide loading dye. Make a high percentage acrylamide (12–19%); the volume of acrylamide and water is dependent upon the gel percentage required to resolve the RNA (Table 1). To prepare the gel solution, dissolve 10.5 g of urea in 5 ml of 5× TBE

(see Note 5) and add 40% acrylamide and RNase-free water for the desired gel percentage resulting in a final volume of 25 ml. These gel solution volumes are sufficient to pour a gel of 185 × 200 mm with 0.5 mm spacers. Once the urea is dissolved filter the gel solution through a 0.45 μm syringe filter using a 50 ml syringe. Once filtered add 40 μl of TEMED and 40 μl of 25% ammonium persulfate, stir and pour into gel casting apparatus as described in (a) above. Leave to set for at least 30 min.

3. Once the gel has set, remove the bulldog clips then the comb. Immediately wash out the wells with 1× TBE buffer to remove any unpolymerized gel solution. This is performed by attaching a 19 gauge needle to a clean 50 ml syringe and washing out the wells after the comb has been removed. Remove the packaging tape before assembling gel in gel apparatus.

4. Run the gel at a constant Wattage depending on the gel apparatus used and for the time required to allow the RNA to migrate approximately 2/3 of the way through the gel using the dyes as indicators.

5. Carefully pry apart the gel plates with a spatula and sandwich the gel between two pieces of Saran Wrap then visualize the RNA by UV shadowing (see Note 6).

6. Excise the band from the gel with a clean scalpel or razor blade and either passive elute or electroelute the RNA from the gel slice:

   (a) *To passively elute the RNA from the gel slice*: cut the gel slice into pieces measuring roughly 4 × 4 mm, transfer into a microcentrifuge tube and cover completely with sufficient passive elution solution. Incubate overnight at room temperature. Remove elution solution from the tube making sure to leave behind any gel slices.

   (b) *To electroelute the RNA from the gel slice*: follow the manufacturer's instructions for the electroelution device.

7. Precipitate the RNA by adding 1 μl of glycogen and 2.5× volumes of absolute ethanol. Briefly vortex to mix.

8. Precipitate for at least 30 min at −20°C.

9. Centrifuge for 5 min at maximum speed in a bench-top centrifuge, carefully remove the ethanol and discard leaving a small white pellet of RNA/glycogen behind (see Note 3).

10. Resuspend the RNA in a small volume (10 μl) RNase-free water and quantify by measuring the OD_{260} (see Note 7).

3.3. Preparation of the 5′ End of the 3′ RNA Used for a Typical Two-Way RNA Ligation

Successful ligation requires the 3′ RNA to possess a single phosphate at its 5′ end. This single phosphate can be a ^{32}P or an unlabeled phosphate. Depending on how the 3′ RNA was produced for the ligation reaction there are a number of different treatments that may, or may not, need to be carried out before the 3′ RNA is capable of being ligated to a 5′ RNA. A 3′ RNA that contains a single phosphate, for example an RNA from an in vitro transcription reaction primed with GMP, can be directly ligated to a 5′ RNA. A synthetic 3′ RNA or a 3′ RNA primed with XpG or guanosine requires a 5′ phosphate group added to it to allow ligation. 3′ RNA molecules that contain a single or tri-phosphate 5′ end can also be dephosphorylated (see Note 8) to then allow a single phosphate to be added. The protocol below describes a small scale reaction where a ^{32}P is introduced at the ligation junction, but other variations on this protocol are possible (see Note 9).

1. To 5′-end label the 3′ RNA with a single ^{32}P, mix 1 μl of 20 μM 3′ RNA without a 5′ phosphate with 1 μl of RNase-free water, 1 μl of 10× PNK buffer, 6 μl of γ-^{32}P-ATP (3,000 Ci/mmole; see Note 10), 0.5 μl (20 units) of RNasin, and 0.5 μl (5 units) of T4 PNK in either a 0.2 ml, a 0.5 ml PCR tube (dependent upon thermocycler block size locally available, see Note 11), or a microcentrifuge tube. Incubate at 37°C for 1 h.

2. Heat to 65°C for 20 min to inactivate the T4 PNK.

3. Next, hybridize the DNA oligonucleotide bridge to the 5′ and 3′ RNAs. To the radiolabeling reaction, add 1.1 μl of 5′ RNA at 20 μM, 0.8 μl of 25 μM DNA oligonucleotide bridge, and 8.1 μl of RNase-free water. Heat to 90°C and cool slowly to 25°C (see Note 11).

4. To ligate the 5′ and 3′ RNAs together add 1 μl of 10× ligase buffer, 0.5 μl (20 units) of RNasin, and 1 μl (2,000 units) of high-concentration T4 DNA ligase to the hybridization mixture. Incubate at 37°C for at least 1 h. Longer incubations of 2–4 h may result in a slight increase in ligation efficiency but risks RNA degradation.

5. After incubation add 1 μl of 0.5 M EDTA pH 8 to stop the reaction. If the reaction has been performed in a 0.2 or 0.5 ml PCR tube transfer it to a 1.7 ml microcentrifuge tube. Add 80 μl of RNase-free water and 100 μl of phenol:chloroform:isoamyl alcohol then vortex for 2 min and centrifuge at maximum speed in a bench-top centrifuge.

6. Remove 100 μl of the upper, aqueous phase into a new 1.7 ml microcentrifuge and add 20 μl of 5 M ammonium acetate, 1 μl of 1 mg/ml tRNA and 300 μl of absolute ethanol. Briefly vortex and precipitate at −20°C for at least 30 min.

3.4. Purification of Ligated RNA

1. Make a gel of the appropriate percentage (see Table 1) as described in Subheading 3.2 (steps 1 and 2).

2. Centrifuge the microcentrifuge tube containing the precipitated ligated RNA for 5 min at maximum rpm in a bench-top centrifuge. Remove ethanol and discard in the correct manner

if this ethanol is radioactive. Resuspend in 6 μl of formamide loading dye and heat the sample at 80°C for 2–5 min prior to loading onto the acrylamide gel.

3. Run the gel at constant Wattage depending on the gel apparatus used and for the time required to allow the RNA to migrate approximately 2/3 of the way through the gel (see Note 12).

4. If the ligated RNA is radiolabeled then it is possible to visualize the 3′ RNA and ligated RNA using X-ray film. Remove one gel plate then cover the gel with Saran Wrap, attach two Glogo Autorad Markers to Saran Wrap on both sides of gel and place gel plate in an autoradiography cassette. Expose gel to X-ray film. The exposure time is dependent on the activity of the radiolabeled RNA, if highly active then a 5 min exposure will suffice. Develop the film and cut around the band on the film representing the ligated RNA. Align the film to the gel using the two Glogo markers and using the film as a mask, excise the ligated RNA.

5. If the ligated RNA is not radiolabeled then visualize by UV shadowing (see Note 5).

6. Electroelute or passively elute the ligated RNA as described in Subheading 3.2 (steps 6–10).

4. Notes

1. Ammonium persulfate works best fresh but it can be stored for up to 1 week at 4°C.

2. EDTA is added following the transcription reaction as in some cases the transcription reaction becomes cloudy as it contains precipitated pyrophosphates released during the incorporation of NTPs by the polymerase. The EDTA solubilizes these pyrophosphates.

3. It may be difficult to see this pellet so it helps to take note of the side of the tube the pellet is likely to be on after centrifugation. This can be easily done by centrifuging with the hinge of the centrifuge tube placed to the outside of the centrifuge and therefore the pellet will stick to the wall of the tube on the same side as the hinge of the tube.

4. When casting the gel using a 50 ml syringe, tilt the gel slightly away from you, holding the glass plates in one hand and the syringe in your dominant hand. Gently compress the syringe to slowly fill the casting apparatus. As you pour the gel it is possible to tap the glass where bubbles have formed and encourage them to move up and out of the gel, this works as long as the gel front is less than 10 mm away from the bubble.

5. Dissolving urea is an endothermic reaction. It will therefore take some time to completely dissolve as all the urea will not go into solution until the mixture has reached room temperature. Although it is tempting to heat the mixture to encourage the urea to dissolve this is inadvisable as this will greatly accelerate the rate at which the gel sets and it is possible for the gel solution to set before it has been introduced into the casting apparatus. Allow time in your protocol to dissolve the urea at room temperature.

6. To identify the position of the RNA, the gel, sandwiched between Saran Wrap, is placed on an intensifying screen or TLC plate and short wave UV light is shined directly on the gel from above. The outline of the shadow of RNA is then marked on the Saran Wrap with a Sharpie ultra fine point permanent marker pen.

7. The concentration of RNA in µM can be roughly calculated by using the equation: OD_{260} divided by length of RNA multiplied by 0.01.

8. An in vitro transcribed RNA can be dephosphorylated by inserting additional steps into the protocol in Subheading 3.1. You will lose a small amount of the total RNA by adding these steps. During **step 5**, resuspend the RNA in 87 µl of RNase-free water, add 10 µl of New England Biolabs restriction enzyme Buffer 3 (10×: 500 mM Tris–HCl pH 7.9, 100 mM $MgCl_2$, 1 M NaCl, and 10 mM dithiothreitol), 2 µl (80 units) of RNasin, and 1 µl (10 units) of calf intestinal alkaline phosphatase. Incubate for 1 h at 37°C. Add 100 µl of phenol:chloroform:isoamyl alcohol (25:24:1) then vortex for 2 min and centrifugation in a bench-top microcentrifuge for 2 min at maximum speed. Remove 95 µl of the upper aqueous layer to a new microcentrifuge tube and add 19 µl of 5 M ammonium acetate, 285 µl of absolute ethanol then mix by vortexing. Resuspend this RNA pellet in 10 µl of RNase-free water and 20 µl of formamide loading dye. Purify RNA as described in Subheading 3.2.

9. The ligation protocol can be varied to ligate more than one RNA by the method described. In addition, if the concentrations of the RNAs to be ligated are increased 25 times with a corresponding increase in bridging oligonucleotide concentration the ligation reaction can be visualized by UV shadowing and remove the requirement for labeling with [32]P.

10. Although this quantity of radioactivity provides the highest specific activity, and will yield the greatest amount of radiolabeled RNA, lower amounts of radioactive γ-^{32}P-ATP between 1 and 5 µl can be used.

11. Using a thermocycler (PCR machine) to perform the labeling, hybridization, and ligation enables close temperature control. During the hybridization step it is possible, using a thermocycler, to reduce the temperature of the reaction slowly from 90 to 25°C (0.1°C per second) in a highly controlled manner.

12. When attempting a new ligation it is usually helpful to run a labeled 3' RNA on its own to distinguish unligated from ligated RNA and to determine what gel % is appropriate for separation of unligated from ligated product. A good efficiency of ligation is 50% or above, however lower than this is useable.

Acknowledgments

This work was supported by the Biotechnology and Biological Sciences Research Council (BBSRC) and The Wellcome Trust.

References

1. Moore MJ, Sharp PA. Site-specific modification of pre-mRNA: the 2'-hydroxyl groups at the splice sites. Science. 1992;256:992–7.
2. O'Keefe RT, Newman AJ. Functional analysis of the U5 snRNA loop 1 in the second catalytic step of yeast pre-mRNA splicing. EMBO. 1998;17:565–74.
3. Juzumiene DI, Wollenzien P. Arrangement of the central pseudoknot region of 16S rRNA in the 30S ribosomal subunit determined by site-directed 4-thiouridine crosslinking. RNA. 2001;7:71–84.
4. O'Keefe RT, Norman C, Newman AJ. The invariant U5 snRNA loop 1 sequence is dispensable for the first catalytic step of pre-mRNA splicing in yeast. Cell. 1996;86:679–89.
5. Dix I, Russel CS, O'Keefe RT, Newman AJ, Beggs JD. Protein-RNA interactions in the U5 snRNP of Saccharomyces cerevisiae. RNA. 1998;4:1675–86.
6. Alvi RK, Lund M, O'Keefe RT. ATP-dependent interaction of yeast U5 snRNA loop1 with the 5' splice site. RNA. 2001;7:1013–23.
7. McGrail JC, Tatum E, O'Keefe RT. Mutation in the U2 snRNA influences exon interactions of the U5 snRNA loop 1 during pre-mRNA splicing. EMBO. 2006;25:3813–22.
8. McGrail JC, O'Keefe RT. The U1, U2 and U5 snRNAs crosslink to the 5' exon during yeast pre-mRNA splicing. Nucleic Acids Res. 2008;36:814–25.
9. Tzakos AG, Easton LE, Lukavsky PJ. Perparation of large RNA oligonucleotides with complementary isotope-labeled segments for NMR structural studies. Nat Protoc. 2007;2:2139–47.
10. Kleppe K, van de Sande JH, Khorana HG. Polynucleotide ligase-catalyzed joining of deoxyribo-oligonucleotides on ribopolynucleotide templates and of ribo-oligonucleotides on deoxyribopolynucleotide templates. Proc Natl Acad Sci USA. 1970;67:68–73.
11. Fareed GC, Wilt EM, Richardson CC. Enzymatic breakage and joining of deoxyribonucleic acid. J Biol Chem. 1971;246: 925–32.
12. Sano H, Feix G. Ribonucleic acid ligase activity of deoxyribonucleic acid ligase from phage T4 infacted *Escherichia coli*. Biochemistry. 1974;13: 5110–5.

INDEX

A

Acetylated bovine serum albumen (BSA) 50, 71, 73, 140, 200, 204
Adenosine 5'(γ-thio)triphosphate (ATPγS) 182
Affi-gel 234, 238
Affinity capture/immobilization 114, 123
Agarose gel electrophoresis (AGE)
    DNA extraction 24, 31, 40, 161, 162
    TAE 24, 28–30, 39, 71
AGE. See Agarose gel electrophoresis (AGE)
Annealing (of RNA) 45, 52, 66, 158, 164, 168
Antibiotic
    ampicillin 2–4, 10, 25, 33, 73, 89, 93, 140, 160–161, 163
    kanamycin 10, 13, 125
ARiBo tag 124, 137–149
Autoradiography 91, 94, 109, 267

B

Bacterial lysis 228, 229, 234, 237–238
Beer–Lambert law ...... 54, 57, 192. See also Ultraviolet (UV), absorbance
Biotin modification (of RNA) 172
γboxB RNA 123, 124, 138
BPB. See Bromophenol blue (BPB)
Bromophenol blue (BPB) 10–12, 24, 48, 61, 67–68, 72, 74, 79, 90, 104, 127, 133, 141, 150, 162, 172, 179, 200, 206, 208, 216, 223, 250, 261, 264

C

Calf intestinal phosphatase (CIP) 141, 153
Cap (m^7G cap) 178
Centrifugal concentration device 61, 64, 72
Chromatography, liquid
    FPLC (see Fast protein liquid chromatography (FPLC))
    HPLC (see High performance liquid chromatography (HPLC))
CIP. See Calf intestinal phosphatase (CIP)
Colony PCR 32, 33

Competent cells (bacterial)
    chemical 25, 32, 70, 73, 140
    electroporation 2
Conformational dynamics 228

D

DEPC. See Diethylpyrocarbonate (DEPC)
Desalting column 72, 75
Dialysis 17, 47, 51, 124, 126, 130
Diethylpyrocarbonate (DEPC) 34, 60, 114, 259
DNA-affinity chromatography 113–120
DNA analysis software 22, 26, 33, 37
DNA labeling 181–192
DNA ligase 32, 40, 71, 73, 89, 93, 161, 166, 173, 177, 257–269
DNA oligonucleotide 9–12, 14–17, 21, 43, 60, 62, 66, 73, 89, 116, 119, 159–164, 166, 167, 173, 182, 186, 199, 201, 258, 260, 266
DNA polymerase 19, 22, 28, 34–35, 38, 40, 89, 93, 107, 139, 142, 161, 173, 199
DNA purification kit
    Giga 140, 143
    Maxi 25, 33–34, 71, 73, 140, 143
    Miniprep 3, 4, 163
DNA-RNA hybrid 198, 209, 260, 262
DNase I 117, 118, 120, 263
DNAzyme/DNA enzyme/deoxyribozyme 9, 85–86, 113–120
Double-stranded DNA (dsDNA) 19, 21, 27, 31, 35, 38, 50, 60, 62, 66, 73, 102, 105–108, 142, 143, 196, 201
dsDNA. See Double-stranded DNA (dsDNA)

E

Electroelution 48, 53, 261, 262, 265, 267
Electrophoresis apparatus. See Polyacrylamide gel electrophoresis (PAGE)
Electrophoretic mobility shift assay
    (EMSA) 184, 186
Electroporator, cuvette 2

EMSA. *See* Electrophoretic mobility shift assay (EMSA)
End labeling 83, 84, 181–192, 208, 262, 263
Enzymatic phosphorylation.............234–235, 239, 242, 243
Escherichia coli
   BL21(DE3) 6, 10, 13, 67, 125, 133, 240
   DH5α 6, 25, 45, 48, 70, 73, 89, 93, 140, 160, 163
   DL323 .... 229–232, 241
   JM101Tr..2
   K10-1516 ....229–230, 232, 241
   TOP10 70
   XL1 Blue 89, 93
EtBr. *See* Ethidium bromide (EtBr)
Ethanol precipitation
   of DNA 49, 95, 105, 109, 178
   of RNA............................... 4, 5, 51, 96, 109, 265
Ethidium bromide (EtBr) 39, 61, 64, 71, 78, 94, 164, 165, 192, 206

F

Fast protein liquid chromatography (FPLC)
   anion exchange 5, 7, 248
   gel filtration/size exclusion 7, 60–67, 69–80, 113, 114, 120, 138
   glutathione (GSH)-Sepharose....................................124
   hydrophobic interaction..7
   Ni-NTA... 11, 13, 14
   systems
      ÄKTA FPLC... 3, 11, 61
      ÄKTA purifier 75, 78
French press..11, 13, 126, 129

G

Gel extraction 1, 31, 35, 96, 163, 167
Gel filtration. *See* Fast protein liquid chromatography (FPLC)
Gel purification 31, 39, 93, 132, 174, 179, 196, 222–224, 264
Gel-shift...209
GK. *See* Guanylate kinase (GK)
GlcN6P. *See* Glucosamine-6-phosphate (GlcN6P)
Glucosamine-6-phosphate (GlcN6P) 124, 138, 141, 145–152
Guanylate kinase (GK).. 234, 239

H

Hand-held UV lamp 3–5, 12, 15, 48, 91, 200, 203
High performance liquid chromatography (HPLC)
   ion-pair.. 238, 247–255
   reversed phase......................................215, 238, 247–255
Homogeneous 3'-end 45, 70, 76, 99–110
Hydrolysis.. 67, 97, 220, 224, 234, 238, 242, 248, 251, 254

I

In vitro transcription
   DNA template
      linearization.................. 22, 34, 69, 74, 114, 140, 199
      preparation......................................19–40, 43–57, 199
      optimization 94–95, 140–141, 144–147
Ion-pair reversed phase. *See* High performance liquid chromatography (HPLC)
Isopropanol precipitation...96
Isotopic label. *See* Labeling

L

Labeling
   fluorescent..176
   isotopic
      site-specific 230
      uniform.. 227, 247
Ligation...21, 22, 25, 32–33, 35, 36, 39, 40, 73, 79, 83–84, 86, 87, 93, 99, 142, 159–164, 166, 167, 171–175, 177, 179, 257–269
Lyophilizer 26, 38, 215, 221, 223, 238, 239
Lysis 2, 4, 33, 45, 46, 48, 54, 126, 228, 234, 237–238, 241–242, 251
Lysogeny broth/Luria–Bertani medium
   (LB) 10, 13, 25, 32–33, 35, 40, 46, 48, 54, 55, 71, 73, 89, 93, 125, 128, 140, 143, 160, 161, 163, 167, 230, 235–237

M

Mass spectrometry.. 17, 125, 132
MCS. *See* Multiple cloning sites (MCS)
Methanococcus jannaschii....................196, 198, 200–207, 209
Methyltransferase 198
m¹G37 (modified tRNA) 198–200, 204–210
Minimal medium.............................229–233, 235–236, 241
MK. *See* Myokinase (MK)
MLS. *See* Multiple linearization sites (MLS)
Molecular imager...128, 133, 142, 144–146, 150, 250, 254
Molecular weight ladder/marker 29–30, 39, 124, 127, 131–133
Multiple cloning sites (MCS).....................33, 35, 70, 88, 92
Multiple linearization sites (MLS)...................44, 88, 90, 95
Myokinase (MK).. 234, 239

N

Nontemplated nucleotide 44, 83–84, 99, 114, 166, 168
Nuclear magnetic resonance (NMR)
   spectroscopy.............................99, 113, 224, 227, 241, 247–248, 258
Nuclease-free water 23, 26, 28, 30–34, 95, 105

Nuclease P1 .... 57, 234, 238, 254
Nucleoside 5'(α-P-seleno) triphosphate
        (Se-NTP) 213, 214
Nucleoside monophosphate (NMP)
        kinase 207–208, 234, 248–249,
        251–255

O

Oligo affinity support 116, 117, 119

P

Passive elution 53, 261, 262, 265
PEP. *See* Phosphoenolpyruvate (PEP)
Phenol extraction (phenol/chloroform
        extraction) 39, 56–57
Phosphoenolpyruvate (PEP) 234–235, 243
Phosphorimager 90, 175, 208
PK. *See* Pyruvate kinase (PK)
Plasmid DNA
        pUC19, pUC119 .... 24, 25, 33, 35,
        36, 44, 70, 72, 73, 159
Polyacrylamide gel electrophoresis (PAGE)
        denaturing (urea)
            mini/analytical 47–48, 51,
            60–64, 95, 118, 127, 141, 142,
            144, 150, 164, 200, 206, 250, 254
            preparative 43–57, 72, 106, 150, 200, 222
        native 76, 77, 80, 160, 162, 164, 165
        RNA loading dye 172, 174, 200, 203, 206
        SDS-PAGE 10, 12, 16, 17, 127
Polymerase chain reaction (PCR) 19–40, 44,
        73, 88, 89, 91–97, 105–107, 142, 143,
        158–163, 166, 167, 173, 177, 179, 182,
        184, 186, 216, 222, 258–260, 266, 269
Poly(A) tail 171–173, 176–179
Promoter
        lpp 6
        T7 RNA polymerase 44, 60, 72,
        104, 105, 201, 260
Proof reading activity 22
Purification tag 114
Pyrophosphatase
        inorganic (IPP) 61, 67, 90, 140,
        152, 216, 222
        yeast (YIP) 90, 140
Pyruvate kinase (PK) 234, 239

Q

Quick ligation 25, 32

R

Radiolabeled RNA 90, 258, 267
Recursive polymerase chain reaction
        (R-PCR) 20–24, 26–29, 33–40

Restriction endonuclease enzyme 22, 24, 25, 31,
        40, 71–73
Reverse transcriptase (RT) 104, 106–107, 158, 159,
        165–166, 168, 184, 186
Ribonuclease (RNase) 11, 15, 17, 45,
        48–50, 57, 60–62, 70, 79, 85, 90,
        95, 100, 114, 117–119, 125, 129, 132,
        133, 140, 144, 147, 151, 153–154, 172, 174,
        176, 179, 184–185, 198, 216, 221–224,
        258, 259, 261–266, 268
Ribonucleoside monophosphates (rNMP) 228, 229,
        234–235, 238–239, 241–243, 247–255
Ribonucleoside triphosphate (rNTP) 43, 45, 47,
        51, 52, 54–56, 59, 61, 62, 67, 90, 94, 95, 97,
        172–174, 176, 178, 179, 216, 227–243, 258
Ribozyme
        cis-acting 9, 44–45, 83–97, 100, 114
        design 70, 91–92
        glmS 124, 138, 145, 148, 151–153
        hammerhead 86–89, 91–93, 96, 114
        hepatitis delta virus (HDV)
            antigenomic 99–110
            genomic 99–110
        optimization 47, 138, 145
        ribozyme recognition site (RRS) 100, 102, 107
        trans-acting 85–86, 99–110, 114
RNA folding 52, 65, 80, 89, 94, 133, 158, 159
RNA heterogeneity 44, 79, 84, 158, 179
RNA modification, cotranscriptional
        3'-end 76, 173
        5'-end 172–175
        internal 171–173, 175–176
RNA precipitation
        ethanol 4–5, 51, 54, 73,
        96, 106, 109, 175
        isopropanol 96
RNA-protein binding 61, 65–66, 84
RNase. *See* Ribonuclease (RNase)
RNase H 9–17, 85, 86,
        198, 201, 206–210
RNase inhibitor 50, 95, 172, 174, 176
RNA structure prediction 80, 89, 91, 157,
        160, 166, 172, 175, 213
rNMP. *See* Ribonucleoside monophosphates (rNMP)
R-PCR. *See* Recursive polymerase chain
        reaction (R-PCR)
RT. *See* Reverse transcriptase (RT)
RT-PCR 184, 186
Run-off. *See* In vitro transcription

S

S-adenosyl-L-methionine (AdoMet) 198, 200,
        204, 205
Secondary structure 26, 27, 37, 38,
        40, 80, 87, 89, 91, 158, 195, 228

Se-derivatization. *See* Selenium (Se)-derivatization
Selenium (Se)-derivatization 213–224
Sephadex G-25 .... 187, 190
Sequenase 196, 199, 201, 207
Sequence editing software 25
Single-stranded RNA (ssRNA) 57, 65
S1 nuclease 248, 249, 251, 254, 255
Sonicator 11, 13, 126, 129
Spin column 35, 40, 178, 187, 201, 205, 208
Splint ligation 175, 257–269
ssRNA. *See* Single-stranded RNA (ssRNA)
Stains-all 10, 12–13, 15–17
Structure cassette 157–168
Structure probing 157–168
Studier medium 233–235, 237, 241
Superdex 75/Superdex 200 .... 7, 61–66, 72, 75–77, 117, 118
SYBR Gold 128, 133, 138, 142, 144–146, 148–150, 250, 254

T

TB. *See* Terrific broth (TB)
Terrific broth (TB) 46, 48
Thin-layer chromatography (TLC) 104, 106, 179, 203, 214, 215, 217, 218, 220–222, 224, 242, 243, 249, 251, 268
TLC. *See* Thin-layer chromatography (TLC)
Toluidine blue 72, 74, 77, 117, 118, 120
Transcript heterogeneity 84–85
Transfer RNA (tRNA)
    chimera/scaffold 1–7, 9–17
    modification 197, 198, 200–201
Transformation, bacterial 89
Triphosphate, 5'-end 84

tRNA. *See* Transfer RNA (tRNA)
tRNA-Lys3 5
tRNA-Met 5
T4 Polynucleotide Kinase (T4 PNK) 84, 86, 161–163, 166, 173, 177, 182, 183, 187–188, 191, 208, 260, 262, 266
T7 RNAP. *See* T7 RNA polymerase (T7 RNAP)
T7 RNA polymerase (T7 RNAP) 1, 36, 43–45, 47, 50–52, 59–62, 67, 69–74, 78, 79, 83–85, 88, 90, 95, 99–101, 103–105, 113–115, 117, 133, 140, 144, 151, 168, 172, 174, 175, 196, 199, 201, 202, 207, 208, 215, 221, 222, 227, 247–248, 250, 253, 258–260, 263
TY medium 2–4

U

Ultraviolet (UV)
    absorbance
        dsDNA concentration determination 31
        ssRNA concentration determination 57
    shadowing 4, 5, 15, 53, 96, 106, 175, 179, 203, 210, 265–268
    spectroscopy 96, 131, 143, 149, 251, 253
    transilluminator (*see* Hand-held UV lamp)
UV. *See* Ultraviolet (UV)

X

XC. *See* Xylene cyanol (XC)
X-ray crystallography 99, 113, 213–224
X-ray film 175, 267
Xylene cyanol (XC) 3, 12, 48, 61, 64, 67–68, 72, 90, 103, 106, 162, 172, 179, 200, 203, 208, 216, 223, 250, 261